T0260430

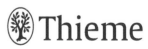

Video Atlas of Spine Surgery

Howard S. An, MD
The Morton International Professor of Orthopaedic Surgery
Department of Orthopaedic Surgery
Rush University Medical Center
Chicago, Illinois, USA

Philip K. Louie, MD
Spine Surgery Fellow
Department of Orthopaedic Surgery
Hospital for Special Surgery
New York, New York, USA

Bryce A. Basques, MD, MHS
Spine Surgery Fellow
Rothman Orthopaedic Institute
Thomas Jefferson University
Philadelphia, Pennsylvania, USA

Gregory D. Lopez, MD
Orthopaedic Surgeon
Department of Orthopaedic Surgery
Rush University Medical Center
Chicago, Illinois, USA

315 illustrations

Thieme
New York • Stuttgart • Delhi • Rio de Janeiro

Library of Congress Cataloging-in-Publication Data is available from the publisher.

Important note: Medicine is an ever-changing science undergoing continual development. Research and clinical experience are continually expanding our knowledge, in particular our knowledge of proper treatment and drug therapy. Insofar as this book mentions any dosage or application, readers may rest assured that the authors, editors, and publishers have made every effort to ensure that such references are in accordance with **the state of knowledge at the time of production of the book.**

Nevertheless, this does not involve, imply, or express any guarantee or responsibility on the part of the publishers in respect to any dosage instructions and forms of applications stated in the book. **Every user is requested to examine carefully** the manufacturers' leafl ets accompanying each drug and to check, if necessary in consultation with a physician or specialist, whether the dosage schedules mentioned therein or the contraindications stated by the manufacturers diff er from the statements made in the present book. Such examination is particularly important with drugs that are either rarely used or have been newly released on the market. Every dosage schedule or every form of application used is entirely at the user's own risk and responsibility. The authors and publishers request every user to report to the publishers any discrepancies or inaccuracies noticed. If errors in this work are found after publication, errata will be posted at www.thieme.com on the product description page.

Some of the product names, patents, and registered designs referred to in this book are in fact registered trademarks or proprietary names even though specifi c reference to this fact is not always made in the text. Therefore, the appearance of a name without designation as proprietary is not to be construed as a representation by the publisher that it is in the public domain.

Thieme Publishers New York
333 Seventh Avenue, New York, NY 10001 USA
+1 800 782 3488, customerservice@thieme.com

Georg Thieme Verlag KG
Rüdigerstrasse 14, 70469 Stuttgart, Germany
+49 [0]711 8931 421, customerservice@thieme.de

Thieme Publishers Delhi
A-12, Second Floor, Sector-2, Noida-201301
Uttar Pradesh, India
+91 120 45 566 00, customerservice@thieme.in

Thieme Publishers Rio de Janeiro,
Thieme Publicações Ltda.
Edifício Rodolpho de Paoli, 25° andar
Av. Nilo Peçanha, 50 – Sala 2508,
Rio de Janeiro 20020-906 Brasil
+55 21 3172-2297

Cover design: Thieme Publishing Group
Typesetting by TNQ Technologies, India

Printed in USA by King Printing Company, Inc.

ISBN 978-1-68420-005-4

Also available as an e-book:
eISBN 978-1-68420-006-1

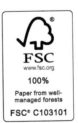

FSC
www.fsc.org
100%
Paper from well-managed forests
FSC® C103101

Contents

8   Degenerative Spondylolisthesis..   68
Craig Forsthoefel and Kris Siemionow

9   Spinal Cord Injury   79
Jakub Sikora-Klak, Ryan O'Leary, and R. Todd Allen

10   Cervical Spine Injuries..   88
Azeem Tariq Malik, Nikhil Jain, Jeffery Kim, and Safdar N. Khan

11 Thoracolumbar Spine Injuries 111

Andrew Sinensky, William T. Li, Matthew Meade, Mayan Lendner, Barrett Boody, Dhruv K.C. Goyal, and Mark Kurd

16 Spinal Infections

Harish Kempegowda and Chadi Tannoury

17 Inflammatory Spinal Disorders

Garrett K. Harada, Jannat M. Khan, and David F. Fardon

Videos

Foreword

In this first edition of *Video Atlas of Spine Surgery*, Dr. Howard S. An has done an incredible job cultivating some of the best minds in the field of spinal care to contribute to this comprehensive, cutting-edge text for managing the majority of spine cases encountered by spinal care physicians on a daily basis. As a master spine surgeon and academic leader, Dr. An has worked tirelessly to improve the field of spine surgery by also serving as a dedicated professor of the craft he loves so much. This is yet another contribution to the education of residents, fellows, and young attendings who share the same aspirations and dedication toward advancing spine care.

In this comprehensive text, Dr. An and his colleagues share a multitude of expert tips on surgical approaches involving the cervical, thoracic, and lumbar spine. The text is all-inclusive and consists of 19 chapters describing the complete workup and nonoperative and operative managements for the most commonly encountered spinal conditions. Dr. An and his team have presented a well-organized way of facilitating the learning of fine details of a multitude of surgical procedures. The book begins with a simple discussion of useful physical examination maneuvers used to accurately diagnose specific spinal pathology and then continues with an extensive set of surgical techniques useful in direct management of degenerative cervical and lumbar cases. The book finishes with an array of more complicated clinical scenarios one may encounter in the field (e.g., thoracolumbar spine injuries, spinal tumors, etc.). Each of these detailed chapters contains an introduction to the spinal pathology, its workup, management, and complications which one may encounter in the care of a patient with the spinal condition. At the end of each section, there is a set of recommended pearls, case examples, and board-style questions to optimize one's understanding of the material presented. What makes this book particularly unique is that, it also contains a myriad of extra resources to maximize learning—including detailed diagrams and illustrations, spinal imaging and photographs, and high-quality videos describing each case.

Spine surgery care has gone through a series of paradigm shifts throughout the past few decades, with vastly complex techniques being proposed at an astoundingly rapid pace. In order for the newer generation of spine surgeons to stay afloat and thrive in this new and innovative era of spine surgery, it is imperative for each individual to be exposed to a variety of different learning tools—including video-based learning. Dr. An, a true visionary, has recognized the importance of this particular avenue for learning and, thus, has accomplished an incredibly important feat in the advancement of spine training. I am pleased to have the opportunity in congratulating Dr. An and his colleagues in this endeavor—one which will serve well in educating the future generations of spine surgeons to come.

Alexander R. Vaccaro, MD, PhD, MBA
Richard H. Rothman Professor and Chairman
Department of Orthopaedic Surgery
Professor of Neurosurgery
Co-director, Delaware Valley Spinal Cord
Injury Center
Co-chief of Spine Surgery
Sidney Kimmel Medical Center
Thomas Jefferson University
President, Rothman Institute
Philadelphia, Pennsylvania, USA

Contributors

Junyoung Ahn
Resident Physician
Department of Orthopaedic Surgery
Rush University Medical Center
Chicago, Illinois, USA

R. Todd Allen, MD, PhD
Associate Professor of Orthopaedic Surgery
Spine Fellowship Director
Department of Orthopaedic Surgery
UC San Diego Health
San Diego, California, USA

Howard S. An, MD
The Morton International Professor of
  Orthopaedic Surgery
Department of Orthopaedic Surgery
Rush University Medical Center
Chicago, Illinois, USA

Jacob R. Ball, MS
MD Candidate
Department of Orthopaedics
Rutgers–New Jersey Medical School
Newark, New Jersey, USA

Bryce A. Basques, MD, MHS
Clinical Spine Fellow
Rothman Orthopaedic Institute
Thomas Jefferson University
Philadelphia, Pennsylvania, USA

Mark Berkowitz, BS
Spine Research Fellow
MD Candidate Class of 2023
New York Medical College
Valhalla, New York, USA

Alexander Beschloss, BS
MD Candidate
Perelman School of Medicine
University of Pennsylvania
Philadelphia, Pennsylvania, USA

Barrett Boody, MD
Orthopedic Spine Surgeon
Indiana Spine Group;
Assistant Professor of Clinical Orthopedic Surgery
Indiana University School of Medicine
Indianapolis, Indiana, USA

Patrick J. Cahill, MD
Robert M. Campbell Jr. Endowed Chair
Director of Wyss/Campbell center for
  Thoracic Insufficiency Syndrome
Perleman School of Medicine
University of Pennsylvania
Children's Hospital of Philadelphia
Philadelphia, Pennsylvania, USA

Thomas D. Cha, MD, MBA
Assistant Chief of Orthopaedic Spine Center
Assistant Professor
Department of Orthopaedic Surgery
Massachusetts General Hospital
Harvard Medical School
Boston, Massachusetts, USA

Matthew W. Colman, MD
Assistant Professor
Department of Orthopaedic Surgery
Rush University Medical Center
Chicago, Illinois, USA

Patrick K. Cronin, MD
Chief Resident
Harvard Orthopaedic Residency Program
Brigham and Women's Hospital
Boston, Massachusetts, USA

Peter B. Derman, MD, MBA
Spine Surgeon
Texas Back Institute
Plano, Texas, USA

Christopher J. DeWald, MD
Assistant Professor
Department of Orthopaedic Surgery;
Director
Section of Spinal Deformity
Rush University Medical Center
Chicago, Illinois, USA

Hicham Drissi, PhD
Professor and Vice Chair of Research
Department of orthopaedics
Emory University School of Medicine
Atlanta, Georgia, USA

David F. Fardon, MD
Assistant Professor, Emeritus
Spine Section
Department of Orthopedics
Rush University Medical Center
Chicago, Illinois, USA

Craig Forsthoefel, MD
Orthopedic Surgery Resident
Department of Orthopedic Surgery
University of Illinois College of Medicine
Chicago, Illinois, USA

Dhruv K.C. Goyal, BA
Spine Research Fellow
Rothman Orthopaedic Institute
Philadelphia, Pennsylvania, USA

Garrett K. Harada, MD
Orthopaedic Spine Surgery Research Fellow
Department of Orthopaedic Surgery
Midwest Orthopaedics at Rush
Chicago, Illinois, USA

Colin B. Harris, MD
Assistant Professor
Department of Orthopaedics
Spine Division
Rutgers–New Jersey Medical School
Newark, New Jersey, USA

Hamid Hassanzadeh, MD
Associate Professor
Department of Orthopaedic Surgery;
Director, Spine Fellowship
Co-director, Spine Center
University of Virginia Health System
Charlottesville, Virginia, USA

Steven T. Heidt, BS
Medical Student
Rush Medical College
Chicago, Illinois, USA

Nikhil Jain, MD
Spine Research Fellow
Department of Orthopaedics
The Ohio State University Wexner Medical Center
Columbus, Ohio, USA

Khaled Kebaish, MBBCh, MD, MS
Professor of Orthopaedic Surgery
Department of Orthopaedic Surgery;
Division Chief, Orthopaedic Spine Surgery;
Director, Spine Fellowship Program;
Professor of Neurosurgery
Department of Neurosurgery
Johns Hopkins University
Baltimore, Maryland, USA

Harish Kempegowda, MD
Attending Physician
Department of Orthopaedics and Spine Surgery
Heartland Regional Medical Center/Crossroads
Community Hospital
Marion, Illinois, USA

Jannat M. Khan, MD
Resident Physician
Department of Orthopaedic Surgery
William Beaumont Hospital
Royal Oak, Michigan, USA

Safdar N. Khan, MD
The Benjamin R. and Helen Slack Wiltberger
Endowed Chair in Orthopaedic Spine Surgery
Associate Professor and Chief
Division of Spine Surgery
Department of Orthopaedic Surgery;
Associate Professor
Department of Integrated Systems Engineering;
Clinical Co-director
Spine Research Institute
The Ohio State University Wexner Medical Center
Columbus, Ohio, USA

Jeffery Kim, MD
Assistant Professor
Division of Spine Surgery
Department of Orthopaedics
The Ohio State University Wexner Medical Center
Columbus, Ohio, USA

Mark Kurd, MD
Associate Professor
Department of Orthopaedic Surgery
Thomas Jefferson University
Rothman Orthopaedic Institute
Philadelphia, Pennsylvania, USA

Lawal A. Labaran, MD
Spine Research Fellow
Department of Orthopaedic Surgery
University of Virginia
Charlottesville, Virginia, USA

Michael J. Lee, MD
Professor Orthopaedic Spine Surgery
Department of Orthopaedic Surgery and
 Rehabilitation
University of Chicago Medical Center
Chicago, Illinois, USA

Mayan Lendner, BS
Research Fellow
Department of Spine Surgery
Rothman Orthopaedics
Philadelphia, Pennsylvania, USA

William T. Li, BS
Clinical Research Fellow
Rothman Orthopaedics,
Philadelphia, Pennsylvania, USA

Gregory D. Lopez, MD
Orthopaedic Surgeon
Department of Orthopaedic Surgery
Rush University Medical Center
Chicago, Illinois, USA

Philip K. Louie, MD
Spine Surgery Fellow
Department of Orthopaedic Surgery
Hospital for Special Surgery
New York, New York, USA

Azeem Tariq Malik, MBBS
Spine Research Fellow
Department of Orthopaedics
The Ohio State University Wexner Medical Center
Columbus, Ohio, USA

Michael H. McCarthy, MD, MPH
Spine Surgery Fellow
Department of Orthopaedic Surgery
Hospital for Special Surgery
New York, New York, USA

Matthew Meade, BA
Medical Student
Philadelphia College of Osteopathic Medicine
Philadelphia, Pennsylvania, USA

Nabil Mehta, MD
Orthopaedic Surgery Resident
Department of Orthopaedic Surgery
Rush University Medical Center
Chicago, Illinois, USA

Daniel J. Miller, MD
Attending Orthopaedic Surgeon
Division of Orthopaedic Surgery
Gillette Children's Specialty Healthcare
St. Paul, Minnesota, USA

Isaac L. Moss, MDCM, MASc, FRCSC
Chairman and Associate Professor
Department of Orthopedic Surgery
UConn Health Musculoskeletal Institute;
Co-director
UConn Comprehensive Spine Center;
Director
UConn Spine Surgery Fellowship
University of Connecticut Health Center
Farmington, Connecticut, USA

Ryan O'Leary, MD
Orthopaedic Surgery Resident
Department of Orthopaedics
UC San Diego Health
San Diego, California, USA

Steven M. Presciutti, MD
Assistant Professor of Orthopaedic Surgery
Director
Whitesides Orthopaedic Research Laboratory
Emory University
Atlanta, Georgia, USA

Alim F. Ramji, MD
Orthopaedic Surgery Resident
University of Connecticut Health Center
Farmington, Connecticut, USA

Comron Saifi, MD
Assistant Professor of Orthopaedic Surgery
Division of Spine Surgery
Director of Clinical Orthopaedic Spine Research
Senior Fellow–Leonard Davis Institute
Perelman School of Medicine
University of Pennsylvania
Philadelphia, Pennsylvania, USA

Francis Shen, MD
Warren G. Stamp Endowed Professor
Department of Orthopaedic Surgery
University of Virginia
Charlottesville, Virginia, USA

Kris Siemionow, MD, PhD
Chief of Spine Surgery
Assistant Professor of Orthopaedics and
  Neurosurgery
University of Illinois
Chicago, Illinois, USA

Jakub Sikora-Klak, MD
Orthopaedic Surgery Resident
Department of Orthopaedics
UC San Diego Health
San Diego, California, USA

Andrew Sinensky, BS
Clinical Research Fellow
Rothman Orthopaedic Institute
Philadelphia, Pennsylvania, USA

Chadi Tannoury, MD, FAOA
Medical Director of Orthopaedic
  Ambulatory Clinic
Director of Spine Research
Associate Professor of Orthopaedic
  Surgery
Boston University Medical Center
Boston, Massachusetts, USA

Carol Wang, BS, BSE
MD Candidate
Perelman School of Medicine
University of Pennsylvania
Philadelphia, Pennsylvania, USA

1 Physical Examination

Jannat M. Khan, Nabil Mehta, Philip K. Louie, and Howard S. An

Abstract

A stepwise approach to history collection can lead to a cost-effective and efficient process of treating the patient. The clinician must determine whether the pain is mechanical or nonmechanical and axial or radicular. Paresthesias, numbness, or weakness that follow a dermatomal distribution and are associated with tension signs are more indicative of radicular pain. If the patient has difficulty characterizing the pain, then myelopathy must be considered. To avoid missing important aspects, follow the classic order of physical examination: inspection, palpation, movement, neurological examination, and other special exams. Prior to starting physical examination, look for walking aids the patient may use for mobility, while assessing for coronal or sagittal imbalance. Check for normal ranges of cervical and thoracolumbar motion by examining flexion, extension, lateral flexion, and rotation. Sensory testing will differentiate between spinal root pathology (dermatomal pattern of sensory dysfunction) versus neuropathy (glove/stocking distribution). Muscle strength is graded from 0 to 5, ranging from no evidence of contractility to normal. A series of additional special tests can be applied based on clinical suspicion: thoracic outlet syndrome (Adson test), sacroiliac tests (Patrick test, Gaenslen test, Thigh trust, anterior superior iliac spine (ASIS) distraction, sacral compression test), tension signs (straight leg raise [SLR], opposite SLR, reverse SLR, sitting SLR tests), upper motor neuron signs (Hoffman reflex, clonus, Babinski reflex, ulnar finger escape, grip-and-release test, inverted brachioradialis reflex, pronator drift, Romberg sign), ankylosing spondylitis, and Waddell signs.

Keywords: Spine physical exam, dermatomal patterns, neurological exam, upper motor neuron signs

1.1 Introduction

The incidence of back pain and subsequent spine surgeries is rising, as are the accompanying postoperative complications. In 2008, spine-related complaints ranked among top six reasons for medical office visits, but that number climbed to top three by 2010. Approximately 80% of the population experience low back pain, affecting patients of all ages. Considering the costs and risks that the patient is undertaking, careful measures must be taken during history collection and physical examination to determine the most appropriate treatment course tailored to the patient's needs.

1.2 History

Collecting a comprehensive history is imperative for generating differential diagnoses to guide the patient through the appropriate physical examinations and diagnostic tests. A stepwise approach to history collection can lead to a cost-effective and efficient process of treating the patient.

1.2.1 Degenerative Spine Disorders

For patient with possible degenerative spine conditions, the patient's pain history is an important component. The clinician must determine whether the pain is mechanical or nonmechanical and axial or radicular (▶ Table 1.1).

Table 1.1 Pain associated with degenerative disorders of spine

Mechanical vs. nonmechanical	Mechanical	Nonmechanical
	• Rest is palliative • Pain worsens progressively throughout the day	• Rest/immobilization is not palliative • Pain is worse at night, independent of activity

Axial vs. Radicular	Axial
	
	• Pain is diffuse
	• Referred pain patterns
	  — Cervical spine disorders: scapula or
	     shoulder
	  — Lumbar spine disorders: buttock or
	     posterior thigh
		Radicular
		
		• Pain presents in dermatomal distribution
		• Associated with paresthesia, numbness, or
		  weakness
		• Pain is associated with tension signs

Pain and symptom severity throughout the day can differentiate between mechanical versus non-mechanical pain. Pain relief with rest and pain worsening throughout the day indicate mechanical pain. If rest is not palliative and the pain worsens at night independent of activity, then nonmechanical pain is higher on the differential.

Localization and radiation differentiate axial versus radicular pain (▶ Table 1.1). Diffuse pain associated with referred pain patterns outlined in ▶ Table 1.2 is a clue of axial pain. Paresthesia, numbness, or weakness that follows a dermatomal distribution and is associated with tension signs is more indicative of radicular pain (▶ Fig. 1.1).

If the patient has difficulty characterizing the pain, then myelopathy must be considered. Pain secondary to myelopathy either follows a cervical dermatomal pattern or is nondermatomal when pain is associated with the neck, arm, or leg. Other motor symptoms include a slow and broad-based gait, signs of poor upper extremity motor functions, and other pathological long tract signs. An early sign of upper extremity motor dysfunction is the patient experiencing trouble fastening buttons. Later in the course, bowel and bladder dysfunction may be noted.

1.2.2 Spinal Deformity

Spinal deformity presenting with pain is especially crucial to examine in pediatric patients. Spinal cord or bony tumor, Scheuermann disease, and spondylolisthesis are among some of the possible etiologies to include in differentials. Obtain medical history, pertinent family history, menarche age of onset, time of curve detection with progression for patients presenting with adolescent scoliosis (▶ Fig. 1.2).

Table 1.2 Points of palpation

Bones	Soft tissue
• Spinous processes • Posterior superior iliac spines • Scapula and ribs • Iliac crests • Sacrum and coccyx • Trochanter • Ischial tuberosity	• Trapezius muscle • Rhomboid/levator muscles • Gluteus muscles • Piriformis muscle • Sciatic nerve

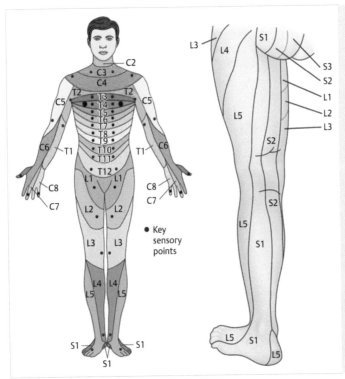

Fig. 1.1 Dermatomal distribution.

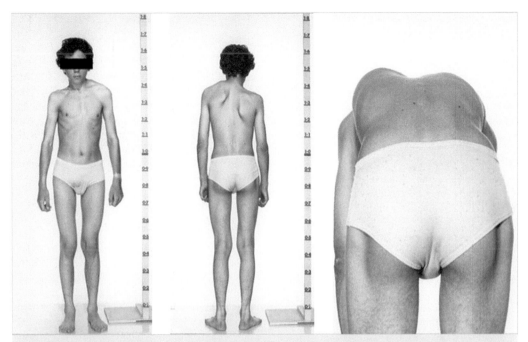

Fig. 1.2 Inspection for spinal deformity. To perform an Adam's forward bending test, ask the patient to stand upright with their feet together and knees extended with both arms at the side. Ensure that the head is in a neutral position. Evaluate for asymmetry in the shoulder or waist alignment as well as any obvious prominence of the scapula or ribs. Make note of the location and laterality of the asymmetry. Next, instruct the patient to place their palms together, tuck the head down, and bend forward (in a diving position). As the examiner, place your eyes at the level with the spine from behind and observe for any differences in the scapula, rib cage, or paraspinous muscles. If a scoliometer is utilized, 5 to 7 degrees is considered the minimum for positive screening.

1.3 Physical Examination

To avoid missing important aspects, follow the classic order of physical examination: inspection, palpation, movement, neurological examination, and other special exams.

1.3.1 Inspection

• Prior to starting physical examination, look for walking aids the patient may use for mobility
• Look for skin lesions (e.g., scars, cafe au lait spots), abnormal hair growth (e.g., occult spinal dysraphism), muscle atrophy (e.g., chronic immobility, neurologic impairment)
• Inspect the patient in coronal and sagittal planes for visible deformities (▶ Table 1.3)

1.3.2 Palpation

See ▶ Table 1.1.

Table 1.3 Features of coronal and sagittal plane examination

Coronal plane examination	Sagittal plane examination

• Scoliosis
• Pelvic obliquity
• Shoulder imbalance
• Scapular protuberance
• Rib prominence
	• Note normal spinal curves
	  – Cervical lordosis: 20–40 degrees
	  – Thoracic kyphosis: 20–45 degrees
	  – Lumbar lordosis: 40–60 degrees

1.3.3 Movement

• Check for normal ranges of cervical and thoracolumbar motion by examining flexion, extension, lateral flexion, and rotation (▶ Table 1.4).

Table 1.4 Normal range of motion

Cervical spine	Thoracolumbar spine
• Flexion: 45 degrees (chin to chest) • Extension: 75 degrees • Lateral flexion: 40 degrees • Rotation: 75 degrees	• Flexion: 80 degrees • Extension: 40 degrees • Lateral flexion: 40 degrees • Rotation: 45 degrees

1.3.4 Neurological Examination

- Sensory testing differentiates between spinal root pathology (dermatomal pattern of sensory dysfunction) and neuropathy (glove/stocking distribution).
  - Pain perception: test with defined anatomic pathways in the spinal cord
  - Light touch: test with cotton swab
  - Temperature: can use two test tubes filled with either a hot or cold solution
  - Proprioception: begin distally (distal phalanx, great toe) and proceed proximally to respective larger joint
- Motor tests
  - Muscle strength is graded from 0 to 5, ranging from no evidence of contractility to normal
    - Grade 5: normal
    - Grade 4: weak against resistance
    - Grade 3: motion against gravity
    - Grade 2: motion with gravity eliminated
    - Grade 1: evidence of contractility
    - Grade 0: no evidence of contractility
  - Motor root reflexes
    - Scapulo-humeral (upper cord): obtained by tapping the tip of the spine of the scapula in a caudal direction
    - Biceps (C5): elicited by placing your thumb on the biceps tendon and striking your thumb with the reflex hammer
    - Brachioradialis (C6): tested by directly striking the brachioradialis tendon approximately 8 to 10 cm above the wrist
    - Triceps (C7): identified by tapping just above the triceps tendon at its insertion on the olecranon while holding the patient's arm with your other hand
    - Patella (L4): examined by striking the patella tendon directly while the lower leg is hanging freely off the edge of the patient's bed
    - Achilles (L5): produced by holding the relaxed foot with one hand and striking the Achilles tendon

1.3.5 Special Tests

- Adson test
  - Tests for thoracic outlet syndrome
  - While feeling the radial pulse, have the patient abduct, extend, and externally rotate the arm. Also have the patient rotate head toward the testing arm
  - Positive test: radial pulse disappears with reproduction of symptoms
- Sacroiliac tests
  - Patrick test
    - Flex, abduct, and externally rotate hip
    - Positive test: referred pain from sacroiliac joint
  - Gaenslen test
    - Have patient extend hip (drop leg on the exam table)
    - Positive test: pain in ipsilateral sacroiliac joint
  - Thigh thrust/Femoral shear
    - Flex hip to 90° with slight adduction (but avoid excessive adduction) while placing one hand over patient's sacrum. Apply axial force on femur as 3–6 high velocity thrusts with increasing pressure
    - Positive test: pain is reproduced in sacroiliac joint/lower back
  - ASIS distraction test (supine)
    - Apply vertically oriented posteriorly directed force to both ASIS
    - Positive test: pain in lumbar spine/sacroiliac joint may indicate sprain of anterior sacroiliac joint ligaments or sacroiliac joint dysfunction
  - Sacral compression test (lateral)
    - Place hand on S2 with fingers pointed in the cranial direction while standing on the symptomatic side and apply 3–6 high velocity thrusts with increasing pressure
    - Positive test: pain is reproduced in the sacroiliac joint
- Tension signs
  - Straight leg raise (SLR) test
    - Position supine without a pillow under his/ her head, the hip medially rotated and adducted, and the knee extended
    - Passively lift the symptomatic leg by the posterior ankle, while keeping the knee extended
    - Positive test: elevation of the leg can cause radicular leg pain (not back pain) and pain is often reproduced at less than 60 degree of flexion

- Cross SLR (opposite leg) test
  - With the patient still supine, passively lift the symptomatic leg by the posterior ankle, while keeping the knee extended
  - Positive test: recreation of back pain or leg pain on the affected side may be a sign of sequestered or large, extruded herniated disc
- Reverse SLR test
  - With the patient prone, lift the hip into extension while keeping the knee straight or bending the knee in order to place the L1–L4 nerve roots under tension
- Positive test: pain over the anterior thigh suggests an upper lumbar disc problem, usually above L4–L5. This test would also be markedly positive in a patient with a condition that involves inflammation of the iliopsoas or appendicitis
- Sitting SLR test

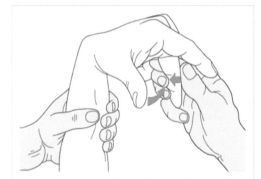

Fig. 1.3 Hoffman exam. Hold the patient's middle finger extended and suddenly extend the distal interphalangeal (DIP) joint of that finger. An alternative method is to flick the DIP joint of that extended digit. The test is considered positive if finger and thumb flexion is observed.

- Distract the patient's attention away from the back by asking whether the patient has knee problems and then lift the foot and extend the knee to evaluate sciatic tension
- Positive test: straightening the knee to full extension on either sides causes the patient to lean back, then significant sciatic tension is present
- Upper motor neuron (UMN) signs and long tract signs
  - Hoffman reflex or sign
    - Hold the middle finger extended and suddenly extend the distal interphalangeal (DIP) joint of that finger. Alternative method: flick the DIP joint
    - Positive test: Finger and thumb flexion indicates presence of myelopathy (▶ Fig. 1.3)
  - Clonus
    - Rapidly dorsiflex the ankle to induce an immediate stretch of the gastrocnemius
    - Positive test: rhythmic, involuntary movements of the ankle more than three beats defined as sustained clonus (▶ Fig. 1.4)
  - Babinski reflex
    - Gentle stimulus applied to the lateral aspect of the sole of the foot, starting over the heel extending towards the 5th digit normally results in flexion of toes
    - Positive test: initial dorsiflexion of the great toe and spreading of the other toes (▶ Fig. 1.5)
  - Ulnar finger escape or Wartenberg sign
    - Ask the patient to extend their fingers and keep their fingers in full extension
    - Positive test: small finger may gradually flex and abduct, indicating weakness of the intrinsic muscles

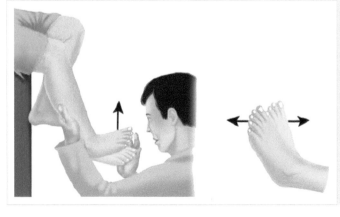

Fig. 1.4 Ankle clonus. Rapidly dorsiflex the ankle to induce an immediate stretch of the gastrocnemius. The test is considered positive (sustained clonus) if rhythmic, involuntary movements of the ankle of more than three beats are observed.

- Grip-and-release test
  - Patients make a fist and release 20 times in 10 seconds
  - Positive test: inability to complete this task in 10 seconds is indicative of myelopathy
- Inverted brachioradialis reflex
  - Tapping of the distal brachioradialis tendon produces spastic ipsilateral finger flexion instead of the normal extension of the wrist
  - Positive test: positive reflex suggests spinal cord compression at the C6 region

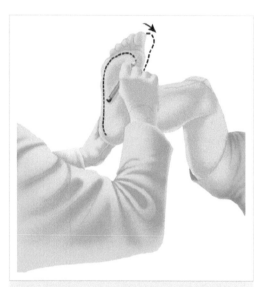

Fig. 1.5 Babinski reflex. Gentle stimulus applied to the lateral aspect of the sole of the foot, starting over the heel extending towards the 5th digit normally, results in flexion of toes. The test is considered positive if initial dorsiflexion of the great toe and spreading of the other toes is observed.

- Pronator drift
  - Patients hold hands in front of them and spread their fingers apart and close their eyes
  - Positive test: one arm will drift down and pronate within 10 seconds which would suggest UMN weakness
- Romberg sign
  - Patient stands with arms held forward and eyes closed
  - Positive test: loss of balance consistent with posterior column dysfunction
- Shober test
  - Tests for ankylosing spondylitis
  - When patient is standing erect, mark 10 cm from the posterior superior iliac spine level. Measure the distance upon forward flexion
  - Positive test: measured distance less than 15 cm (normal lumbar excursion is greater than 5 cm)
- Waddell sign
  - Tests for suggestive signs of malingering
  - Positive test: three or more of the following signs
    - Disproportionate superficial tenderness or nonanatomical exam findings
    - Overreaction
    - Weakness and sensory findings that do not follow appropriate anatomical pattern
    - Simulated tests: Flip test; negative leg extension in sitting position, but markedly positive straight leg raise on supine position; patient-reported pain with the following maneuvers - have patient stand with feet together and rotate the pelvis or compress on the top of the head

Pearls

- Gaenslen test may be difficult to perform in patients with knee pathology. If this is present, reposition hand to flex hip from under knee rather than on top.
- When performing ASIS distraction in the supine position, some authors advocate for 30 seconds of continuous force then repetitive thrusts. However, others do not specify a time limit. This high variability in technique leads to a lower reliability of the test.
- If you are having difficult eliciting the patellar reflex, ask the patient to hold their hands in an attempt to relax a bit more.
- When having difficulty performing the Hoffman reflex by extending the DIP joint of the middle finger while holding that finger in extension, try the alternative method of flicking the DIP joint.

Suggested Readings

An HS, Singh K. Synopsis of spine surgery. New York, NY: Thieme; 2016

Miller MD, Thompson SR. Miller's review of orthopaedics. New York, NY: Elsevier; 2016

2 Patient Positioning—Spine Surgery

Peter B. Derman

Abstract

Careful attention to patient positioning is paramount in order to facilitate operative efficiency, optimize outcomes, and minimize complications. In this chapter, the details of how to properly position patients for a variety of spinal procedures are reviewed. Anterior cervical, anterior lumbar, lateral thoracic and lumbar, posterior cervical, and posterior thoracic and lumbar positions are discussed. Familiarity with these concepts is a prerequisite to performing successful spine surgeries.

Keywords: patient positioning, spine surgery, cervical, thoracic, lumbar

2.1 Introduction

Patient positioning is generally considered to be among the most important aspects of any surgery. It is critical to properly position the patient before surgery to ensure efficiency, adequate visualization of the operative field, and safety of the patient.

2.2 Anterior Cervical Spine Positioning

For anterior cervical procedures, a standard flat OR table is employed. A long, folded sheet is laid over the table prior to positioning the patient. This will be used to help secure the upper extremities. Thigh-high compression stockings and sequential compression devices are placed on the patient to prevent venous stasis. The patient is transferred onto the operating table in a supine position, and a blanket followed by a safety strap is placed across the pelvis. Pillows are placed under the patient's knees to provide support and gentle flexion; a donut pillow is placed under the head. The heels are protected with gel pads or any compressible material. It is important to examine the patient's cervical range of motion preoperatively and avoid deviating from this during induction of anesthesia and patient positioning. Awake endotracheal intubation with pre- and postpositional motors may be advisable in the setting of myelopathy. The anesthesiologist should be instructed to tape the endotracheal tube to the side contralateral to the surgical approach so that the tube is not in the way.

After induction of anesthesia, a Foley catheter and neuromonitoring leads may be placed. Gardner–Wells tongs are used by some surgeons to provide intraoperative axial traction. If tongs are being used, then it can be placed at this time. The pins should be inserted on either side of the head in line with the external auditory meatus approximately 1 centimeter (cm) above the pinna and below the equator of the head to prevent migration. Pins placed too far anteriorly may injure the temporalis muscle as well as the temporal artery and vein. Before placing the pins, scrub the sites with an antiseptic and place antibiotic ointment onto the pins themselves. The screw mechanism should be tightened until the indicator pin protrudes 1 millimeter (mm) from flush; the securing nuts are tightened.

If it can be tolerated by the patient based on preoperative range of motion, a small bump fashioned from a 1 liter (L) saline bag and a towel is positioned in a transverse orientation under the patient's cervico-thoracic junction. Foam padding may be used to provide additional cushion for bony prominences in the cubital tunnel to prevent compression of the ulnar nerve. Keep the patient's thumbs oriented upward and hands relatively accessible so that the anesthesia team can access their intravenous (IV) lines if needed. Next, use heavy cloth tape to tape the shoulders down to the far end of the table. This helps with exposure and radiographic visualization. However, overzealous traction should be avoided as it may lead to loss of neuromonitoring signals and neurologic compromise.

The bed is placed in slight reverse Trendelenburg position to decrease bleeding. If a Foley catheter was placed, then the bag should be brought to the head of the table for access by anesthesia, and the tube should be secured to the table so as not to be accidentally pulled by intraoperative fluoroscopy coming in and out. If Gardner-Wells traction is being used, an anesthesia endotracheal tube holder, also called a Christmas tree, is placed at the head of the bed with the long end positioned under the patient's head pad. Fifteen pounds (lbs) of weight is then suspended from the Gardner–Wells tongs using the endotracheal tube holder as a fulcrum. Drapes were then used to square up the operative field, making sure to leave plenty of room to avoid draping oneself out. The neck is shaved with clippers as needed. A warming device is placed over the patient distal to the operative field to prevent hypothermia during the procedure. Anteroposterior (AP) fluoroscopy may be taken at this point to confirm visualization and neutral rotation, and lateral fluoroscopy can be taken for level localization. The patient is then prepped and draped in the standard sterile fashion.

2.3 Anterior Lumbar Spine Positioning

For lumbar spine procedures performed via an anterior approach, a standard OR table is used. Various retractor systems are available for this procedure. Regardless of which is used, any attachment clamps may be secured to the outer rim of the OR table at this point. Thigh-high compression stockings and sequential compression devices are placed on the patient to prevent venous stasis. The patient is transferred onto the operating table in a supine position, and a blanket under the patient's knees followed by a safety strap is placed across the pelvis. Pillows were placed under the patient's knees to provide support and gentle flexion; a doughnut pillow was placed under the head. The heels are protected with gel pads or a compressible material. After induction of anesthesia, a small bump fashioned from a 1-L saline bag and a towel is positioned in a transverse orientation under the patient's sacrum. This provides improved access to the lumbosacral spine. Neuromonitoring leads and a Foley catheter may be placed at this time. If the L4–L5 level is being approached as part of the procedure, a pulse oximetry monitor is placed onto the patient's left great toe to provide advanced notice of any hypoperfusion related to retraction of the great vessels. This is not necessary if L5–S1 alone is being approached, as the operative window at this level is between the vessels and therefore requires less retraction. The table is placed in slight Trendelenburg position so that gravity assists in pulling abdominal contents cranially and to improve the working angle, given the orientation of the L4–L5 and L5–S1 disc spaces.

The upper extremities are then positioned. Various techniques exist for this. The arms may be extended out from the patient's sides or folded over the patient's chest. Regardless of the arm position chosen, the arms should be out of the way, and all bony prominences and potential sites of peripheral nerve compression should be well-padded. Clear U drapes are then used to isolate the operative field, and the region is shaved using clippers if needed.

The Foley bag should be brought to the head of the table for access by anesthesia, and the tube should be secured to the table so as to not be accidentally pulled by intraoperative fluoroscopy coming in and out. A warming device is placed over the patient's lower extremities to prevent hypothermia during the procedure. An AP fluoroscopy shot is taken to confirm adequate visualization as well as neutral rotation of the spine. Small adjustments can be made by rolling the operating table to one side or the other via the table's adjustment mechanisms. However, anything greater should trigger repositioning of the patient as excessive rolling of the table can lead to an unstable patient and potential injury. Once the AP fluoroscopy is optimized, a lateral fluoroscopy shot should be taken to localize for the surgical incision which is then marked. The patient is then prepped and draped in the standard sterile fashion.

2.4 Lateral Thoracic and Lumbar Spine Positioning

For direct lateral approaches to the lumbar and thoracic spine, a standard OR table is used but rotated 180 degrees so that the normal head of the table will be at the foot. This allows for intraoperative imaging unimpeded by the base of the OR table. A table extender is placed at the end where the patient's head will rest so that the table is sufficiently long. Thigh-high compression stockings and sequential compression devices are placed on the patient to prevent venous stasis. The patient is transferred onto the OR table in a supine position, and a blanket followed by a safety strap is placed across the pelvis.

After induction of anesthesia, a Foley catheter and neuromonitoring leads may be inserted. The patient is then carefully rolled into the lateral position with the greater trochanter just distal to the break in the table. For thoracic cases it may be helpful to place a bump under the level of interest to improve surgical access. The patient's back should lie close to the edge of table so that the surgeon does not have to lean over as far during the operation. This position is particularly important if the procedure requires percutaneous pedicle screw insertion from the lateral position otherwise the table will block your angle for cannulating the pedicles on the down side. Blankets are then placed beneath the patient's head to support it in a neutral position. An axillary roll was placed just caudal to the axilla on the downside, and additional gel or foam padding is used on the down leg to protect bony prominences and peripheral nerves such as the peroneal nerve. The hips should be flexed 45 degrees to minimize traction across the lumbar plexus and the knees are flexed to 90. A blanket or pillow is placed between the knees to pad them. An arm board is attached to the table anterior to the patient onto which both arms rest. Blankets and foam padding are used between and around the arms. Heavy cloth tape is then wrapped circumferentially around the patient and table to secure the patient's pelvis and chest. A towel should be placed over the chest to prevent direct adhesive contact to the nipple. Some surgeons prefer a kidney post at the patient's sacrum for additional support while others do not. The arms are then secured with heavy cloth tape. The lower extremities are then taped as well–starting at the greater trochanter on the up side, extending along the thigh to the anterior corner of the table, looping around the foot of the table, and then coming back up along the leg to the side of the table just anterior to the greater trochanter. This forms an "X" or figure-8 formation. Make sure the knee and ankle are padded with foam in the regions under the tape. The table was then flexed as needed to improve access to the levels of interest, but excessive "jack knifing" of the table may place undue stress on the lumbar plexus and predispose the patient to neurologic injury.

Clear U drapes are then used to isolate the operative field; make sure the drapes are sufficiently wide to avoid draping yourself out, especially if using a two-incision technique. If a fixed retractor is being used, make sure that any associated bracket is snugly fixed to the table in the appropriate position. The Foley bag should be brought to the head of the table for access by anesthesia, and the tube should be secured to the table so as not to be accidentally pulled by intraoperative fluoroscopy coming in and out. The surgeon typically stands posterior to the patient, and the C-arm comes in from the patient's anterior. Unless a wide-open approach as planned, these procedures rely heavily on fluoroscopic imaging, and it is extremely important to achieve good fluoroscopic views with the spinal level of interest position perfectly perpendicular to the floor. First, obtain a perfect AP fluoroscopy shot at the level of interest with the beam parallel to the floor. This is to ensure that the patient isn't rotated. If the rotation is slightly off, small adjustments can be made by rolling the operating table from one side to the other via the table's adjustment mechanism. But anything greater should trigger repositioning of the patient,

as excessive rolling of the table can lead to an unstable patient and potential injury. A lateral fluoroscopy shot is then taken. Adjust the table flexion and Trendelenburg position so that you have a clear view working straight down the disc space of interest. Then localize and mark the surgical incision. To prevent hypothermia during the procedure, a warming device may be placed over the patient's upper body or lower extremities as dictated by the spinal region be approached. The patient is then prepped and draped in the standard sterile fashion.

2.5 Posterior Cervical

For posterior cervical procedures, a standard OR table with a Mayfield skull clamp attached may be used. Large gel bolsters are placed longitudinally on each side of the table flush with its head. A long-folded sheet is laid over the bolsters prior to positioning the patient. This will be used to help secure the upper extremities. Additional gel pads are placed distally to pad the patient's knees. Another option is to use an open Jackson frame with posts. Thigh-high compression stockings and sequential compression devices are placed on the patient to prevent venous stasis. It is important to examine the patient's cervical range of motion preoperatively and avoid deviating from this during induction of anesthesia and patient positioning. Awake endotracheal intubation with pre- and postpositional motors may be advisable in the setting of myelopathy.

After induction of anesthesia, a Foley catheter and neuromonitoring leads can be placed. The Mayfield tongs are also placed ensuring that the main arc of the device has sufficient clearance over the patient's forehead and face. Before pin placement, scrub the sites with antiseptic and place antibiotic ointment onto the pins themselves. The pins are positioned with a single pin on one side of the head and two pins on the other, all of which are placed over the region where a sweatband might lie if the patient were wearing one. Pressure of 60 lbs is applied. The patient is then carefully rolled prone onto the operating table. The Mayfield tongs are firmly attached to the bed making sure that the neck is appropriately positioned. This typically means that it is straight in the coronal plane, and in the sagittal plane, the neck is flexed throughout with the chin tucked to aid in exposure. For fusion procedures, this position can be modified intraoperatively prior to locking down the final cervical alignment.

A blanket is placed across the legs, and a safety strap secured over it. The upper extremities are then positioned. Foam padding can be used to provide additional cushion at bony prominences and over the cubital tunnel. The down sheet is wrapped over the arms and may be tucked under the patient on either side or secured on top of the patient with tape or clamps. The patient's arms should be straight with the thumbs oriented downward. If a Wilson frame is being used, another option is to rest the arms, positioned by the patient's sides, on arm boards. The hand should be relatively accessible so anesthesia can access their IV's if needed. Next, use heavy cloth tape to tape the shoulders down to the far end of the table. This helps with exposure and radiographic visualization. Overzealous traction should be avoided however, as it may lead to loss of neuromonitoring signals and neurologic compromise. In obese patients, additional strips of tape can be used to pull down on the thoracic soft tissue to aid in visualization. The bed is placed in slight reverse Trendelenburg position to decrease bleeding. The knees should be slightly flexed and legs supported with pillows. The foot of the table can also be flexed up slightly to support the legs and prevent the patient from sliding down the table. Shave the patient's neck and posterior hairline as needed, depending on the spinal levels to be approached. Apply clear drapes to square out the field. If a Foley catheter was placed, the bag should be brought to the head of the table for access by the anesthesiologist, and the tube should be secured to the table so as not to be accidentally pulled by intraoperative fluoroscopy coming in and out. A warming device is placed distal to the operative field so as to prevent hypothermia during the procedure. Fluoroscopy shots can be taken at this point to confirm adequate radiographic visualization and appropriate positioning. The patient is then prepped and draped in the standard sterile fashion.

2.6 Posterior Thoracic and Lumbar Spine Positioning

Posterior thoracic and lumbar procedures are typically performed on an open Jackson frame, although a Wilson frame or a standard OR table with chest bolsters are also options. In this section, positioning on a Jackson frame will be described. Padded chest and pelvic pads are placed onto the frame bilaterally. For isolated decompressions, the lower extremities are typically supported in a sling to flex and therefore open up the posterior aspect of the spine. For procedures involving fusion, the lower extremities are placed on a padded flat board

and a Wilson frame is not used to maximize lumbar lordosis and prevent fusion in a kyphotic position. Thigh-high compression stockings and sequential compression devices are placed onto the patient to prevent venous stasis.

After induction of anesthesia, a Foley catheter and neuromonitoring leads may be inserted. The patient is carefully rolled into the prone position on the operating table. The patient's head rests on a foam face pad with great care taken to ensure that there is no pressure on the eyes. For longer procedures such as spinal deformity correction, some surgeons utilize Gardner–Wells tongs and axial traction to support the head and offload the face. If being used, the tongs should be placed after the induction of anesthesia, but prior to rolling the patient onto the Jackson frame. The pins should be located at the patient's head, in line with the external auditory meatus approximately 1 cm above the pinna and below the equator of the head to prevent migration. Pins placed too far anteriorly may injure the temporalis muscle as well as the temporal artery and vein. Before pin placement, scrub the sites with antiseptic and place antibiotic ointment onto the pins themselves. The screw mechanism should be tightened until the indicator pin protrudes 1 millimeter (mm) from flush; the securing nuts are then tightened. Once the patient is flipped onto the operating frame, 15 to 20 lbs of axial traction is applied. Some surgeons allow the face to be freely suspended while others use the foam face pad in addition to traction.

Chest pads should be located just caudal to, but not impinging on the axilla, to prevent injury to the brachial plexus. The breasts are tucked medially. Pelvic pads should be situated at the anterior superior iliac spine or even slightly below. This allows the abdomen to hang free which decreases venous back bleeding and serves to maximize lordosis for fusion cases. For male patients, make sure that the genitals hang free with no sources of external pressure. The upper extremities are placed on adjustable arm boards such that the shoulders are abducted and the elbows are bent at 90 degrees. Additionally, the shoulders should be forward flexed slightly such that they rest in a comfortable position. Make sure that the arm boards are slid as cranially as possible while still maintaining appropriate patient positioning so that they allow as much working room as possible for the surgeon, especially if working in the thoracic spine. Foam cradles are placed under the upper extremities to provide additional padding of bony prominences and peripheral nerves such as the ulnar nerve at the cubital tunnel. Make sure that the wrists are in neutral position to prevent iatrogenic median nerve compression. If a Foley catheter was placed, the bag should be brought to the head of the table for access by anesthesia, and the tube should be secured to the table so as not to be accidentally pulled by intraoperative fluoroscopy coming in and out. Clear drapes are then used to isolate the operative field, in the region is shaved with clippers if needed. To prevent hypothermia during the procedure, a warming device is placed over the patient's upper back or lower extremities as dictated by the surgical region to be approached. Fluoroscopic shots can then be taken to localize for the surgical incision at this time. The patient was then prepped and draped in the standard sterile fashion.

Pearls

- When positioning for an anterior cervical spine procedure, make sure to examine the patient's cervical range of motion preoperatively and avoid deviating from this during induction of anesthesia and patient positioning.
- For anterior lumbar spine procedure, the table is placed in slight Trendelenburg position so that gravity assists in pulling abdominal contents cranially and to improve the working angle given the orientation of the L4–L5–S1 disc spaces.
- After lateral thoracic and lumbar spine positioning, obtain perfect AP and lateral fluoroscopic images at the level of interest with the beam parallel and perpendicular to the floor, respectively, to ensure that the patient is not rotated and that the disc level is oriented in a vertical position.
- During posterior cervical spine positioning, use heavy cloth tape to tape the shoulders down to the far end of the table. This helps with exposure and radiographic visualization. Overzealous traction should be avoided however, as it may lead to loss of neuromonitoring signals and neurologic compromise.
- When positioning for posterior lumbar procedures involving fusion, a Wilson frame is not used, and the lower extremities are placed on a padded flat board rather than in a sling to maximize lumbar lordosis and prevent fusion in a kyphotic position.
- For posterior thoracic spine positioning, be diligent to slide the arm boards as cranially as possible while still maintaining appropriate patient positioning so that they allow as much working room as possible for the surgeon.

2.7 Board-style Questions

1. When positioning for a procedure utilizing the posterior cervical approach, overzealous traction should be avoided to prevent which of the following?
   a) Abrasions
   b) Difficulty with intra-operative imaging
   c) Post-operative dysphagia
   d) Loss of neuromonitoring signals and neurologic compromise

2. During the positioning for an anterior lumbar spine procedure, table is placed in Trendelenburg position for which of the following reasons?
   a) Decrease bleeding
   b) Pull abdominal contents cranially
   c) Improve the working angle for L4–L5–S1 disc spaces
   d) a & c
   e) b & c
   f) a & b

3. For posterior lumbar fusion procedures, lower extremities are placed on a padded flat board to achieve which of the following?
   a) Maximize lumbar lordosis

b) Prevent fusion in lordosis
c) Prevent fusion in kyphosis
d) a & c
e) a & b
f) b & c

4. The hips and knees are flexed when positioning for a lateral approach to prevent which of the following?
   a) Stress on the peroneal nerve on the asymptomatic side
   b) Pressure on femoral nerve on the asymptomatic side
   c) Stress on the lumbar plexus
   d) Stress on the sciatic nerve on the asymptomatic side
   e) Stress on the femoral nerve on the symptomatic side

Answers

1. d
2. e
3. d
4. c

3 Cervical Radiculopathy

Philip K. Louie, Michael H. McCarthy, and Howard S. An

Abstract

There are two main etiologies of cervical radiculopathy: (1) degenerative cervical spondylosis and (2) disc herniation. Many conditions can present with symptoms similar to those observed in cervical radiculopathy. A careful examination should be carried out to identify the pathologic nerve root level. However, it is important to remember that there can be a cross-over between myotomes and dermatomes in presentation. Nonsurgical/Conservative management is generally the first line of treatment as the natural history of cervical radiculopathy is generally considered favorable, without progression to myelopathy. Patients are generally indicated for operative intervention if conservative treatment has failed to relieve neurologic deficits or radicular symptoms or if there are signs of progressive root/cord dysfunction. Depending on the pathology, surgery can be addressed either anteriorly or posteriorly. Anterior cervical surgery allows for a muscle-sparing approach, allows for direct removal of anterior pathology without direct retraction of neural structures, and can be utilized in patients with a kyphotic deformity. However, complications include dysphagia, hoarseness, vertebral/carotid artery injury, dural tears, or esophageal/tracheal injury. The posterior approach can be performed through minimally invasive techniques. It allows for direct access to the posterior longitudinal ligament (PLL), and for decompression-only procedures without significant destabilization of the cervical spine. With either an anterior or posterior approach, success rates are high when decompressing cervical nerve roots for radiculopathy.

Keywords: Cervical radiculopathy, disc herniation, cervical spondylosis, anterior cervical discectomy fusion, posterior cervical decompression and fusion

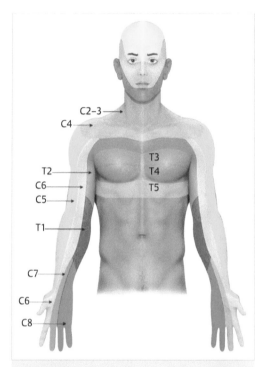

Fig. 3.1 Cervical and thoracic nerve root dermatomal distribution.

3.1 Introduction

Cervical radiculopathy presents as sensory and/or motor deficits in the upper extremities, with a reported incidence of 83 per 100,000 adults. Symptoms often follow a dermatomal distribution of cervical and/or thoracic nerve roots (▶ Fig. 3.1).

There are two main etiologies of cervical radiculopathy: (1) degenerative cervical spondylosis and (2) disc herniation (▶ Fig. 3.2).

3.2 History and Examination

Disc herniation generally presents in individuals younger than age 50, with an equal distribution between males and females. The symptoms are often predominantly in the upper extremities in a single dermatomal distribution and tend to present acutely. Concomitant neck pain is common, whereas myelopathic symptoms (secondary to spinal cord compression) are less common. Patients presenting with cervical spondylosis often are older than 50 years old with a male predominance. Onset of symptoms tends to be more insidious in nature with pain evenly distributed between the neck and upper extremities over multiple myotomes/dermatomes. Concomitant

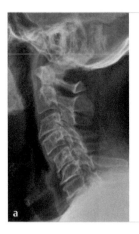 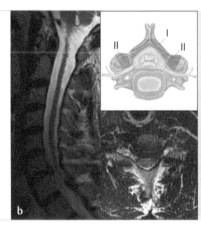

Fig. 3.2 (a) Lateral plain radiograph of the cervical spine demonstrates multilevel cervical spondylosis. (b) T2-weighted magnetic resonance (MR) imaging in a patient presenting with C6 radicular symptoms in the left upper extremity revealing a left-sided disc protrusion at C6–C7, causing left-sided foraminal stenosis.

Table 3.1 Cervical spine muscle and reflex testing

Nerve root	Pain/Sensory loss distribution	Motor function involved	Reflex
C2–C3	Temporal Occipital headaches Retroauricular	–	–
C4	Neck base Trapezial	–	–
C5	Shoulder Lateral arm	Deltoid	Biceps
C6	Forearm (radial) Thumb, index fingers	Biceps Brachioradialis Wrist extension	Brachioradialis
C7	Medial scapula Dorsum forearm Middle finger	Triceps Wrist flexion Finger extension	Triceps
C8	Forearm (ulnar) Ring and small fingers	Finger flexion	–
T1	Upper arm (medial)	Hand intrinsics	–

myelopathy is more common in this patient population compared to those presenting with an acute disc herniation. Patients may complain of numbness, paresthesias, weakness, and/or hyporeflexia in the affected dermatomes. Additionally, patients may also present with occipital headaches or interscapular/trapezial pain, especially if the upper cervical nerve roots are compressed.

A careful examination should be carried out to identify the pathologic nerve root level. However, it is important to remember that there can be a cross-over between myotomes and dermatomes in presentation. The sensory exam should evaluate at least one function from the dorsal columns (joint position, light touch) as well as the spinothalamic tract (temperature sensation, pain). The motor exam should grade strength on a standard 0 to 5 scale. Specific muscle and reflex testing is summarized in ▶ Table 3.1. Additionally, provocative tests can be performed to reproduce radicular symptoms. A positive Spurling sign is observed when radicular pain is exacerbated by neck extension and rotation towards the symptomatic side. A shoulder abduction relief sign may also be present. This is exhibited by the improvement of radicular pain by shoulder abduction (most often observed in the setting of a soft disc herniation). Concomitant myelopathy should be assessed for by evaluating upper motor neuron signs: gait instability, Hoffmann sign, clonus, inverted brachioradialis reflex, and Babinski sign.

Table 3.2 Cervical radiculopathy differential diagnosis

Pathology	Differential diagnosis
Shoulder	Rotator cuff disease/injury Impingement syndrome Adhesive capsulitis Glenoid cyst
Trauma	Muscular strain Brachial plexus injury Instability secondary to trauma
Infection	Osteomyelitis Diskitis Soft tissue abscess
Tumor	Spinal cord tumors Horner syndrome Pancoast tumor Primary bone tumor Metastatic disease
Neurologic	Guillain–Barre syndrome Other demyelinating diseases Amyotrophic lateral sclerosis
Vascular	Epidural varicose veins Vertebral artery dissection
Inflammatory	Ankylosing spondylitis Rheumatoid arthritis
Visceral	Coronary artery disease Cholecystitis
Others	Tendinopathies shoulder, elbow, wrist Thoracic outlet syndrome Multiple sclerosis Acute brachial neuritis Angina pectoris Reflex sympathetic dystrophy Peripheral nerve entrapments

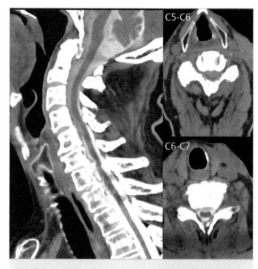

Fig. 3.3 Computed tomography (CT) myelogram sagittal and axial cuts of the cervical spine demonstrating multilevel degenerative. There is a C4–C5 disc extrusion, along with buckling and calcification of the ligamentum flavum. Visible foraminal narrowing bilaterally.

3.2.1 Differential Diagnosis

Many conditions can present with symptoms similar to those observed in cervical radiculopathy (▶ Table 3.2). A thorough history and physical exam must be obtained to rule out alternative pathology.

3.2.2 Diagnostic Imaging

The first line of imaging is plain radiographs (anteroposterior [AP], lateral, and oblique views). In patients with spondylosis, the radiographs may reveal osteophyte formation or decreased disc height at the pathologic levels compared to adjacent levels (▶ Fig. 3.2a). These patients may also present with degenerative changes in the zygaphophyseal joints and forminal narrowing (seen on oblique views). Advanced imaging allows for better visualization of neural anatomy and associated pathology. Magnetic resonance imaging (MRI) is the modality of choice to further evaluate cervical spine radiculopathy when symptoms are severe or not improving with conservative measures (▶ Fig. 3.2b). It is important to remember that there is MRI evidence of nerve root compression in 19% of asymptomatic individuals, so correlation with clinical symptoms is critical. MRI is essential for evaluation of the space available for the cord (less than 13 mm is relative stenosis, less than 10 mm is critical stenosis). Additionally, this imaging is useful to visualize and rule out spinal cord lesions (i.e., tumors, myelomalacia, syringomyelia). For patients who are unable to obtain an MRI or if instrumentation is present, a computed tomography (CT) may be helpful. In rare cases, myelo-CT can be performed. This is an invasive study, involving intradural injections with radiopaque dye that allows for visualization of mechanical blocks to cerebrospinal fluid (CSF) (▶ Fig. 3.3). CT myelogram may also be useful to detect foraminal stenosis and discern if the nerve root compression is caused by soft or hard disc pathology. A regular CT scan without myelogram is adequate for the majority of patients to further evaluate the osseous anatomy (▶ Fig. 3.4).

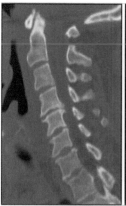
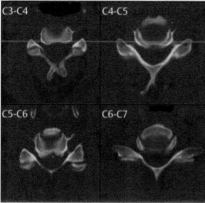

Fig. 3.4 Computed tomography (CT) sagittal and axial cuts of the cervical spine demonstrating multilevel degenerative changes.

C3-C4

C4-C5

C5-C6

C6-C7

Table 3.3 Initial conservative treatment for cervical radiculopathy

Phase	Treatment modality
Acute (first 2 weeks)	Nonsteroidal anti-inflammatory drugs/medications (NSAIDs)
	Short-term analgesia (limit use of narcotics)
	Oral steroids
	Application of heat or ice
	Activity modification
	Immobilization—soft collar
	Home traction
Intermediate (3–4 weeks)	Stretching
	Isometric exercises
	Formal physical therapy—various modalities if not improving
	Epidural injections (if persistent radicular pain)
Rehabilitation (>4 weeks)	Cardiovascular conditioning
	Vigorous strengthening exercise program

3.2.3 Treatments

Nonsurgical/Conservative management is generally the first line of treatment as the natural history of cervical radiculopathy is generally considered favorable, without progression to myelopathy. Literature establishes that 70 to 85% of patients describe resolution of symptoms following 2 to 3 months of a conservative treatment (▶ Table 3.3).

Patients are generally indicated for operative intervention if conservative treatment has failed to relieve neurologic deficits or radicular symptoms or if there are signs of progressive root/cord dysfunction. If the patient experiences resolution of radicular symptoms, but continues to describe axial neck pain, conservative treatment should be continued as long as possible, because surgical outcomes are less predictable when radicular symptoms are no longer present.

Depending on the pathology, surgery can be addressed either anteriorly or posteriorly (▶ Table 3.4). Anterior cervical surgery allows for a muscle-sparing approach, allows for direct removal of anterior pathology without direct retraction of neural structures, and can be utilized in patients with a kyphotic deformity. However, complications include dysphagia, hoarseness, vertebral/carotid artery injury, dural tears, or esophageal/tracheal injury. Anterior cervical discectomy and fusion (ACDF) has been associated with successful outcomes for a variety of degenerative conditions of the cervical spine via neural decompression and stabilization. Allograft with local autograft can be used in instrumentation for fusion. Previous off-label use of recombinant human bone morphogenetic protein-2 (rhBMP-2) has declined following concerns of dysphagia and soft tissue swelling causing airway compromise. Interbody cage devices can be used to hold graft material, maintain foraminal height, and provide additional structural integrity. An increased use of polyetheretherketone (PEEK) cages has replaced titanium and carbon fiber cages, due to several beneficial properties: radiolucent cage, similar modulus of elasticity to bone, nonabsorbable and biocompatible, with a reduced risk of subsidence (▶ Fig. 3.5). Use of anterior plates is generally recommended for patients undergoing single-level fusion with allograft, multilevel interbody fusion, and high-risk patients (smokers, revision). Cervical disc arthroplasty (CDA) was designed as a motion-preserving device to reduce the risk of adjacent segment degeneration (ASD). Rates of revision and re-operations as well as rates of ASD have been controversial in the setting of author and industry bias. The indications for CDA include radiculopathy

Table 3.4 Operative options for cervical radiculopathy

Approach	Procedure	Indication(s)
Anterior	Anterior cervical discectomy and fusion (ACDF)	Bilateral radiculopathy at same level Unilateral soft disc herniation Central soft disc herniation Kyphosis
	Cervical disc arthroplasty (CDA)	*Purpose:* motion-sparing device to reduce ASD
Posterior	Laminoforaminotomy	Minimal axial neck pain • Unilateral soft disc herniation • Foraminal stenosis Ossification of the PLL Neutral or lordotic sagittal alignment Desire motion preservation
	Laminoplasty (+/– instrumentation)	Same as Laminoforaminotomy, except not as effective for foraminal stenosis
	Laminectomy and instrumented fusion	Same as Laminoforaminotomy, except: • Bilateral foraminal stenosis • Significant axial neck pain • Instability present

Abbreviations: ASD, adjacent segment degeneration; PLL, posterior longitudinal ligament.

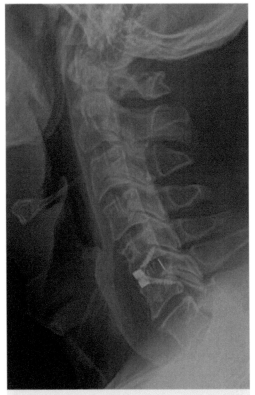

Fig. 3.5 Stand-alone polyetheretherketone (PEEK) cage with integrated screw fixation.

due to herniated nucleus pulposus (HNP) or foraminal stenosis without significant facet arthritis, and disc space narrowing greater than 50%. The segment also should have motion on flexion/extension and lateral bending radiographs. The posterior approach can be performed through minimally invasive techniques. It allows for direct access to the posterior longitudinal ligament (PLL), and for decompression-only procedures without significant destabilization of the cervical spine. A laminoforaminotomy is a motion-preserving procedure that is indicated for cervical radiculopathy (with foraminal pathology) and minimal axial neck symptoms (▶ Fig. 3.6).

Postoperatively, a rigid collar is generally not necessary if an instrumented fusion has been performed. Soft collars can be applied for comfort. The patient can generally begin range of motion activities in the immediate post-operative period.

3.2.4 Outcomes

With either an anterior or posterior approach, success rates are high when decompressing cervical nerve roots for radiculopathy. Outcomes of arm pain relief as well as improvements in motor and sensory function have been shown to be 80 to 90%. The current literature does not well establish which patients and when patients should undergo operative intervention. Many comparative studies suffer from a selection bias and lack randomization.

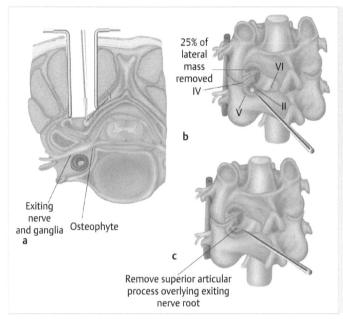

Fig. 3.6 Posterior cervical foraminotomy. (**a**) A cutting burr is used to thin out the lamina (labeled I). (**b**) Approximately 25% of the lateral mass is removed, which exposes the lamina (II), superior articular process of the inferior lamina (V), facet joint (IV), and ligamentum flavum (VI). (**c**) A curette is then utilized to remove the superior articular process overlying the nerve root.

Pearls

- Differential diagnosis should include intrinsic shoulder pathology, peripheral nerve entrapment syndrome, and double crush syndrome.
- Upper cervical radiculopathy (C4 and rarely C3) due to foraminal stenosis is not uncommon, and they present with unilateral neck pain over the trapezius muscle.
- C8 radiculopathy and cubital tunnel syndrome present with similar findings of intrinsic muscle weakness and decreased sensation of the small finger, but differentiating examination findings for C8 radiculopathy include decreased sensation over the medial forearm and weakness of the EPL or EDL of the index finger. T1 radiculopathy is rare but can occur due to HNP or foraminal stenosis at T1–T2.
- Foraminal stenosis due to bony osteophytes can be assessed by oblique radiographs and 45-degree oblique reconstruction CT images. Direct oblique MRI can be done as well.
- In the absence of severe or progressive neurologic symptoms, conservative therapies should be trialed for most patients presenting with cervical radiculopathy.
- The key to laminoforaminotomy is adequate decompression while preserving stability. The average amount of facet excision is 50% but the amount of facet excision depends on the patient's pathoanatomy. At the end of laminoforaminotomy, a Woodson should pass through the foramen and palpation of the pedicle above and below.
- During ACDF, anterior osteophytes should be removed to the level of vertebral body for better discectomy and plating flush to the vertebral body. For anterior foraminotomy, a burr is usually recommended to thin the uncovertebral joint, followed by microcurett or 1-mm Kerrison rongeur to complete decompression of the nerve root. A nerve hook should pass into the foramen after adequate decompression of the foramen.
- The key to fusion success is the preparation of the endplates and adequate sized graft or cage with optimal distraction. Distraction of 2 mm is recommended to improve the size of the foramen and to provide compression between the graft and the endplate after release of the distraction. Distraction can be achieved by tongs, laminar spreader or Caspar pins. A 3-mm burr holes are made in the middle of the endplates to enhance vascularity and bone marrow content to infuse the graft.

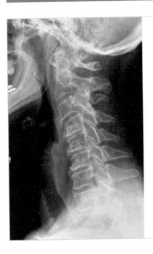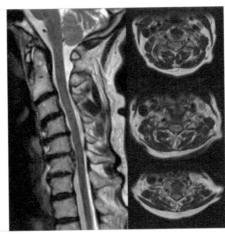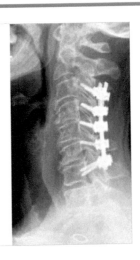

3.3 Case Examples

3.3.1 Case 1

This is a 78-year-old female with a long-standing history of axial neck pain and bilateral upper extremity radicular symptoms. She trialed various conservative treatments for 15 months, including: anti-inflammatory medications, traction, epidural injections, physical therapy, and narcotic pain medications. However, she did not experience any improvement of symptoms. Plain radiographs of the cervical spine showed multilevel degenerative changes (*left image*). MRI demonstrated multilevel cervical stenosis at the multiple bilateral foramina with degenerative disc disease (*middle image*). She subsequently underwent right C3–C4 and C4–C5 hemilaminectomies with foraminotomies, bilateral C5–C6 hemilaminectomies with foraminotomies, and a C3–C7 posterolateral instrumented fusion with fixation using lateral mass screws (see the above images).

3.3.2 Case 2

This is a 47-year-old female who presented with a several month history of axial neck pain and numbness/tingling and weakness down the right upper extremity in the C6 and C7 nerve root distributions. Plain radiographs of the cervical spine were consistent with degenerative changes at C5–C6 and C6–C7 with loss of lordosis (*left image*). MRI and CT demonstrated significant foraminal stenosis at C5–C6 and C6–C7 with degenerative disc changes (*middle two images*). She attempted multiple conservative measures including: traction, anti-inflammatory medications, activity modification, epidural injections, and narcotic medications. However, the symptoms all persisted. She subsequently underwent an ACDF at C5–C6 and C6–C7 with cortico-cancellous allograft and a rigid, locking anterior plate. Her symptoms improved over the next several weeks following surgery (see the images on next page).

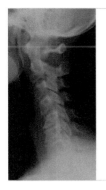 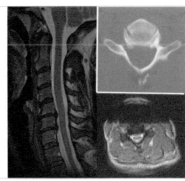 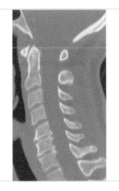 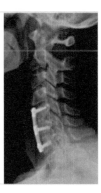

3.4 Board-style Questions

1. A 28-year-old man describes left upper extremity pain and tingling that radiates from the left side of his neck down his arm, to the dorso-radial aspect of the forearm, to the thumb and index fingers. At which level is he most likely to have a left-sided cervical disc herniation?
   a) C3–C4
   b) C4–C5
   c) C5–C6
   d) C6–C7
   e) C7–T1

2. A 42-year-old female is diagnosed with a herniated nucleus pulposus at C6–C7; what is the most likely distribution of symptoms?
   a) Posterior neck, scapula, and clavicle; weakness of head-and-neck extensor muscles
   b) Pain at the wrist; tingling at the ring and small fingers, weak finger flexors
   c) Pain at the elbow; tingling at the thumb and index finger, weakness of biceps and wrist extensors
   d) Pain at the forearm and hand; numbness of the middle finger; weakness of the triceps and finger extensors
   e) Pain and numbness around the shoulder; weakness of the deltoid

3. A 56-year-old male mechanic presents with 4 months of pain at the hypothenar region of his left hand. He states, that over the past few weeks, he has noticed worsening of the pain and weakness of his grip in the left hand. Thinking through the differential, which of the following exam findings would be most suggestive of cervical pathology?
   a) Atrophy of the hypothenar musculature
   b) Positive Tinel sign at the levator scapulae
   c) Ulnar nerve subluxation with elbow range of motion
   d) Relief of symptoms with shoulder abduction over the head
   e) Hyperflexion of the next and rotation to the contralateral side recreates the symptoms

4. What is the preferred screw placement technique during a posterior cervical fusion at the C7 vertebral body?
   a) Pedicle; due to the thin anatomy of the lateral mass
   b) Lateral mass; due to the thin anatomy of the pedicle
   c) Lateral mass; vertebral artery at greater risk with pedicle screw placement
   d) Pedicle; vertebral artery at greater risk with lateral mass screw placement

e) Lateral mass; pedicle landmarks are increasingly difficult to visualize and palpate at the C7 level

5. Following an anterior cervical discectomy and fusion, the following are radiographic examples of ASD, except:
   a) Anterior vertebral body osteophytes
   b) Disc space narrowing
   c) Calcification of the anterior longitudinal ligament
   d) Progressive spondylolisthesis
   e) Blunting of the endplates

Answers ✓

1. c
2. d
3. d
4. a
5. e

Suggested Readings

Boden SD, Davis DO, Dina TS, Patronas NJ, Wiesel SW. Abnormal magnetic-resonance scans of the lumbar spine in asymptomatic subjects. A prospective investigation. J Bone Joint Surg Am. 1990; 72(3):403–408

Bohlman HH, Emery SE, Goodfellow DB, Jones PK. Robinson anterior cervical discectomy and arthrodesis for cervical radiculopathy: long-term follow-up of one hundred and twenty-two patients. J Bone Joint Surg Am. 1993; 75(9):1298–1307

Bono CM, Ghiselli G, Gilbert TJ, et al. North American Spine Society. An evidence-based clinical guideline for the diagnosis and treatment of cervical radiculopathy from degenerative disorders. Spine J. 2011; 11(1):64–72

Engquist M, Löfgren H, Öberg B, et al. Surgery versus nonsurgical treatment of cervical radiculopathy: a prospective, randomized study comparing surgery plus physiotherapy with physiotherapy alone with a 2-year follow-up. Spine. 2013; 38(20): 1715–1722

Lees F, Turner JW. Natural history and prognosis of cervical spondylosis. BMJ. 1963; 2(5373):1607–1610

Matz PG, Holly LT, Groff MW, et al. Indications for Anterior Cervical Decompression for the Treatment of Cervical Degenerative Radiculopathy. Vol. 11. American Association of Neurological Surgeons; 2009:174–182

Phillips FM, Geisler FH, Gilder KM, Reah C, Howell KM, McAfee PC. Long-term outcomes of the US FDA IDE prospective, randomized controlled clinical trial comparing PCM cervical disc arthroplasty with anterior cervical discectomy and fusion. Spine. 2015; 40(10):674–683

Radhakrishnan K, Litchy WJ, O'Fallon WM, Kurland LT. Epidemiology of cervical radiculopathy: a population-based study from Rochester, Minnesota, 1976 through 1990. Brain. 1994; 117 (Pt 2):325–335

Rao R. Neck pain, cervical radiculopathy, and cervical myelopathy: pathophysiology, natural history, and clinical evaluation. J Bone Joint Surg Am. 2002; 84(10):1872–1881

Rhee JM, Yoon T, Riew KD. Cervical radiculopathy. J Am Acad Orthop Surg. 2007; 15(8):486–494

Schoenfeld AJ, George AA, Bader JO, Caram PM, Jr. Incidence and epidemiology of cervical radiculopathy in the United States military: 2000 to 2009. J Spinal Disord Tech. 2012; 25 (1):17–22

Wang TY, Lubelski D, Abdullah KG, Steinmetz MP, Benzel EC, Mroz TE. Rates of anterior cervical discectomy and fusion after initial posterior cervical foraminotomy. Spine J. 2015; 15(5):971–976

4 Cervical Myelopathy

Michael J. Lee

Abstract

Cervical myelopathy refers to pathology of the spinal cord in the cervical spine. Clinically, patients often present with decreasing dexterity and increased clumsiness of the upper extremities, sensory changes, motor changes, and balance difficulties. Radiographically, cord compression is often present on advanced imaging. While it is possible for cervical myelopathy to exist in the absence of cord compression (ex radiation myelopathy), neuro-compressive etiologies are the most common causes of cervical myelopathy. In advanced cases, cord signal change may be observed on T2 images. Unlike the treatment of cervical radiculopathy, when myelopathy is clinically evident and correlating cord compression is radiographically confirmed, surgery is often recommended even in the absence of prior nonoperative care. Clinically, the goal of surgical care of cervical myelopathy is to prevent progression of neurological deterioration. While neurological improvement can and often does occur, it does so variably. The technical goals of surgery are to achieve decompression of the spinal cord while maintaining spinal stability.

Keywords: cervical myelopathy, spinal stenosis, laminectomy, myelomalacia

4.1 Introduction

Cervical myelopathy is a progressive injury to the cervical spinal cord characterized by cord compression and resulting ischemia. This pathology results in a constellation of clinical symptoms that include long tract signs, loss of fine motor skills, and gait imbalance. While myelopathy can be seen in the setting of trauma, tumor, infection, hypermobility, or congenital disorders, it most commonly occurs in the degenerative spine. Degenerative cervical myelopathy is an overarching term representing the common clinical entities that result from age-related degeneration of the cervical spine such as disc herniation, spondylosis, ligament hypertrophy, or ligament ossification.[1] Current prevalence estimates range from 1.6 to 4.04 per 100,000 persons.[2,3] Once diagnosed, it is generally considered an operative disorder given the progressive nature of the symptoms and disease.

4.2 History

Patients can present to the clinician with a wide range of symptoms from mild pain and subtle fine motor abnormalities to gross extremity weakness and quadriplegia. Axial neck pain is a common and nonspecific symptom in many patients and may overlap with findings in nonmyelopathic patients. Patients may complain of pain in the neck, subscapular region, shoulder, or arms. Pain that is specifically located in the posterior neck and that worsens with flexion may be related to myofascial pain, whereas pain in the anterior neck exacerbated by rotation may be more related to the sternocleidomastoid muscle. Posterior neck pain worsened by extension and rotation to one side may be related to a spondylosis (discogenic component or facet joint).[4] Given its lack of specificity, axial neck pain is a low-yield discriminatory factor when evaluating patients for cervical myelopathy. Arm pain is a common symptom found in patients with cervical radiculopathy and myelopathy; both conditions may be present in the same patient.

Patients presenting with myelopathy may describe both upper and lower extremity symptoms. In the upper extremity, they may describe the insidious onset of hand numbness, clumsiness, and loss of fine motor skills. Examples of difficulty with fine motor skills include trouble with buttons, handwriting, and clasping/gripping objects.[5] Lower extremity symptoms may include sciatica-like leg pain, or generalized weakness resulting in increasing difficulty with gait as well as trouble maintaining balance. Sciatica-like leg pain caused by cervical myelopathy is referred to as funicular leg pain, and is a false localizing presentation caused by compression of the ascending spinothalamic tract.[6] Urinary urgency, hesitation, and increased frequency are also common complaints, whereas frank urinary incontinence is a rarer presenting symptom.

4.3 Physical Examination

A thorough head-to-toe musculoskeletal and neurological examination of the upper and lower extremities is important in the evaluation of myelopathy. Examination involves inspection, palpation, range of motion, motor testing of key muscle groups, sensory examination, and provocative tests (▶ Table 4.1). On inspection, patients may present with

Table 4.1 Spine motor, sensory, reflex exam

Root	Motor	Sensory	Reflex
C5	Shoulder abduction	Lateral shoulder	Biceps
C6	Elbow flexion, wrist extension	Radial forearm, thumb	Brachioradialis
C7	Elbow extension, wrist flexion	Index, long, ring fingers	Triceps
C8	Finger flexion	Ulnar forearm, small finger	
T1	Finger abduction	Ulnar elbow	
L2–L3	Hip flexion, adduction	Medial thigh	
L4	Knee extension, ankle flexion	Lateral thigh, anterior knee, medial leg	Patellar
L5	Toe flexion, hip extension, abduction	Lateral leg, dorsal foot	
S1	Foot plantar flexion	Lateral malleolus, posterolateral leg	Achilles
S2	Toe plantar flexion	Plantar hindfoot, posteromedial leg	

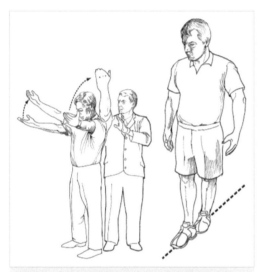

Fig. 4.1 Romberg test: Static Romberg (*left*) is performed by having the patient stand with their eyes closed and arms outstretched. A positive test is loss of balance or upward drift and/or pronation of the upper extremities. Dynamic Romberg (*right*) is performed by having the patient ambulate in a straight line in a heel-to-toe fashion. A positive test is an unsteady gait. (Reproduced with permission from Todd J. Albert, Alexander R. Vaccaro. Physical Examination of the Spine. 1st Edition, Thieme; 2005.)

muscle wasting in the upper and/or lower extremities. Sensory examination to light touch, pain, temperature, proprioception, and vibration may all be affected. Gait is assessed by having the patient attempt to walk normally first, followed by the ability to heel-to-toe walk. On motor strength testing, they may display diffuse weakness of upper and lower extremity motor groups. The finger escape sign describes the abduction of the small finger when the patient is asked to keep fingers extended and adducted, due to the weakness of the hand intrinsic muscles and overpowering of the extensor digitorum minimi. The Romberg test is also performed to assess for posterior column dysfunction (▶ Fig. 4.1).

Provocative signs include hyperreflexia, sustained clonus (> 3 beats), Hoffman sign, inverted brachioradialis reflex, Babinski reflex, grip-and-release test, scapulohumeral reflex (Shimizu reflex), and Lhermitte sign. The latter three represent pathologic spinal cord reflexes. Hoffman sign is best described as flicking of the distal phalanx of the long finger, resulting in abnormal flexion of the ipsilateral thumb and/or index finger (▶ Fig. 4.2).[7] The inverted brachioradialis reflex is elicited by tapping the brachioradialis, resulting in a lack of contraction of the brachioradialis muscle and a hyperactive response of the finger flexor muscles (▶ Fig. 4.3).[8] This reflex corresponds to the C5–C6 level. The Babinski reflex is a pathologic reflex resulting in activation of the toe extensors when the skin of the sole of the foot is stroked and a lack of response by the toe flexors (▶ Fig. 4.4).[9] The grip-and-release test is another provocative where the patient may have difficulty making a closed fist and releasing in rapid succession. A patient without myelopathy can typically do this 20 times in 10 seconds. The scapulohumeral reflex is described by Professor T. Shimiz,[10] and the positive response is elicited by tapping the spine of the scapula that elevates the scapula or the humerus, which suggests spinal cord compression at the craniovertebral or high cervical region. Lhermitte sign is characterized by an electric shock–like sensation radiating down the spine that occurs with neck flexion (▶ Fig. 4.5).

4.4 Differential Diagnosis

Due to the overlapping symptoms and presentation, cervical myelopathy can be confused with

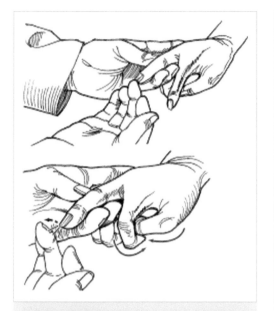

Fig. 4.2 Hoffman sign: The test is performed by flicking the distal phalanx of a relaxed long finger. A positive test is flexion of the ipsilateral thumb or index finger. (Reproduced with permission from Todd J. Albert, Alexander R. Vaccaro. Physical Examination of the Spine. 1st Edition, Thieme; 2005.)

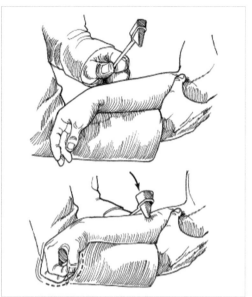

Fig. 4.3 Inverted brachioradialis reflex: The test is performed by tapping the brachioradialis at the musculotendinous junction. A positive test is finger flexion with no wrist extension. (Reproduced with permission from Todd J. Albert, Alexander R. Vaccaro. Physical Examination of the Spine. 1st Edition, Thieme; 2005.)

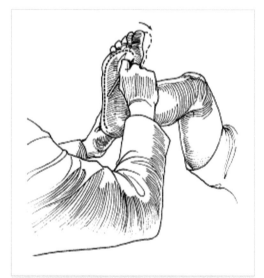

Fig. 4.4 Babinski reflex: The test is performed by stroking the plantar forefoot. A positive test is extension of the great toe. (Reproduced with permission from Todd J. Albert, Alexander R. Vaccaro. Physical Examination of the Spine. 1st Edition, Thieme; 2005.)

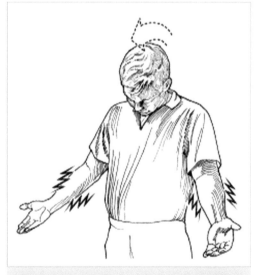

Fig. 4.5 Lhermitte sign: The test is performed by having the patient actively forward flex at the neck. A positive test is pain and/or paresthesias in the upper extremities. (Reproduced with permission from Todd J. Albert, Alexander R. Vaccaro. Physical Examination of the Spine. 1st Edition, Thieme; 2005.)

Table 4.2 Differential diagnoses for cervical spondylotic myelopathy

Compressive	Infectious	Inflammatory, immune	Other
Trauma	Poliomyelitis	Diskitis	Cord infarction
Epidural abscess	Tabes dorsalis (syphilis)	Osteomyelitis	NPH
Intramedullary tumor	Tropical spastic paraparesis	Radiation myelopathy	AVM/AVF
Metastases	HIV associated myelopathy	Sarcoidosis	Syringomyelia
Epidural hematoma	Other acute infectious myelitis	ALS	Subacute combined degeneration (B12 deficiency)
Hematomyelia	Postinfectious myelitis	MS	Hereditary spastic paraplegia
Chiari malformation		RA	Congenital abnormalities of C1–C2, occiput
Thoracic cord compression		SLE	Klippel–Feil syndrome
		SS	Os odontoideum
		PLS	Hereditary spastic paraplegia
		NMO	Adrenomyeloneuropathy
		Transverse myelitis	Peripheral neuropathy
		GBS	

Abbreviations: ALS, amyotrophic lateral sclerosis; AVF, arteriovenous fistulas; AVM, arteriovenous malformations; GBS, Guillain–Barré syndrome; HIV, human immunodeficiency virus; MS, multiple sclerosis; NMO, neuromyelitis optica; NPH, normal pressure hydrocephalus; PLS, primary lateral sclerosis; RA, rheumatoid arthritis; SLE, systemic lupus erythematosus; SS, Sjögren syndrome.

several other clinical diagnoses. These include multiple sclerosis, amyotrophic lateral sclerosis (ALS), various cervical cord disorders (transverse myelitis, viral myelitis, epidural abscess, cord infarction, syringomyelia, subacute combined degeneration, epidural metastasis, intramedullary tumor, and vascular malformation), Guillain–Barré syndrome, normal pressure hydrocephalus, and peripheral neuropathy (▶ Table 4.2). Therefore, a thorough clinical assessment with history and physical examination must be performed to rule out other diagnoses.

4.5 Diagnostic Imaging

Imaging plays a central role in the diagnosis and management of cervical myelopathy. Plain radiographs, computed tomography (CT) and magnetic resonance imaging (MRI) are used separately and in complement to evaluate the pathology and determine the overall treatment plan.[11]

Plain radiographs are usually the initial modality of imaging used to assess the cervical spine. They are simple to obtain, ubiquitous, and provide information in a 2D plane regarding overall alignment, segmental disease, or other bony abnormalities. In addition, radiographs can be obtained with the cervical spine in flexion and extension to delineate areas of instability under physiologic loads.[11] The Pavlov ratio is a gross radiographic marker used to evaluate for developmental canal stenosis which may be a precursor to development of myelopathy (▶ Fig. 4.6). It is calculated by dividing the anteroposterior diameter of the spinal canal with the anteroposterior diameter of the vertebral body. A value < 0.8 suggests developmental canal stenosis (normal value = 1.0).[4]

CT is a modality that also uses x-ray absorption but uses high-resolution cross-sectional imaging to provide 3D views. CT highlights mineralization and bony anatomy with excellent detail, which can be useful to identify pathology (e.g., ossification of the posterior longitudinal ligament [OPLL]) and help with preoperative planning for instrumentation. CT is better than MRI for assessing foraminal stenosis due to osteophytes, and 45-degree oblique reconstruction view is particularly helpful. However, it is limited for the evaluation of soft tissues and is typically obtained in a supine position, rendering it inadequate for assessment of instability. CT myelography can be considered as an adjunct, where a contrast dye can be injected into the cerebrospinal fluid (CSF) prior to CT imaging to outline the spinal cord and identify areas of compression (▶ Fig. 4.7). However, in this current era, this modality is often used in patients who have contraindications for MRI.

MRI is the preferred imaging modality to assess for cervical myelopathy given its superior resolution

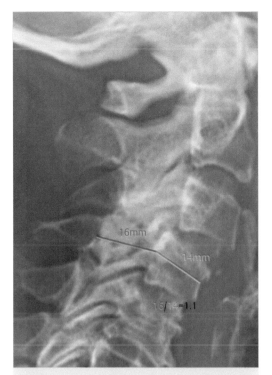

Fig. 4.6 The Pavlov ratio is calculated by dividing the diameter of the spinal canal by the diameter of the vertebral body. A value < 0.8 suggests developmental canal stenosis (normal value = 1.0).

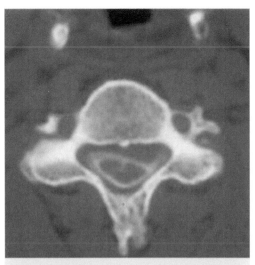

Fig. 4.7 CT myelogram shows a left-sided C5–C6 disc herniation with compression of the spinal cord and left C6 nerve root. (Reproduced with permission from Acquired Functional and Structural Abnormalities of the Spine. In: Hosten N, Liebig T, Hrsg. CT of the Head and Spine. 1st Edition. Thieme; 2001.)

for soft tissues and its lack of ionizing radiation (▶ Fig. 4.8). Unlike radiographs and CT, MRI can outline any compression of the spinal cord in relation to the surrounding CSF. The morphology of the spinal cord can also be assessed at different levels, such as narrowing or flattening. While increased T2-signal hyperintensity within the spinal cord is representative of cord edema, its clinical significance is unclear. Increased T2-signal intensity in combination with decreased T1-signal intensity correlates with late stages of myelopathy and is indicative of a more severe pathologic condition with possible irreversible cord injury. Dynamic MRI is a newer technique that can be employed to identify instability.[11]

4.6 Treatment

Cervical myelopathy is a progressive disease characterized by periods of stability mixed with periods of neurological decline. Given this stepwise functional deterioration, surgery is generally recommended when there are unequivocal findings on history, physical examination, and diagnostic imaging. However, for certain patients with significant comorbidities or those with mild disease and no functional impairment, surgery may be delayed with close follow-up.

Nonoperative treatment can include the use of a cervical collar, home exercises, anti-inflammatory medications, intermittent bedrest, cervical traction, and avoidance of risky activities (e.g., physical overloading, slippery surfaces, etc.).[12] Physical therapy for gait training and balance may be of benefit. Patients should be closely monitored for neurological progression.

Operative management of cervical myelopathy varies based on the type and location of pathology as well as the number of segments involved. Sources of anterior cord pathology include disc herniation, osteophytes, or OPLL, whereas posterior cord pathology involves hypertrophy or ossification of the ligamentum flavum. Typically, anterior cervical surgery is recommended when there is compression from one to three levels or if there is presence of cervical kyphosis. This includes anterior cervical discectomy and fusion (ACDF), anterior cervical corpectomy and fusion (ACCF), a combined ACDF and ACCF, or less commonly cervical disc arthroplasty. Posterior decompression with laminectomy or laminoplasty is used when there is compression at greater than three levels or if the anterior

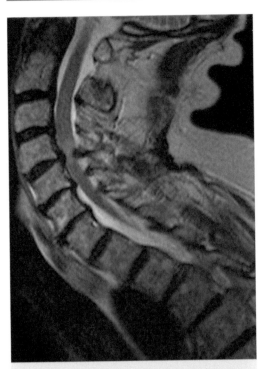

Fig. 4.8 Sagittal T2 MRI shows cervical spinal stenosis and C4–C5 disc protrusion with cord signal hyperintensity consistent with cervical myelopathy. (Reproduced with permission from Spinal Stenosis. In: Forsting M, Jansen O, Hrsg. MR Neuroimaging: Brain, Spine, Peripheral Nerves. 1st Edition. Thieme; 2016.)

column has already undergone fusion. The success of the posterior approach relies on the presence of cervical lordosis and posterior drift of the cervical cord after decompression is completed. ACDF and ACCF are performed using muscle-sparing approach as originally described by Smith and Robinson.[13] ACDF involves removal of the disc material and osteophytes at the affected levels with placement of graft at the interspace with additional instrumentation using an anterior plate for support. Cervical disc arthroplasty is an alternative to conventional ACDF, where the disc space is replaced by motion-preserving prosthesis; however, long-term studies are still ongoing and unequivocal superiority with this technique has not been established.[14] ACCF uses the same approach; however, it involves resection of the vertebral body at the affected levels with incorporation of a large strut graft. This technique is useful when the pathology involves the entire vertebral body rather than just the disc space.

Posterior cervical laminectomy and fusion is a useful technique for multilevel decompression when there is existing cervical lordosis. It involves a midline posterior approach with removal of the lamina and instrumented fusion with lateral mass screw fixation in the subaxial spine and occasionally pedicle screws in the upper thoracic spine. Laminectomy without instrumented fusion is generally not commonly recommended due to the high incidence of post-laminectomy kyphosis. Laminoplasty is a canal-expanding procedure developed to decompress the cervical cord by hinging the posterior arch open. The majority of laminoplasty is performed by sparing the large C2 and C7 spinous processes, which helps maintain the soft tissue arch-and-wound closure. It is a technically demanding, yet useful procedure for decompression in patients with preserved cervical lordosis. The choice between laminoplasty and laminectomy and fusion is largely dependent on the surgeon's training and preference, but laminectomy and fusion is preferred if the patient has significant neck pain, myeloradiculopathy that requires bilateral foraminotomies, and if there is need for alignment correction.

4.7 Outcomes

Outcomes in surgery for myelopathy is closely related to the preoperative neurological status of the patient including functionality, gait impairment, age, and duration of symptoms.[15] In addition, the pattern of signal changes observed on MRI and the specific pathology being addressed during operative intervention, all contribute to overall outcomes. Anterior or posterior approaches both have satisfactory outcomes when properly indicated in consideration with sagittal alignment and location of pathology.

Common complications of cervical surgery include persistent radiculopathy or myelopathy, recurrent laryngeal nerve palsy, dysphagia, hematoma, Horner syndrome, and axial neck pain and stiffness following multilevel surgery. Adjacent segment degeneration is also a concern with a reported rate of 25% of symptomatic disease at 10 years.[16]

4.8 Case Examples

4.8.1 Case 1

This is a 71-year-old male who presented with 9 months of right-sided neck pain and right arm radicular pain and hand weakness. Imaging reveals multilevel stenosis at C3–C7. The patient underwent a C3–C7 laminectomy and C2–T2 instrumented fusion (lateral mass screws C3–C6, pedicle screws C2, T1–T2) (see images on next page).

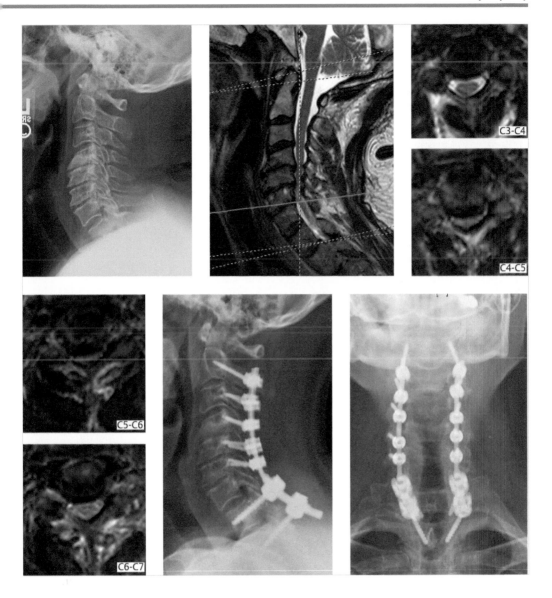

4.8.2 Case 2

This is a 61-year-old female who presented with 3 years of neck pain, right arm radicular pain, hand clumsiness, and an unsteady gait. Imaging reveals central stenosis and grade I anterolisthesis at C3–C4. The patient underwent a C3–C4 anterior cervical decompression and fusion (see images on next page).

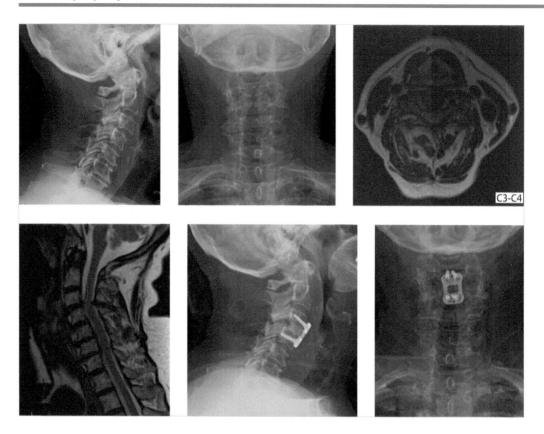

- The primary factors to consider when determining the optimal surgical approach are the patient's sagittal balance and number of affected levels. For either anterior or posterior approach, patient positioning is important to avoid iatrogenic injury, maintain alignment, and correct deformity.
- When performing multilevel ACDFs, all the levels should be decompressed first and then fused with grafts or cages. If a graft is inserted first at one level, the decompression of the adjacent level is more challenging because distraction of the disc space at the fused level affects the adjacent level to be less distracted. The graft should be inserted at the more severe level first. If all the levels are similarly affected, the graft should be inserted at the caudad segment first so that the larger graft gives more biomechanical strength in the caudad segment. Over-distraction of the disc space should be avoided as it can contribute to endplate fracture, subsidence, graft collapse, facet joint overloading, etc. The ideal amount of disc space distraction for graft placement is no more than 2 mm beyond the preoperative disc height.
- The uncovertebral joint is a reliable landmark that can be used to establish the midline when utilizing an anterior cervical plate. Another landmark for the midline identification is the convex contour of the vertebral body. A vertical line can be drawn on the vertebral body for midline identification.
- Avoiding excessive retraction can mitigate the risk of postoperative dysphagia and vascular injury during ACDF.
- During a posterior approach, avoid dissecting lateral to the facet joints to minimize soft tissue bleeding. For laminectomy and fusion cases, preoperative assessment of symptomatic and asymptomatic foraminal stenosis is important, as neck positioning in the operating room can affect the nerve roots in the foramen. Foraminotomy should be performed first, followed by laminectomy to prevent inadvertent injury to the spinal cord or dura. For posterior approach, meticulous soft tissue closure using multiple layer stitches is important to prevent myofascial dehiscence from the midline and postoperative neck pain.

4.9 Board-style Questions

1. What physical exam finding is not consistent with a diagnosis of cervical myelopathy?
   a) Spontaneous abduction of the small finger when fingers are adducted and extended
   b) Decreased sensation to pinprick
   c) Spontaneous finger flexion when the distal phalanx of the long finger is flicked
   d) Finger paresthesias when pressure is applied over the anterior scalene muscle
   e) Great toe extension when the sole of the foot is stroked

2. What radiographic finding would be considered a contraindication to laminoplasty?
   a) Fixed kyphosis of 16 degrees at C3–C7
   b) Ligamentum flavum hypertrophy
   c) Ossification of the posterior longitudinal ligament
   d) Cervical lordosis of 33 degrees
   e) Stenosis affecting C2–C7

3. What is the typical course of symptomatic cervical myelopathy?
   a) Progressive deterioration at a constant rate
   b) Rarely progresses beyond symptoms present at time of initial visit
   c) Progressive deterioration punctuated by periods of improved neurological function
   d) Progressive deterioration punctuated by periods of stable neurological function
   e) Progression is dependent on site of compression

4. Postsurgical kyphosis is most likely to occur following what surgical technique?
   a) Laminoplasty
   b) Laminectomy
   c) Laminectomy and fusion
   d) Anterior decompression and fusion
   e) Corpectomy and strut grafting

5. Nerve root palsy after posterior cervical decompression typically occurs at what level?
   a) C4
   b) C5
   c) C6
   d) C7
   e) C8

Answers

1. d
2. a
3. d
4. b
5. b

References

[1] Nouri A, Tetreault L, Singh A, Karadimas SK, Fehlings MG. Degenerative cervical myelopathy: epidemiology, genetics, and pathogenesis. Spine. 2015; 40(12):E675–E693

[2] Wu JC, Ko CC, Yen YS, et al. Epidemiology of cervical spondylotic myelopathy and its risk of causing spinal cord injury: a national cohort study. Neurosurg Focus. 2013; 35(1):E10

[3] Boogaarts HD, Bartels RH. Prevalence of cervical spondylotic myelopathy. Eur Spine J. 2015; 24 Suppl 2:139–141

[4] Rao RD, Currier BL, Albert TJ, et al. Degenerative cervical spondylosis: clinical syndromes, pathogenesis, and management. J Bone Joint Surg Am. 2007; 89(6):1360–1378

[5] Rao R. Neck pain, cervical radiculopathy, and cervical myelopathy: pathophysiology, natural history, and clinical evaluation. J Bone Joint Surg Am. 2002; 84(10):1872–1881

[6] Chan CK, Lee HY, Choi WC, Cho JY, Lee SH. Cervical cord compression presenting with sciatica-like leg pain. Eur Spine J. 2011; 20 Suppl 2:S217–S221

[7] Glaser JA, Curé JK, Bailey KL, Morrow DL. Cervical spinal cord compression and the Hoffmann sign. Iowa Orthop J. 2001; 21:49–52

[8] Estanol BV, Marin OS. Mechanism of the inverted supinator reflex: a clinical and neurophysiological study. J Neurol Neurosurg Psychiatry. 1976; 39(9):905–908

[9] van Gijn J. The Babinski reflex. Postgrad Med J. 1995; 71 (841):645–648

[10] Shimizu T, Shimada H, Shirakura K. Scapulohumeral reflex (Shimizu): its clinical significance and testing maneuver. Spine. 1993; 18(15):2182–2190

[11] Martin AR, Tadokoro N, Tetreault L, et al. Imaging evaluation of degenerative cervical myelopathy: current state of the art and future directions. Neurosurg Clin N Am. 2018; 29(1):33–45

[12] Badhiwala JH, Wilson JR. The natural history of degenerative cervical myelopathy. Neurosurg Clin N Am. 2018; 29(1):21–32

[13] Smith GW, Robinson RA. The treatment of certain cervical-spine disorders by anterior removal of the intervertebral disc and interbody fusion. J Bone Joint Surg Am. 1958; 40-A(3):607–624

[14] Kato S, Fehlings M. Degenerative cervical myelopathy. Curr Rev Musculoskelet Med. 2016; 9(3):263–271

[15] Tetreault LA, Kopjar B, Vaccaro A, et al. A clinical prediction model to determine outcomes in patients with cervical spondylotic myelopathy undergoing surgical treatment: data from the prospective, multi-center AOSpine North America study. J Bone Joint Surg Am. 2013; 95(18):1659–1666

[16] Hilibrand AS, Carlson GD, Palumbo MA, Jones PK, Bohlman HH. Radiculopathy and myelopathy at segments adjacent to the site of a previous anterior cervical arthrodesis. J Bone Joint Surg Am. 1999; 81(4):519–528

5 Intervertebral Disc: Form, Biomechanics, Biology, and Pathology

Steven M. Presciutti and Hicham Drissi

Abstract

The intervertebral disc (IVD) is an avascular fibro-cartilaginous organ that facilitates load transmission and bestows multiaxial flexibility to the spine. This chapter discusses the embryology, form, and function of the healthy, nondegenerate adult human IVD. The biomechanics and unique biologic features of the IVD are also discussed. Understanding these features of the disc when it is healthy helps inform future directions for regenerative strategies of a degenerative disc.

Keywords: intervertebral disc, anulus fibrosus, nucleus pulposus, anatomy, embryology, biomechanics, spine

5.1 Introduction

The human spine consists of 33 vertebral bodies which, with the exception of C1–C2 and the sacrum, are separated by an intervertebral disc (IVD).[1] The disc is a specialized structure consisting of three interdependent tissues: the anulus fibrosus (AF) and the nucleus pulposus (NP) are sandwiched in part between two cartilage end plates (CEPs) that are integrated to the adjacent vertebral bodies (▶ Fig. 5.1).[2] The IVD is a highly specialized structure that facilitates load transmission and multiaxial flexibility of the spine while simultaneously resisting high amounts of biomechanical stress in multiple planes. The IVD has a very limited potential for self-repair as it deals with these high biomechanical forces over time, and thus almost inevitably leads to degeneration of the disc over time with natural aging.

Due to the IVD's biomechanical synergy with the posterior facet joints and its close relationship to the neural structures, the association between intervertebral disc degeneration (IDD) and low back pain is not limited solely to discogenic pain.[3] IDD typically results in collapse of disc height, causing abnormal facet loading that can often lead to osteoarthritic changes in the hyaline cartilage surface of the facet joint. In addition, disc height loss and subsequent bulging of the AF, as well as discrete herniations of the NP, can cause compression of the nearby traversing neural structures.

All of these pathologic entities are consequences of IDD, which is a crippling problem that affects the global society both physically and socioeconomically. IDD occurs in 40% of individuals younger than 30 years of age and in more than 95% of those older than 50.[4,5] This is significant because IDD is the major contributor to low back and neck pain, which are the first and fourth leading causes,

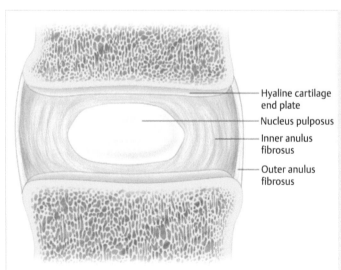

Fig. 5.1 Schematic representation of the anatomic structure of the human intervertebral disc (IVD). Each vertebral end plate is coated with a layer of hyaline articular cartilage (cartilaginous end plate). Adjacent vertebrae are united by a fibrocartilaginous IVD. Concentric, crossing layers of tough fibrous tissue, the anulus fibrosus (AF), make up the outer circumference of the disc, enclosing a central, shock-absorbing gelatinous core, the nucleus pulposus (NP).

Hyaline cartilage end plate

Nucleus pulposus

Inner anulus fibrosus

Outer anulus fibrosus

respectively, of years lived with disability in the United States.[6] The annual cost in terms of lost productivity, medical expenses, and workers' compensation benefits is estimated between $100 and $200 billion annually in the United States alone.

Given the scale of the problem of disc degeneration, it is important for the surgeon and for disc researchers to understand the form and function of the healthy, nondegenerate IVD. This chapter will review these topics as well as the biology and homeostasis of the healthy disc and its specialized compartments. A more complete review of disc degeneration can be found in the following chapter.

5.2 Anatomy and Biomechanics of the Intervertebral Disc

5.2.1 Disc Morphology and Composition

The NP's structure is gelatinous with a high-water content, which allows the NP to resist compression when axially loaded. The NP contains randomly organized networks of loose collagen type II and elastin fibers that encase an aggregating proteoglycan called aggrecan, which imbibe water and provide tensile properties to the tissue (▶ Fig. 5.2). While articular chondrocytes also express aggrecan

and collagen II, the NP matrix can be distinguished from cartilage by a distinct GAG:hydroxyproline ratio. While the GAG:hydroxyproline ratio in juvenile articular cartilage is ~3:1 and decreases to ~2:1 with age in the NP, the ratio is much higher at all ages. In juvenile (2–5 years) and young adult (15–25 years) NP, the ratio is ~25:1 and ~27:1, respectively. Again, the ratio decreases with age and degeneration, but not to the level of articular cartilage, reaching ~5:1 in the elderly (60–80 years).[7] The number of viable cells in the adult NP is estimated to be about $5 \times 10^6/cm^3$.

The main function of the AF is to restrict lateral motion and to prevent extrusion of the NP. To accomplish this, the collagen fibers of the mature anulus are arranged in up to 25 concentric lamellae wrapped around the NP (▶ Fig. 5.2). The lamellae are parallel to one another and traverse between adjacent vertebrae at an angle of 60 degrees to the axis of the spine. The collagen fibers within a single annular lamella are organized in a parallel fashion, whereas the fibers in adjacent layers differ by 30 degrees. The concentration of collagen type I is highest in the anulus and decreases radially toward the NP. Elastin fibers, arranged in a network between the lamellae, contribute to the structure and mechanical functions of the AF. There are more viable cells in the adult human AF than the NP, with about $9 \times 10^6/cm^3$.

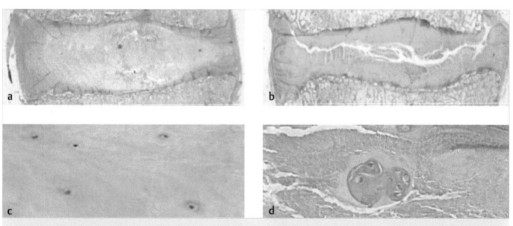

Fig. 5.2 Human intervertebral disc (IVD) histology. Histological images of normal (**a, c**) and degenerate (**b, d**) human IVD stained with hematoxylin and eosin used for grading. Macroscopically normal IVD (**a**) demonstrates matrix integrity and clear demarcation between NP and AF regions, while degenerate IVD demonstrates slits within the NP extending to the AF and a loss of demarcation between NP and AF regions (**b**). Cells in normal IVD are distributed evenly throughout the matrix (**c**), while degenerate tissue shows evidence of cell clusters (**d**). Image magnifications × 1 (**a, c**), × 150 (**b, d**). (Adapted with permission from Richardson SM, Knowles R, Tyler J, Mobasheri A, Hoyland J. Expression of glucose transporters GLUT-1, GLUT-3, GLUT-9 and HIF-1α in normal and degenerate human intervertebral disc. Histochem Cell Biol. 2008;129(4):503–511.)

The IVD is separated from the adjacent vertebral bodies by a distinct CEP, which is considered the third specialized compartment of the IVD. In humans, unlike in most animal species, this end plate acts as the growth plate for the vertebral bodies and has the typical structure of an epiphyseal growth plate.[8] In infancy, this growth plate is thick and occupies a substantial fraction of the disc and is penetrated by cartilage canals and small blood vessels. It thins as growth progresses, however. This thinning is accompanied by the end plate losing its vascularity and the cartilage canals disappearing. By maturity, the end plate consists of a thin (< 1 mm) avascular layer of hyaline cartilage that may become partially calcified at the vertebral body–end plate junction.[8] Under compressive loading, the pressure of the NP pressing against the CEP and bony end plate can cause them to bulge into the vertebral body by up to 1 mm.[9] This bulging increases the volume available to the NP, thereby reducing pressure in the nucleus and shifting some compressive load-bearing from the NP to the AF.[10]

Quantitatively, the major component of the disc is water that contains ions whose concentration is governed by the extracellular matrix (ECM) glycosaminoglycans (GAGs). The nutrients essential for cell survival, and the cell's metabolites that must be removed from the tissue, are transported in the water phase by diffusion. The interstitial water also contains bioactive molecules such as growth factors arising from the blood, soluble factors produced by cells, and degraded ECM fragments, all at very low concentrations in the healthy disc.

The exact concentration of water varies with position in the disc, however, and also with age.[11,12] In general, the NP is the most highly hydrated of the disc's compartments. The water content of the nucleus may be as high as 90% in an infant, falling to around 80% in the nondegenerate disc of a young adult.[13] The water content of the anulus is lower than that of the nucleus, falling to around 65% in the outer anulus in adult humans. In disc degeneration, the water content in the NP falls as the ECM degenerates.

5.2.2 Extracellular Matrix of the Intervertebral Disc

The morphology and function of the disc depend entirely on the organization and properties of its ECM. This matrix has two functions: to endow the tissue with the requisite biomechanical properties and to act as a selective filter, regulating the composition of the extracellular fluid and the rate at which nutrients, metabolites, and perhaps signal molecules can be exchanged between the disc cells and the rest of the body (▶ Fig. 5.3).

Aggrecan, a large aggregating proteoglycan, is one of the major macromolecules of the IVD.[14] Aggrecan is a very large molecule, consisting of a protein core that has around 100 GAG side-chains attached to it in a bottle-brush-like configuration. Many aggrecan molecules covalently attach to hyaluronic acid chains via a globular region (G1 domain) at one end of the protein core, forming large aggregates (hence the name "aggrecan"). These enormous aggregates are trapped in the disc by the surrounding collagen network. The GAGs maintain tissue hydration and determine the ionic composition of the interstitial fluid. They contain anionic groups (SO_3^- and COO^-), which impart a net negative charge to the matrix. Electroneutrality of the tissue is maintained, however, because the interstitial water contains an excess of cations and a deficit of anions. The concentrations of negatively charged solutes, particularly anions such as Cl^- are thus lower than in the plasma, while those of positively charged species are higher. The predominant cation in the body is Na^+ and, in the disc, its concentration is directly related to concentrations of fixed negative charge and hence to GAG concentration.[11] Na^+ is thus highest in the NP and lowest in the outer AF and is proportionately affected by load-induced changes in hydration and by changes in GAG concentration. This high concentration of Na^+ imparts a high osmotic pressure to the tissue, which consequently tends to imbibe water. The ionic osmotic pressure is thus of major functional importance for the IVD, as it governs the swelling pressure and hence the ability of the disc to maintain hydration and turgor under physiologic loading.[15]

These macromolecules of the IVD are synthesized and maintained throughout life by a small population of cells, occupying less than 1% of the volume of the tissue in the NP.[16] Matrix production and turnover is slow in normal and degenerate human discs with aggrecan half-lives being ~12 and ~8 years, respectively and that of collagen > 90 years.[17,18] The disc cells also produce a complex array of proteases, able to degrade all matrix components.[19,20] In the healthy disc, a steady state is maintained between the rates of synthesis and degradation of matrix components, but in degeneration this delicate balance is disturbed.

As we have indicated above, aging and IDD are associated with the proteolysis of matrix macromolecules in the NP. These degraded molecules are

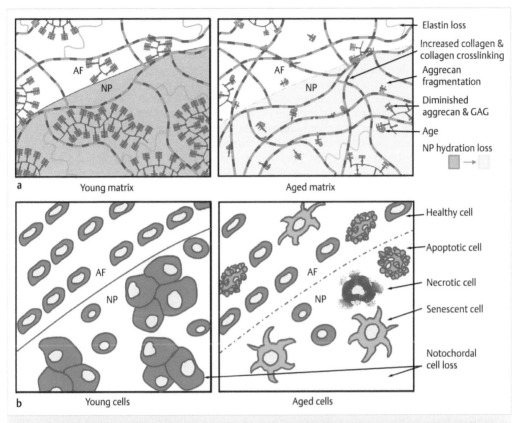

Fig. 5.3 Molecular features of the aging disc. Young and aged extracellular matrix (**a**) and cells (**b**) are schematically compared to summarize important changes that occur during disc aging. (**a**) Young matrix is rich in elastin (*green*, coiled fiber), aggregated aggrecan (*dark blue*, bottle-brush aggregate), and collagen fibers (banded fibers). Aged matrix shows loss of elastin, increased collagen and collagen crosslinking, fragmented aggrecan, diminished GAG quality, reduced aggrecan aggregates, increased accumulation of advanced glycation end-products (AGEs) along with lower hydration. (**b**) Young AF cells are elongated fibrochondrocytes and NP cells are a mixture of large, clustering, notochordal cells and smaller, chondrocyte-like cells. Aged cells show reduced cellularity, loss of notochordal cells, and incidence of senescence, apoptosis, and necrosis. (Reproduced with permission from Vo NV, Hartman RA, Patil PR, et al. Molecular mechanisms of biological aging in intervertebral discs. J Orthop Res. 2016;34(8):1289–1306.)

no longer trapped in the tissue matrix and are able to slowly diffuse out of the disc. The consequent fall in concentration of NP matrix results in a loss of matrix integrity, a failure of appropriate biomechanical responses to load, and ultimately to the morphological features of degeneration. The sequence of cause and effect is still incompletely understood, but the earliest and most marked degradative change in disc composition is loss of GAG,[21] which decreases in parallel with the grade of disc degeneration. Loss of GAG leads to a fall in swelling pressure,[15] loss of hydration and loss of disc height, with adverse effects on the disc's ability to respond appropriately to applied biomechanical loads.

5.2.3 Disc Biomechanics

The unique structure of the IVD facilitates the capacity to absorb shock and transmit high forces from different vectors around the spine. In fact, between 75 and 97% of the compressive load applied to the lumbar spine is carried by the IVDs.[22] The tensile and elastic properties of different components of the disc allow for a state of equilibrium between stability and flexibility. When the NP is compressed, the water that is bound to aggrecan is distorted and is redistributed radially to the AF. This pressure in turn distorts the AF, but the resilience of the AF allows it to recover its shape after the pressure has been removed.

The outer AF is primarily responsible for withstanding tensile stresses (circumferential, longitudinal, and torsion) while the NP is responsible for withstanding compressive stress. The inner anulus withstands a mixture of both of these.[23] The CEP, in turn, resists displacement of the NP tissue into the adjacent vertebral body. Together, these specialized compartments can handle more load than each tissue alone, highlighting the importance of intact and properly integrated structures. Thus, all three compartments are critical to the proper functioning of the disc. With age, however, as the water content of the NP decreases, this fine balance is perturbed and the AF then becomes the main load-bearing structure of the disc.[24]

The IVD is always under load from body weight and muscle activity. During activities of daily living, the human spine normally experiences loads that are both large in magnitude and dynamic in nature. The compressive forces that the IVD experiences have been estimated to be up to ~2,500 N during dynamic lifting,[25] and intradiskal pressures approach 1 MPa during normal daily activities such as climbing stairs (0.5–0.7 MPa) or jogging (0.35–0.95 MPa).[26] The forces that the IVD experiences are expected to be higher under more extreme conditions. To put that in perspective, the force exerted on our body by Earth's gravity is around 0.1 MPa.

Within normal physiologic ranges, this dynamic loading of the IVD is actually critical to the proper functioning of the disc. Dynamic loads play an important role in stimulating biosynthesis of the ECM[27,28,29] as well as promoting molecular transport of nutrients and waste products in and out of the disc.[30,31] In addition, the cells of the NP and AF are tethered to the ECM and are therefore stretched and deformed themselves in response to loading. This allows for the direct transmission of signals from the ECM to the intracellular environment. In addition to direct effects on cells, mechanical strain can also affect the extracellular environment itself. It has been shown that when strain is applied to the disc, it causes changes in water content, pressure, and pH.[32]

Adverse load to the IVD, on the other hand, leads to an increase in the secretion of catabolic enzymes by disc cells as well as apoptotic and inflammatory factors.[33,34] Therefore, while biomechanical factors are essential to proper disc function, adverse loading events in supraphysiologic ranges can itself initiate the process of disc degeneration.

But how are these mechanical signals transduced into the cells of the IVD? This largely occurs through interactions between the matrix-binding proteins integrin and laminin. Several studies have shown that NP cells adhere strongly to these proteins, suggesting their crucial role in cell–matrix interactions.[35] Integrins are mechanically sensitive ion channels that open and close in response to biomechanical stress, initiating signaling cascades with direct effects on cell metabolism, viability, and phenotype. Several studies have shown elevated expression in porcine and human NP cells compared to AF cells of integrins α3, α6, and β4, and laminin α5.[36,37] In addition, the cells of the NP are also known to specifically express laminin –111, –511, and –322.[38] While integrin α6β1 mediates laminin-111 attachment in the porcine NP, this interaction is mediated by integrins α3β1 and α5β1 in the human NP.[39] This interspecies variability suggests that the underlying nature of the adhesion between cells and the ECM may not be a critical determinant of proper IVD cell function.

5.2.4 Nutrient Supply to the Disc

Vascularization of the end plate is supplied by the basivertebral vessel bundles, which enter the vertebral body through the posterior basivertebral foramen and capillary branches from the segmental artery that arises from the anterior spinal artery.[40] Early in postnatal life, the vascular density of the end plate decreases, reducing nutrient supply to the disc. The nondegenerate adult disc is largely avascular and the capillaries form an intricate "mesh" throughout the porous bony end plate and bud in the superficial cartilage layer, providing nutrient delivery and waste exchange with the disc tissue. The density of this network is greatest in the region adjacent to the NP (▶ Fig. 5.4).[41]

In adults, the cartilaginous end plate is a thin (< 1 mm) layer of hyaline cartilage of lower water content and higher cellularity than the adjacent disc.[12] Nutrients can readily diffuse through this cartilage under normal conditions. However, the end plate tends to calcify with age and degeneration, particularly in scoliotic discs.[42] Calcification is a significant barrier to nutrient transport.[43] In fact, modeling studies have confirmed the disastrous effect of end plate calcification, showing that if the effective exchange area between the disc and microcirculation falls below 25% of total area, the concentrations of glucose and oxygen in the disc center fall rapidly.[44]

The other main capillary plexus supplying the IVD exists in the outer AF. This plexus penetrates only a small distance (1–2 mm) into the outer AF, at least in the adult human nondegenerate disc.

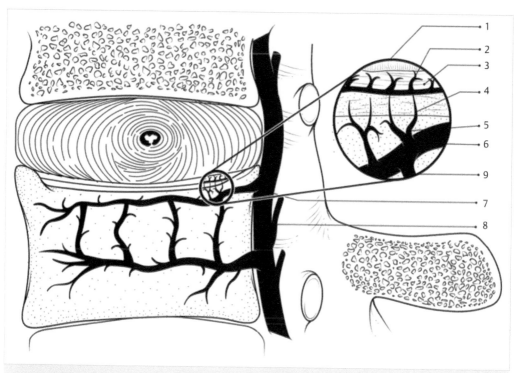

Fig. 5.4 The organization of the venous system in a human vertebral body. The inset shows an enlarged section of the disc–bone interface with the intervertebral disc (IVD) (1), the capillary bed through which nutrients to the disc are provided (2–3), the venous system perforating the subchondral plate and the collecting vein (4–5), and the venous system of the vertebral body (6–9). (Reproduced with permission from Crock HV, Yoshizawa H, Kame SK. Observations on the venous drainage of the human vertebral body. J Bone Joint Surg Br 1973;55(3):528–533.)

The one case in which capillaries are known to extend through the outer anulus and into the inner AF, however, is in the case of IDD. Recent evidence suggests that, in disc degeneration, the route of entry for this nerve and blood vessel in-growth is through the proteoglycan-depleted regions of annular fissures.[45]

The metabolism of disc cells, though similar to the cells of other cartilaginous tissue, is in many respects unusual. They obtain their energy primarily by glycolysis,[46] consuming glucose and producing lactic acid at a high rate. An adequate supply of glucose is essential, as the cells die within 2 to 3 days under low glucose (< 0.5 mM) conditions.[47] Removal of lactic acid, produced by the breakdown of glucose to form adenosine triphosphate (ATP), is also essential to the survival of the cells.[47] The concentration of lactic acid in the ECM can be as high as 6 to 8 mM in the center of the NP, compared with 1 mM in plasma.[46] In addition, there is an inherent attraction of protons into the disc due to the negative fixed charge of the matrix. These conditions cause the extracellular pH in the NP to be slightly acidic (pH 6.9–7.1), even in normal healthy discs.

Failure of the disc's nutrient supply has long been considered a major event in the progression or even initiation of disc degeneration.[48] Cells in the middle of an adult lumbar disc may be as much as 6 to 8 mm from the nearest blood supply, and nutrients passing from the capillaries then have to diffuse through the dense ECM of the disc. Products of metabolism such as lactic acid are removed by the reverse process.[31] The nutritional environment within the disc can be quite variable from region to region because of its size. Concentration gradients of oxygen, glucose, and lactic acid occur across the disc, governed by the balance between the rate of nutrient supply and cellular consumption and the rate of metabolite production and removal. These gradients have been measured in a few instances using needle microelectrodes[49,50,51] and show that in accordance with diffusion theory, the center of the disc has low concentrations of oxygen and glucose and high concentrations of lactic acid when compared to the regions closest to the blood supply.

The factors regulating normal and pathological nutrient supply in the IVD are still not well understood, however, and warrant further study. Although evidence of the effect of blood supply on disc degeneration is indirect, a number of studies have shown that atherosclerosis of the lumbar arteries or disorders such as sickle cell disease, which affect the microcirculation, is highly associated with IDD.[52,53]

5.3 Development of the Intervertebral Disc

Understanding the embryology and origin of a tissue and its cells, particularly a heterogeneous structure like the IVD, is instructive in understanding the degenerative process as well as in informing regenerative strategies. If one can understand the molecular signals that cue a particular tissue like the disc to form in the first place, it may be possible to leverage those same signals in the degenerative state in order to prompt regeneration.

5.3.1 Embryology of the Disc

The embryonic origins of the IVD can be traced back to the third week of embryonic development (▶ Fig. 5.5). By the end of the third week, the mesoderm, from which most connective tissues originate, undergoes a subdivision into axial mesoderm (notochord), paraxial mesoderm (somites), intermediate mesoderm, and lateral plate mesoderm. The notochord is positioned in the dorsal region of the embryo along the anteroposterior axis and consists of a flexible core of glycoprotein with high osmotic potential surrounded by a sheath of fibrous connective tissue.[54] The notochord is an important source of signals for patterning of the developing embryo, specifically axis determination in both dorso-ventral and left–right planes.[55,56]

During week 4, the notochord induces the somites to readopt mesenchymal characteristics, enabling their cells to migrate. This migration causes the cells to divide into two distinct populations: (1) those that migrate peripherally constitute the dermatomyotome, which later form the dermis and muscle; and (2) the ones that migrate toward and encircle the notochord and neural tube constitute the sclerotome, which will later form the spinal skeleton.[57]

By the beginning of week 7, the sclerotomal cells have a distinct segmented shape with highly condensed cell regions intercalating with looser cell regions. Occupying the most central part along the axis of the fetus is a continuous row of large vacuolated notochordal cells. Between the seventh and ninth week, the sclerotomal-derived segments containing the more loosely organized cells will push against the notochord; conversely, the more densely arranged sclerotomal-derived segments expand (becoming even denser) to accommodate the notochord that is being pushed away from the adjacent segments.

After week 10, the segments containing the more loosely organized cells have completely pushed the notochord from their center and will become the vertebral body; the denser sclerotomal-derived cells have expanded even further and will become the AF, which encircles the notochord-derived NP.[58,59] Within the IVD, notochordal cells proliferate and accumulate a gelatinous, GAG-rich ECM, which separates the original cell mass into a network of small cell clusters.

5.3.2 Ontogeny of Disc Cells

There is a long-held debate over the ontogeny of the cells that make up the human adult nondegenerate NP. Early anatomical studies recognized a morphological heterogeneity of cells within the NP.[60] A population of larger (25–85 mm), vacuolated cells have long been considered "notochordal" because of their resemblance to embryonic notochord cells, whereas a population of smaller (10 mm), rounder cells has been considered "chondrocyte-like" (▶ Fig. 5.6). Fluorescence-activated cell sorting of these two different populations has revealed differential expression of certain genes.[61] Although the human embryonic notochord and juvenile NP possess populations of "notochordal" cells, these cells gradually disappear or change their appearance and are replaced by the "chondrocyte-like" cells in the adult.[62,63]

Some investigators believe that notochordal cells die and are replaced by a new population of cells migrating from adjacent tissues.[64] Favoring this hypothesis are the histological observations of rabbit notochordal NP cells being gradually replaced by chondrocytes migrating in a centripetal manner from the end plate[65] or from the AF.[64] Chemotactic signals derived from notochordal cells have been implicated as being the driving forces for this migration.[66]

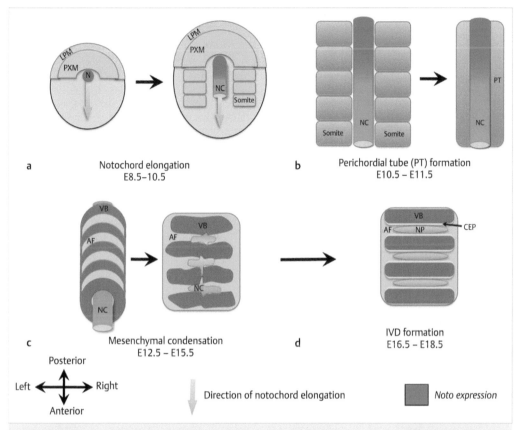

Fig. 5.5 Schematic representation of the main stages in axial skeletogenesis. (**a**) Formation of the node (N) and elongation of the notochord (NC). LPM, lateral plate mesoderm; PXM, paraxial mesoderm. (**b**) Aggregation of the somatic mesenchyme around the notochord leads to formation of a continuous perichordal tube (PT). Localization of Noto expression at these time points is indicated in green. (**c**) Condensation of the axial mesenchyme leads to spine segmentation and perichordal disc formation. (**d**) Formation of IVDs is associated with the disappearance of the notochord within the vertebral bodies, and its expansion within the IVD. (Used with permission from McCann MR, Tamplin OJ, Rossant J, Séguin CA. Tracing notochord-derived cells using a Noto-cre mouse: implications for intervertebral disc development. Dis Model Mech. 2012;5:73–82.)

Other authors, however, argue that the smaller adult NP cells, despite their distinct morphology, are derived from the original population of larger notochordal cells. Recent fate-mapping studies in mice using notochord-specific Cre recombinase, driven by either the sonic hedgehog (Shh)[67] or Noto[68] promoters, have convincingly revealed that all cells of the adult NP derive from the embryonic notochord. Additionally, notochordal cells of porcine,[69] rabbit,[70] and mouse[71] NP have been shown to transition into "chondrocyte-like" cells both in vitro and in vivo. This transition was favored by both physiological stimuli, such as dynamic loading[69] and standard tissue culture conditions,[70] as well as pathological stimulus like needle puncture injury.[71] Importantly, a robust expression of brachyury, an unequivocal marker of notochord, has been seen in adult human NP tissues.[72] Together, these results strongly suggest that morphological differences between "notochordal" and "chondrocyte-like" cells represent different stages of cellular activity or differentiation, rather than a different lineage.[63,64,65,66,67,68,69,70,71]

5.4 Unique Biology of Intervertebral Disc Cells

The fact that the cells of the NP reside in a unique hypoxic and hyperosmotic niche and derive from

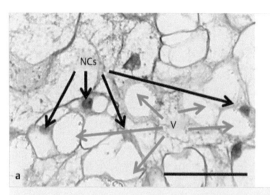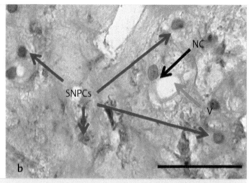

Fig. 5.6 (a, b) Notochordal cells (NCs) are defined phenotypically as having nuclei in direct contact and surrounded by large vacuoles. Chondrocyte-like cells, or small nucleus pulposus cells (SNPCs), are characterized by having nuclei surrounded by matrix with no contact with vacuoles. *Black arrows*, NCs; *blue arrows*, SNPCs. V, vacuoles (*green arrows*). Scale bar = 50 μm. (Adapted from Purmessur D, Guterl CC, Cho SK, et al. Dynamic pressurization induces transition of notochordal cells to a mature phenotype while retaining production of important patterning ligands from development. Arthritis Res Ther. 2013;15(5):R122.)

the embryonic notochord means that these cells are quite unlike any other cell type in the body. As a result, NP cells have developed distinguishing characteristics that are not found in any other cell types in the body. These characteristics allow the cells of the NP to adapt to their unique environment. In this section, we will discuss several unique biologic features of the NP.

In general, cells of the body are able to adapt to survive hypoxic settings through expression of the transcription factors: hypoxia-inducible factor-1a and -2a (HIF-1/2). The cells of the NP, however, constitutively and robustly express HIF-1α and HIF-2α, even when cultured under normoxia.[73] Interestingly, this constitutive expression of HIF-1α in NP is consistent across multiple species.[74] Because NP cells are obligately glycolytic and rely very little on aerobic metabolism even when oxygen is abundant,[75] this constitutive HIF-1α activity in NP cells appears to suggests that HIF-1α strongly drives glycolytic metabolism in NP cells. This is believed to occur through the upregulation of several crucial genes including glucose transporter (GLUT) 1 and 3, glyceraldehyde 3-phosphate dehydrogenase (GAPDH), aggrecan,[76] β-1,3-glucuronyltransferase 1,[77] galectin-3,[78] and vascular endothelial growth factor-A (VEGF-A).[73] In addition, when HIF-1α is conditionally deleted in mouse NP notochordal cells using the Foxa2-driven Cre recombinase, Merceron and colleagues were able to demonstrate that HIF-1α is required for NP cell survival.[79]

Brachyury is a transcription factor that is necessary for development of the embryonic mesoderm as well as the morphogenesis of the notochord. Although previously considered only a notochordal gene and studied in a developmental context, the expression of brachyury has been recently reported in postnatal and mature NP cells.[80,81,82] This is a distinct feature of NP cells in postnatal humans. Studies have shown that, in comparison to non-chondrodystrophic dogs, "chondrocyte-like" cells of the NP in chondrodystrophic breeds show a decrease in brachyury expression relative to notochordal cells with aging and degeneration.[80] Conversely, other reports using human tissue have not found a correlation between brachyury expression and the degree of disc degeneration.[81] Similarly, the transition from notochordal to "chondrocyte-like" morphology in organ-cultured porcine discs by continuous pressurization did not involve a decrease in brachyury expression.[69] Despite the importance of this transcription factor in notochord development and function, the specific role of brachyury in the maintenance of postnatal NP remains unexplored.

Recent studies using chromatin-immunoprecipitation and next-generation sequencing (ChIP-seq) in mouse embryonic stem cells[83] and a human chordoma cell line[84] have given insight into the direct gene targets of brachyury binding. Gene targets of brachyury that are of potential importance to NP physiology include fibroblast growth factor 8, Axin2, and pleiotrophin.[85] Brachyury was also found to regulate the gene expression of connective tissue growth factor (CTGF, also called CCN2), an ECM protein that is necessary for postnatal NP function[86] and is also known to suppress the catabolic effects of IL-1b in

NP cells.[87] Knowing these gene targets for brachyury gives important insight into its transcriptional control network, and thus, provides insight into the mechanism by which it exerts its widespread effects.

Another unique feature of NP cells is their expression of Shh, which is a ligand of the hedgehog family that is expressed specifically in the developing notochord. Conditional deletion of both Smoothened (Smo) and Shh itself has demonstrated that this signaling pathway is required for the formation of the notochordal sheath as well as patterning of the NP.[88,89] Importantly, Shh expression remains active in the postnatal NP, at least for the first few weeks, and is required for proper functioning of NP cells.[90,91] Although Shh expression and signaling are decreased with aging and degeneration, a recent study has demonstrated that overexpression of Shh in aged IVDs can increase expression of brachyury and aggrecan, as well as accumulation of chondroitin sulfate.[92]

It is clear that the recent advancements in understanding disc cell biology and the continued efforts of the scientific community in this direction will have a significant impact on our ability to devise new and exciting therapies for IDD. Understanding the unique features of young, healthy NP cells is important, particularly when devising new stem cell–based strategies to treat IDD.

5.5 Conclusion

Low back pain remains one of the most common causes of disability worldwide.[6] While the exact etiology of back pain remains unknown, it is typically associated with IDD. Our ability to effectively treat disc degeneration is hampered by an incomplete understanding of the biological processes that control IVD development, function, and disease. Further confounding our ability to treat disc degeneration is the lack of correlation between radiological diagnostic criteria and patient symptoms, including pain.[93] Consequently, the clinical management of disc pathologies remains severely limited, with no options yet for early intervention or predictive patient screening.

Revealing the complex biology and biochemistry of the healthy IVD, both for a developmental and homeostasis perspective, is an important first step in better understanding the degenerative process as well as devising new regenerative strategies. While we already know so much about the unique biology of the IVD, we as a research community are only now beginning to scratch the surface. The next wave of disc research should focus on unbiased systems biology approaches to better learn about the biologic changes that occur over time with natural aging and with degeneration.

Pearls i

- The IVD is a highly specialized structure that facilitates load transmission and multiaxial flexibility of the spine while simultaneously resisting high amounts of biomechanical stress in multiple planes.
- The IVD is the largest avascular organ in the human body.
- The NP's structure is gelatinous with a high water and aggrecan content, which allows the NP to resist compression when loaded.
- The concentric lamellar organization of the AF's collagen fibers give it the strength required to restrict lateral motion and to prevent extrusion of the NP.
- The CEP consists of a thin (< 1 mm) avascular layer of hyaline cartilage that allows for the diffusion of nutrition into and waste out of the IVD.
- The macromolecules of the NP are synthesized and maintained throughout life by a small population of cells, occupying less than 1% of the volume of the tissue in the NP.
- The compressive forces that the IVD experiences have been estimated to be up to ~2,500 N during dynamic lifting, and intradiskal pressures approach 1 MPa during normal daily activities such as climbing stairs (0.5–0.7 MPa) or jogging (0.35–0.95 MPa).
- The major nutritional supply of the IVD comes from capillary beds in the vertebral end plate in which metabolites must diffuse across the CEP and into the NP. The other main capillary plexus supplying the IVD exists in the outer AF, with this plexus penetrating only 1 to 2 mm into the outer AF.
- The NP is unique in the human body as it is the only tissue remnant of the embryonic notochord, which gives the cells of the NP several unique biologic features.
- The expression of HIF-1α, brachyury, and Shh are verified markers that distinguish young, healthy NP cells from other cell types in the adult human.

5.6 Board-style Questions

1. What is the main route of nutrition and glucose into the NP?
   a) Capillary beds in the outer anulus fibrosus
   b) Diffusion across the cartilaginous end plate
   c) Capillary beds in the inner anulus fibrosus
   d) Diffusion through the outer anulus fibrosus

2. Which compartment of the IVD originates from the embryonic notochord?
   a) Cartilaginous end plate
   b) Inner anulus fibrosus
   c) Outer anulus fibrosus
   d) Nucleus pulposus

3. What is the predominant type of collagen in the nucleus pulposus?
   a) Collagen I
   b) Collagen IX
   c) Collagen II
   d) Collagen X

4. What is the GAG: hydroxyproline ratio in the young adult intervertebral disc?
   a) 1:1
   b) 5:1
   c) 10:1
   d) 25:1

5. How are the mechanical stresses of the disc transduced into disc cells?
   a) Integrins
   b) Aggrecan
   c) Collagen II
   d) Extracellular water

6. What is the predominant type of collagen in the anulus fibrosus?
   a) Collagen I
   b) Collagen II
   c) Collagen IX
   d) Collagen X

7. What is the main type of mechanical stress that the anulus fibrosus protects the intervertebral disc from during normal loading?
   a) Compression
   b) Shear
   c) Tension
   d) Torsion

8. Which of the following statements about the nucleus pulposus is true?
   a) Notochordal cells and small chondrocyte-like cells share the same ontogeny and represent different phenotypes of the same cell
   b) The major type of proteoglycan in the nucleus pulposus is heparan sulfate

   c) As notochordal cell populations decrease over time, the cells of the adult NP are replaced by cells that migrate from the anulus and/or cartilaginous end plate
   d) The nucleus pulposus usually provides resistance to tension and shear

9. What is the main vascular supply to the vertebral body and cartilaginous end plate?
   a) Anterior spinal artery
   b) Sinuvertebral artery
   c) Basivertebral artery
   d) Artery of Adamkiewicz

10. Which of the following statements about the embryology of the intervertebral disc is true?
   a) The notochord develops from the paraxial mesoderm
   b) The spinal skeleton forms from the dermato-myotome
   c) The formation of the notochord occurs around the 7th week of embryonic development
   d) The cells of the anulus fibrosus form from sclerotomal-derived cells

Answers ✓

1. b
2. d
3. c
4. d
5. a
6. b
7. c
8. a
9. c
10. d

References

[1] Bogduk N. The inter-body joints and the intervertebral discs. In: Bogduk N, eds. Clinical Anatomy of the Lumbar Spine and Sarcum. New York, NY: Churchill Livingstone; 1997:13–31

[2] Hukins DW. Disc structure and function. In: Ghosh P, eds. Biology of Intervertebral Disc. Boca Raton, FL: CRC Press; 1998:2–37

[3] Katz JN. Lumbar disc disorders and low-back pain: socioeconomic factors and consequences. J Bone Joint Surg Am. 2006; 88 Suppl 2:21–24

[4] Andersson GB. Epidemiological features of chronic low-back pain. Lancet. 1999; 354(9178):581–585

[5] Cheung KM, Karppinen J, Chan D, et al. Prevalence and pattern of lumbar magnetic resonance imaging changes in a population study of one thousand forty-three individuals. Spine. 2009; 34(9):934–940

[6] Murray CJ, Atkinson C, Bhalla K, et al. U.S. Burden of Disease Collaborators. The state of US health, 1990–2010: burden of diseases, injuries, and risk factors. JAMA. 2013; 310(6):591–608

[7] Mwale F, Roughley P, Antoniou J. Distinction between the extracellular matrix of the nucleus pulposus and hyaline cartilage: a requisite for tissue engineering of intervertebral disc. Eur Cell Mater. 2004; 8:58–63, discussion 63–64

[8] Bernick S, Cailliet R. Vertebral end-plate changes with aging of human vertebrae. Spine. 1982; 7(2):97–102

[9] Holmes AD, Hukins DW, Freemont AJ. End-plate displacement during compression of lumbar vertebra-disc-vertebra segments and the mechanism of failure. Spine. 1993; 18(1): 128–135

[10] Adams MA. Intervertebral disc tissues. In: Derby B, Akhtar R, eds. Mechanical Properties of Aging Soft Tissues. New York, NY: Springer; 2015:7–35

[11] Urban JPG, Maroudas A. Measurement of fixed charge density and partition coefficients in the intervertebral disc. Biochim Biophys Acta. 1979; 586:166–178

[12] Roberts S, Menage J, Urban JPG. Biochemical and structural properties of the cartilage end-plate and its relation to the intervertebral disc. Spine. 1989; 14(2):166–174

[13] Antoniou J, Steffen T, Nelson F, et al. The human lumbar intervertebral disc: evidence for changes in the biosynthesis and denaturation of the extracellular matrix with growth, maturation, ageing, and degeneration. J Clin Invest. 1996; 98 (4):996–1003

[14] Johnstone B, Bayliss MT. The large proteoglycans of the human intervertebral disc: changes in their biosynthesis and structure with age, topography, and pathology. Spine. 1995; 20(6):674–684

[15] Urban JP, McMullin JF. Swelling pressure of the intervertebral disc: influence of proteoglycan and collagen contents. Biorheology. 1985; 22(2):145–157

[16] Maroudas A, Stockwell RA, Nachemson A, Urban J. Factors involved in the nutrition of the human lumbar intervertebral disc: cellularity and diffusion of glucose in vitro. J Anat. 1975; 120(Pt 1):113–130

[17] Sivan SS, Tsitron E, Wachtel E, et al. Age-related accumulation of pentosidine in aggrecan and collagen from normal and degenerate human intervertebral discs. Biochem J. 2006; 399(1):29–35

[18] Sivan SS, Wachtel E, Tsitron E, et al. Collagen turnover in normal and degenerate human intervertebral discs as determined by the racemization of aspartic acid. J Biol Chem. 2008; 283(14):8796–8801

[19] Melrose J, Ghosh P, Taylor TK. Neutral proteinases of the human intervertebral disc. Biochim Biophys Acta. 1987; 923 (3):483–495

[20] Roberts S, Caterson B, Menage J, Evans EH, Jaffray DC, Eisenstein SM. Matrix metalloproteinases and aggrecanase: their role in disorders of the human intervertebral disc. Spine. 2000; 25(23):3005–3013

[21] Lyons G, Eisenstein SM, Sweet MB. Biochemical changes in intervertebral disc degeneration. Biochim Biophys Acta. 1981; 673(4):443–453

[22] Yang KH, King AI. Mechanism of facet load transmission as a hypothesis for low-back pain. Spine. 1984; 9(6): 557–565

[23] Simon SR, Buckwalter JA, Einhorn TA. Kinesiology. In: Simon SR, ed. Orthopedic Basic Science. Park Ridge, IL: American Academy of Orthopedic Surgeons; 1994: 558–68

[24] Adams MA, Bogduk N, Burton K, Dolan P, eds. The Biomechanics of Back Pain. 2nd ed. London, England: Churchill Livingstone; 2006

[25] Marras WS, Davis KG, Ferguson SA, Lucas BR, Gupta P. Spine loading characteristics of patients with low back pain compared with asymptomatic individuals. Spine. 2001; 26(23): 2566–2574

[26] Wilke HJ, Rohlmann A, Neller S, Graichen F, Claes L, Bergmann G. ISSLS prize winner: a novel approach to determine trunk muscle forces during flexion and extension—a comparison of data from an in vitro experiment and in vivo measurements. Spine. 2003; 28(23): 2585–2593

[27] Chan SC, Ferguson SJ, Gantenbein-Ritter B. The effects of dynamic loading on the intervertebral disc. Eur Spine J. 2011; 20(11):1796–1812

[28] Korecki CL, MacLean JJ, Iatridis JC. Dynamic compression effects on intervertebral disc mechanics and biology. Spine. 2008; 33(13):1403–1409

[29] Maclean JJ, Lee CR, Alini M, Iatridis JC. Anabolic and catabolic mRNA levels of the intervertebral disc vary with the magnitude and frequency of in vivo dynamic compression. J Orthop Res. 2004; 22(6):1193–1200

[30] Huang CY, Gu WY. Effects of mechanical compression on metabolism and distribution of oxygen and lactate in intervertebral disc. J Biomech. 2008; 41(6):1184–1196

[31] Urban JP, Smith S, Fairbank JC. Nutrition of the intervertebral disc. Spine. 2004; 29(23):2700–2709

[32] McMillan DW, Garbutt G, Adams MA. Effect of sustained loading on the water content of intervertebral discs: implications for disc metabolism. Ann Rheum Dis. 1996; 55(12): 880–887

[33] Alkhatib B, Rosenzweig DH, Krock E, et al. Acute mechanical injury of the human intervertebral disc: link to degeneration and pain. Eur Cell Mater. 2014; 28:98–110, discussion 110–111

[34] Gawri R, Rosenzweig DH, Krock E, et al. High mechanical strain of primary intervertebral disc cells promotes secretion of inflammatory factors associated with disc degeneration and pain. Arthritis Res Ther. 2014; 16(1):R21

[35] Gilchrist CL, Chen J, Richardson WJ, Loeser RF, Setton LA. Functional integrin subunits regulating cell-matrix interactions in the intervertebral disc. J Orthop Res. 2007; 25(6): 829–840

[36] Chen J, Jing L, Gilchrist CL, Richardson WJ, Fitch RD, Setton LA. Expression of laminin isoforms, receptors, and binding proteins unique to nucleus pulposus cells of immature intervertebral disc. Connect Tissue Res. 2009; 50(5): 294–306

[37] Nettles DL, Richardson WJ, Setton LA. Integrin expression in cells of the intervertebral disc. J Anat. 2004; 204(6): 515–520

[38] Gilchrist CL, Francisco AT, Plopper GE, Chen J, Setton LA. Nucleus pulposus cell-matrix interactions with laminins. Eur Cell Mater. 2011; 21:523–532

[39] Bridgen DT, Gilchrist CL, Richardson WJ, et al. Integrin-mediated interactions with extracellular matrix proteins for nucleus pulposus cells of the human intervertebral disc. J Orthop Res. 2013; 31(10):1661–1667

[40] Raj PP. Intervertebral disc: anatomy-physiology-pathophysiology-treatment. Pain Pract. 2008; 8(1):18–44

[41] Crock HV, Goldwasser M. Anatomic studies of the circulation in the region of the vertebral end-plate in adult Greyhound dogs. Spine. 1984; 9(7):702–706

[42] Roberts S, Menage J, Eisenstein SM. The cartilage end-plate and intervertebral disc in scoliosis: calcification and other sequelae. J Orthop Res. 1993; 11(5):747–757

[43] Roberts S, Urban JPG, Evans H, Eisenstein SM. Transport properties of the human cartilage endplate in relation to its composition and calcification. Spine. 1996; 21(4):415–420

[44] Grunhagen T, Wilde G, Soukane DM, Shirazi-Adl SA, Urban JP. Nutrient supply and intervertebral disc metabolism. J Bone Joint Surg Am. 2006; 88 Suppl 2:30–35

[45] Lama P, Le Maitre CL, Harding IJ, Dolan P, Adams MA. Nerves and blood vessels in degenerated intervertebral discs are confined to physically disrupted tissue. J Anat. 2018; 233(1):86–97; [Epub ahead of print]

[46] Holm S, Maroudas A, Urban JP, Selstam G, Nachemson A. Nutrition of the intervertebral disc: solute transport and metabolism. Connect Tissue Res. 1981; 8(2):101–119

[47] Bibby SR, Urban JP. Effect of nutrient deprivation on the viability of intervertebral disc cells. Eur Spine J. 2004; 13(8):695–701

[48] Nachemson A, Lewin T, Maroudas A, Freeman MAF. In vitro diffusion of dye through the end-plates and the annulus fibrosus of human lumbar inter-vertebral discs. Acta Orthop Scand. 1970; 41(6):589–607

[49] Bashir A, Gray ML, Hartke J, Burstein D. Nondestructive imaging of human cartilage glycosaminoglycan concentration by MRI. Magn Reson Med. 1999; 41(5):857–865

[50] Bartels EM, Fairbank JCT, Winlove CP, Urban JPG. Oxygen and lactate concentrations measured in vivo in the intervertebral discs of scoliotic and back pain patients. Spine. 1998; 23:1–8

[51] Bibby SR, Fairbank JC, Urban MR, Urban JP. Cell viability in scoliotic discs in relation to disc deformity and nutrient levels. Spine. 2002; 27(20):2220–2228, discussion 2227–2228

[52] Kauppila LI, McAlindon T, Evans S, Wilson PW, Kiel D, Felson DT. Disc degeneration/back pain and calcification of the abdominal aorta: a 25-year follow-up study in Framingham. Spine. 1997; 22(14):1642–1647, discussion 1648–1649

[53] Jones JP. Subchondral osteonecrosis can conceivably cause disk degeneration and "primary" osteoarthritis. In: Urbaniak JR, Jones JP, eds. Osteonecrosis. Park Ridge, IL: American Academy of Orthopedic Surgeons; 1997:135–142

[54] Pazzaglia UE, Salisbury JR, Byers PD. Development and involution of the notochord in the human spine. J R Soc Med. 1989; 82(7):413–415

[55] Johnson RL, Laufer E, Riddle RD, Tabin C. Ectopic expression of Sonic hedgehog alters dorsal-ventral patterning of somites. Cell. 1994; 79(7):1165–1173

[56] Beckers A, Alten L, Viebahn C, Andre P, Gossler A. The mouse homeobox gene Noto regulates node morphogenesis, notochordal ciliogenesis, and left-right patterning. Proc Natl Acad Sci U S A. 2007; 104(40):15765–15770

[57] Hay ED. The mesenchymal cell, its role in the embryo, and the remarkable signaling mechanisms that create it. Dev Dyn. 2005; 233(3):706–720

[58] Peacock A. Observations on the prenatal development of the intervertebral disc in man. J Anat. 1951; 85(3):260–274

[59] Aszódi A, Chan D, Hunziker E, Bateman JF, Fässler R. Collagen II is essential for the removal of the notochord and the formation of intervertebral discs. J Cell Biol. 1998; 143(5):1399–1412

[60] Trout JJ, Buckwalter JA, Moore KC, Landas SK. Ultrastructure of the human intervertebral disc. I. Changes in notochordal cells with age. Tissue Cell. 1982; 14(2):359–369

[61] Chen J, Yan W, Setton LA. Molecular phenotypes of notochordal cells purified from immature nucleus pulposus. Eur Spine J. 2006; 15 Suppl 3:S303–S311

[62] Gilson A, Dreger M, Urban JP. Differential expression level of cytokeratin 8 in cells of the bovine nucleus pulposus complicates the search for specific intervertebral disc cell markers. Arthritis Res Ther. 2010; 12(1):R24

[63] Weiler C, Nerlich AG, Schaaf R, Bachmeier BE, Wuertz K, Boos N. Immunohistochemical identification of notochordal markers in cells in the aging human lumbar intervertebral disc. Eur Spine J. 2010; 19(10):1761–1770

[64] Butler WF. Comparative anatomy and development of the mammalian disc. In: Ghosh P, eds. The Biology of the Intervertebral Disc. Boca Raton, FL: CRC Press; 1989:83–108

[65] Kim KW, Lim TH, Kim JG, Jeong ST, Masuda K, An HS. The origin of chondrocytes in the nucleus pulposus and histologic findings associated with the transition of a notochordal nucleus pulposus to a fibrocartilaginous nucleus pulposus in intact rabbit intervertebral discs. Spine. 2003; 28(10):982–990

[66] Kim KW, Ha KY, Lee JS, et al. Notochordal cells stimulate migration of cartilage end plate chondrocytes of the intervertebral disc in in vitro cell migration assays. Spine J. 2009; 9(4):323–329

[67] Choi K-S, Cohn MJ, Harfe BD. Identification of nucleus pulposus precursor cells and notochordal remnants in the mouse: implications for disk degeneration and chordoma formation. Dev Dyn. 2008; 237(12):3953–3958

[68] McCann MR, Tamplin OJ, Rossant J, Séguin CA. Tracing notochord-derived cells using a Noto-cre mouse: implications for intervertebral disc development. Dis Model Mech. 2012; 5(1):73–82

[69] Purmessur D, Guterl CC, Cho SK, et al. Dynamic pressurization induces transition of notochordal cells to a mature phenotype while retaining production of important patterning ligands from development. Arthritis Res Ther. 2013; 15(5):R122

[70] Kim JH, Deasy BM, Seo HY, et al. Differentiation of intervertebral notochordal cells through live automated cell imaging system in vitro. Spine. 2009; 34(23):2486–2493

[71] Yang F, Leung VYL, Luk KDK, Chan D, Cheung KM. Injury-induced sequential transformation of notochordal nucleus pulposus to chondrogenic and fibrocartilaginous phenotype in the mouse. J Pathol. 2009; 218(1):113–121

[72] Risbud MV, Shapiro IM. Notochordal cells in the adult intervertebral disc: new perspective on an old question. Crit Rev Eukaryot Gene Expr. 2011; 21(1):29–41

[73] Agrawal A, Gajghate S, Smith H, et al. Cited2 modulates hypoxia-inducible factor-dependent expression of vascular endothelial growth factor in nucleus pulposus cells of the rat intervertebral disc. Arthritis Rheum. 2008; 58(12):3798–3808

[74] Risbud MV, Guttapalli A, Stokes DG, et al. Nucleus pulposus cells express HIF-1 alpha under normoxic culture conditions: a metabolic adaptation to the intervertebral disc microenvironment. J Cell Biochem. 2006; 98(1):152–159

[75] Agrawal A, Guttapalli A, Narayan S, Albert TJ, Shapiro IM, Risbud MV. Normoxic stabilization of HIF-1alpha drives glycolytic metabolism and regulates aggrecan gene expression in nucleus pulposus cells of the rat intervertebral disk. Am J Physiol Cell Physiol. 2007; 293(2):C621–C631

[76] Rajpurohit R, Risbud MV, Ducheyne P, Vresilovic EJ, Shapiro IM. Phenotypic characteristics of the nucleus pulposus:

expression of hypoxia inducing factor-1, glucose transporter-1 and MMP-2. Cell Tissue Res. 2002; 308(3):401–407

[77] Gogate SS, Nasser R, Shapiro IM, Risbud MV. Hypoxic regulation of β-1,3-glucuronyltransferase 1 expression in nucleus pulposus cells of the rat intervertebral disc: role of hypoxia-inducible factor proteins. Arthritis Rheum. 2011; 63(7): 1950–1960

[78] Zeng Y, Danielson KG, Albert TJ, Shapiro IM, Risbud MV. HIF-1 alpha is a regulator of galectin-3 expression in the intervertebral disc. J Bone Miner Res. 2007; 22(12):1851–1861

[79] Merceron C, Mangiavini L, Robling A, et al. Loss of HIF-1α in the notochord results in cell death and complete disappearance of the nucleus pulposus. PLoS One. 2014; 9(10):e110768

[80] Smolders LA, Meij BP, Riemers FM, et al. Canonical Wnt signaling in the notochordal cell is upregulated in early intervertebral disk degeneration. J Orthop Res. 2012; 30(6):950–957

[81] Minogue BM, Richardson SM, Zeef LA, Freemont AJ, Hoyland JA. Transcriptional profiling of bovine intervertebral disc cells: implications for identification of normal and degenerate human intervertebral disc cell phenotypes. Arthritis Res Ther. 2010; 12(1):R22

[82] Maier JA, Lo Y, Harfe BD. Foxa1 and Foxa2 are required for formation of the intervertebral discs. PLoS One. 2013; 8(1): e55528

[83] Evans AL, Faial T, Gilchrist MJ, et al. Genomic targets of Brachyury (T) in differentiating mouse embryonic stem cells. PLoS One. 2012; 7(3):e33346

[84] Nelson AC, Pillay N, Henderson S, et al. An integrated functional genomics approach identifies the regulatory network directed by brachyury (T) in chordoma. J Pathol. 2012; 228 (3):274–285

[85] Risbud MV, Schoepflin ZR, Mwale F, et al. Defining the phenotype of young healthy nucleus pulposus cells: recommendations of the Spine Research Interest Group at the 2014 annual ORS meeting. J Orthop Res. 2015; 33(3):283–293

[86] Bedore J, Sha W, McCann MR, Liu S, Leask A, Séguin CA. Impaired intervertebral disc development and premature disc degeneration in mice with notochord-specific deletion of CCN2. Arthritis Rheum. 2013; 65(10):2634–2644

[87] Tran CM, Schoepflin ZR, Markova DZ, et al. CCN2 suppresses catabolic effects of interleukin-1β through α5β1 and αVβ3 integrins in nucleus pulposus cells: implications in intervertebral disc degeneration. J Biol Chem. 2014; 289:7374–7387

[88] Choi K-S, Harfe BD. Hedgehog signaling is required for formation of the notochord sheath and patterning of nuclei pulposi within the intervertebral discs. Proc Natl Acad Sci U S A. 2011; 108(23):9484–9489

[89] Choi K-S, Lee C, Harfe BD. Sonic hedgehog in the notochord is sufficient for patterning of the intervertebral discs. Mech Dev. 2012; 129(9–12):255–262

[90] Dahia CL, Mahoney E, Wylie C. Shh signaling from the nucleus pulposus is required for the postnatal growth and differentiation of the mouse intervertebral disc. PLoS One. 2012; 7(4):e35944

[91] Dahia CL, Mahoney EJ, Durrani AA, Wylie C. Intercellular signaling pathways active during intervertebral disc growth, differentiation, and aging. Spine. 2009; 34(5): 456–462

[92] Winkler T, Mahoney EJ, Sinner D, Wylie CC, Dahia CL. WNT signaling activates Shh signaling in early postnatal intervertebral discs, and re-activates Shh signaling in old discs in the mouse. PLoS One. 2014; 9(6):e98444

[93] Takatalo J, Karppinen J, Niinimäki J, et al. Does lumbar disc degeneration on magnetic resonance imaging associate with low back symptom severity in young Finnish adults? Spine. 2011; 36(25):2180–2189

Suggested Readings

Classic Articles

Andersson BJ, Ortengren R, Nachemson AL, Elfström G, Broman H. The sitting posture: an electromyographic and discometric study. Orthop Clin North Am. 1975; 6(1):105–120

Bogduk N. The innervation of the lumbar spine. Spine. 1983; 8(3): 286–293

Herkowitz HN, Rothman RH, Simeone FA, eds. The Spine. 4th ed. Philadelphia, PA: Elsevier Health Science; 1998

Urban JP, Smith S, Fairbank JC. Nutrition of the intervertebral disc. Spine. 2004; 29(23):2700–2709

White AA III, Panjabi MM, eds. Clinical Biomechanics of the Spine. 2nd ed. Philadelphia, PA: Lippincott; 1990

Current Research

Dudli S, Sing DC, Hu SS, et al. ISSLS Prize in Basic Science 2017: intervertebral disc/bone marrow cross-talk with Modic changes. Eur Spine J. 2017; 26(5):1362–1373

Gruber HE, Hoelscher GL, Ingram JA, Zinchenko N, Hanley EN, Jr. Senescent vs. non-senescent cells in the human annulus in vivo: cell harvest with laser capture microdissection and gene expression studies with microarray analysis. BMC Biotechnol. 2010; 10:5–15

Miyazaki S, Diwan AD, Kato K, et al. ISSLS Prize in Basic Science 2018: growth differentiation factor-6 attenuated pro-inflammatory molecular changes in the rabbit anular-puncture model and degenerated disc-induced pain generation in the rat xenograft radiculopathy model. Eur Spine J. 2018; 27(4): 739–751

Purmessur D, Cornejo MC, Cho SK, et al. Intact glycosaminoglycans from intervertebral disc-derived notochordal cell-conditioned media inhibit neurite growth while maintaining neuronal cell viability. Spine J. 2015; 15(5):1060–1069

Zhao K, Zhang Y, Kang L, et al. Epigenetic silencing of miRNA-143 regulates apoptosis by targeting BCL2 in human intervertebral disc degeneration. Gene. 2017; 628:259–266

6 Degenerative Disc Disease and the Herniated Nucleus Pulposus

Alim F. Ramji and Isaac L. Moss

Abstract

Lower back and neck pain assume an enormous global burden of disease and have multifactorial etiologies. One such etiology is considered to be intervertebral disc (IVD) degeneration, which is a complex pathologic process associated with herniation of the nucleus pulposus (NP). The IVD is a specialized heterogeneous tissue composed of an outer rigid fibrous anulus and an inner hydrophilic gelatinous substance known as the NP; it is bounded superiorly and inferiorly by cartilaginous end plates. A great deal of research has been aimed at elucidating the mechanisms behind this degeneration so as to inform clinical treatment strategies. In this chapter we aim to present the current pathophysiologic understanding of IVD degeneration, its clinical presentation with imaging findings, as well as several clinical case examples and treatment pearls. Board-style questions and answers are provided at the end of the chapter to test material comprehension.

Keywords: intervertebral, disc, degeneration, herniation, discectomy

6.1 Introduction

Lower back and neck pain assume an enormous global burden of disease. In 2015 they accounted for the leading cause of disability in most high-income countries, growing 59.5% in terms of disability-adjusted life years (DALYs) compared to 1990.[1] In terms of economic effects, loss of productivity due to absence of work costs the United States roughly 91 billion dollars annually.[2] Back pain holds a strong association with intervertebral disc (IVD) degeneration and associated IVD herniated nucleus pulposus (HNP).[3,4] Given the immense disease burden associated with IVD degeneration and herniation, it is crucial for physicians and scientists to work to further elucidate the mechanisms and behaviors that connect them. In this chapter, we aim to present a summary of the available recent literature regarding lumbar IVD degeneration and HNP, as well as to provide clinical correlates for physicians.

The IVD connects adjacent vertebrae in the spine and functions to transmit and absorb the mechanical load that is created during activities of daily living. The disc itself is a complex tissue composed of an external, highly organized fibrous ring known as the anulus fibrosus (AF) and an inner hydrophilic gel known as the nucleus pulposus (NP). The AF and NP are confined cranially and caudally by the cartilaginous end plates (CEP).[5] The integrity of these three anatomic regions is critical in ensuring optimal mechanical function of the IVD. However, as the tissue has a low cell density and is principally avascular, it is more vulnerable to age-related degeneration than other tissues in the body.[6] The outer AF is assembled by fibroblast-rich colonies to allow for lamellae of primarily type 1 collagen oriented based on anatomic location within the spinal column.[5] Its rigid fibrous composition allows for a pressurized containment of the inner NP, which is made of a mixture of type II collagen and aggrecan-rich proteoglycans that allow for a very hydrophilic local environment. Nutrition and oxygen are transmitted to the IVD via diffusion through the CEPs ~600 micrometer layers of specialized hyaline cartilage situated near vasculature supplying the vertebral body.[6] The collagen fibers within this interface run parallel to the vertebral bodies and are continuous with those within the AF.[4]

In the healthy young adult, the IVD exhibits multiple formative characteristics that differentiate it from those in later adulthood. The AF collagen fibers exist in a multidimensional tensioned state by both the homogenous inner NP and the superior-inferior pull by the CEP.[7] The oblique collagen fibers alternate regularly with proteoglycan substrates forming concentric, regular lamellae that maintain a rigid structural integrity. The NP retains a high saturation of proteoglycans that allow the well-hydrated gel to evenly distribute forces along the two parallel end plates.[4,7] The CEP acts as a uniform cartilaginous anchor that both confines the NP and allows for an even, regular diffusion of nutrients.

6.2 Pathogenesis of Disc Degeneration

Degeneration of the IVD is a complex process that has continued to gain more attention in recent years. For the purposes of this chapter, we will focus mainly on age-related degeneration.

During the process of skeletal maturity, the disc loses much of its peripheral vascularity and approaches a near avascular state.[8] With further aging, all three distinct anatomic regions of the IVD begin to undergo a process of disarray as their collagen architecture becomes more disorganized. The extracellular matrix, so fundamental in maintaining the rigid structural integrity of the IVD, loses its ability to maintain functioning homeostasis. Even in infancy and childhood, the extracellular matrix is a dynamic tissue continuously being turned over by a mixture of metalloproteinases and aggrecanases, while simultaneously being synthesized by fibroblast-rich cell colonies.[9,10] This homeostatic balance is altered with aging. With an imbalance in production and degradation of various collagen molecules, there follows a natural declination of cellular viability; this activity leads to an upregulation of the inflammatory cascade and cytokine concentration that results in proteoglycan breakdown and eventual dehydration within the IVD.[4,5,9] This is coupled with sclerotic changes seen within the CEP that are thought to decrease the efficiency of nutrient diffusion by losing vascular permeability and contact, further leading to an increase in oxidative stress.[6] Additionally, loss of proteoglycan reduces the osmotic potential and effective net negative charge within the IVD. Without an ability to recruit and retain water molecules, the intradiskal pressure gradient drops and the vital tensioning of the outer AF is lost.

Loss of intradiskal pressure can be seen radiographically as a reduction in disc height.[11] As the intradiskal pressure continues to reduce with age and degeneration, the biomechanical function of the IVD also deteriorates. Without the constant tensioning of the outer AF collagen lamellae, interdigitated clefts begin to appear that weaken its structural integrity by causing mechanical heterogeneity.[9] Irregular stress distributions form within the IVD motion segments that lead to excess bending, torsional, and shear stresses within the NP.[7] This often lead to fissuring that begins in the outer AF and traverses toward the inner AF.[12] In the aberrant repair response accompanying these changes, there is an observed increase in both local innervation and inflammatory mediator secretion that can be a source of pain.[12] In animal models, this alteration in biomechanics within the IVD causes an imbalance in catabolic processes that further lead to degenerative changes within the IVD, furthering a vicious cycle that tends toward tissue breakdown and often eventual disc herniation.[7,9,12] Local oxidative stresses that play a paramount role in the degradation of the IVD are amplified by calcific changes within the CEP, limiting both nutrient inflow and metabolic outflow, causing local increases in anaerobic byproducts and lower pH microenvironments.[13]

In addition to the direct tissue damage caused by the accumulation of these metabolic byproducts and the resultant oxidative stress, DNA damage and an alteration of DNA repair mechanisms are also thought to contribute to the pathologic changes within the IVD.[14] In the healthy IVD, the homogenous NP maintains a hypertonic environment preserved by a high concentration of aggrecan side-chains, which in turn induces the NP cells to steadily activate a local protein known as the tonicity enhancer binding protein (TonEBP).[15] Though this protein chiefly acts to maintain the water-binding matrix within the NP, it also functions in an ancillary capacity to initiate DNA damage repair mechanisms and cell-cycle arrest, thereby allowing for fewer aberrant cell lines.[14] As proteoglycan loss ensues with IVD degradation and tonicity drops within the IVD, this pathway for DNA repair is negated and cellular apoptosis and necrosis are more frequently observed.

This process ties in directly to a relatively newer paradigm regarding global disease processes, known as cellular senescence, where biologic stress leads to an irreversible growth arrest within cells.[16] These cells remain metabolically active, but exist in a truncated, vacuolated form and appear to be susceptible to degenerative processes. Senescence is thought to mediate many disease processes associated with aging, such as osteoarthritis and Alzheimer, though the mechanisms are unclear.[9,14] Regardless, senescent cells are observed to accumulate in clusters within a herniated IVD and thought to compromise both the detection of cellular damage and impair local repair mechanisms.[17,18] In some studies, senescent cells are found in 10 × higher numbers within herniated discs than in those normal discs sampled at autopsy.[18] More research is needed to elucidate the mechanisms by which these senescent cells contribute to local tissue breakdown, though a general consensus exists that these cells contribute to the pathophysiologic processes in IVD degeneration.

Lastly, genetic predisposition and lifestyle factors also play a significant role in the progression of IVD degradation. Tissue integrity of the extracellular matrix can be compromised in certain individuals leading to a lower threshold for anulus tears, vertebral end plate sclerosis, and other features associated with IVD degeneration.[7] In a study of monozygotic and dizygotic female twins from the United Kingdom, Modic changes (MCs) were observed in a higher frequency in the monozygotic group compared to the dizygotic group, suggesting a heritable component to end plate degeneration.[19] In a large sample of the Southern Chinese population, magnetic resonance imaging (MRI) changes of lumbar disc were found to have a high variability based on level, but certain single nucleotide polymorphisms were inherited in conserved patterns and were associated with differences in upper versus lower lumbar degeneration.[20] Research in this area is actively ongoing and the search for specific genes predisposing to IVD degeneration may lead to a better understanding of its mechanisms and more targeted therapies.[7,21]

In short, IVD degeneration and herniation are coupled through pathophysiologic cascades of biomechanical stress alterations, local cellular catabolic overload, impaired regeneration, genetic predisposition, and lifestyle factors. While many more processes are likely at play, the simple idea of a progressive feedback loop of the aforementioned factors illustrates the multifaceted nature of degenerative disc disease.

6.3 Nomenclature of the Herniated Nucleus Pulposus

While degeneration can include a variety of nonspecific findings such as disc desiccation, fissuring, and IVD sclerosis, disc protrusion and herniation carry with them specific defining criteria. Broadly speaking, a disc herniation is considered to be a focal displacement of disc material beyond the typical confines of the IVD space; the disc material itself may be heterogeneously composed of AF, nucleus, apophyseal bone or osteophyte.[22] The term "disc bulge" is meant to convey overextension of disc material, generally with an intact AF, beyond the aforementioned apophyseal ring boundaries. This is distinct from a disc herniation, which can only occur once the outer AF is compromised. Herniations are

considered "protrusions" if the measurement of the outward projection of the disc material is less than that of the herniation base's edges and the herniated disc material remains continuous with the NP.[23,24] "Extrusions" present if the aberrant disc material has no inner continuity with the root disc or if the measurement of the outward projection of the aberrant disc material exceeds that of its base.[22] If the disc material has displaced and shares no continuity with its parent disc, then we consider that fragment "sequestered."[22]

6.4 Clinical Presentation of Lumbar Degenerative Disc Disease and HNP

With advanced stages of degeneration leading to abnormal biomechanical forces, inflammatory cascades, and IVD pathology as previously summarized, hypertrophy of posterior soft tissue structures, such as facet joint capsule and ligamentum flavum, as well as osseous narrowing of the canal and foramina can lead to irritation or compression of the neural elements.[7,9,25] This extrinsic pressure can induce an inflammatory response leading to edema of the affected nerve root, fibrosis, release of chemical modulators, and local hyperexcitability, ultimately thought to cause radiculopathy and pain.[26,27]

The constellation of physical exam and imaging findings that present in the setting of degenerative lumbar disease can be variable and dependent on a variety of factors, including genetic, environmental, and behavioral influences. While no formal definition exists regarding lumbar degenerative disc disease, it is generally agreed upon that advanced imaging findings consistent with IVD degeneration can be associated with lumbar back pain, though the relationship is poorly understood.[28,29] In a case-controlled study evaluating adults with and without lower back pain, Teichtahl et al. reported that high fat content in the lumbar paraspinal muscles is closely associated with signs of IVD degeneration at each respective level.[29] Imaging findings were graded using Pfirrmann grading system (▶ Fig. 6.1), which aims to grade the IVD structure, homogeneity, height, signal intensity, and level distinction between anulus and nucleus on a scale of 1 to 5, with higher scores indicative of more advanced degrees of degeneration.[30] Hicks et al. reported that IVD degeneration was most commonly found in the lower lumbar segments with a slight decrease at L5–S1, given

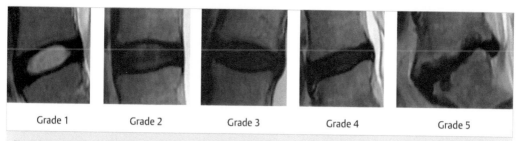

| Grade 1 | Grade 2 | Grade 3 | Grade 4 | Grade 5 |

Fig. 6.1 Stages of the Pfirrmann grading system with sequential loss of disc hydration as seen on T2-weighted imaging with eventual disc collapse and compromise.

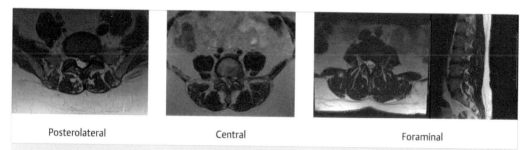

| Posterolateral | Central | Foraminal |

Fig. 6.2 Axial MRI images demonstrating the varying locations for disc herniations. Symptoms and treatment strategies are dependent upon the location of the herniated segment.

that the change in lordosis at that level substitutes shear force for compressive force which may change the degenerative characteristics at that level.[31] Furthermore, they noted that > 95% of their study population showed signs of IVD degeneration, though severe findings were associated with a two-fold greater risk of chronic lower back pain.[31] It is important to note that while this relationship exists, degenerative changes can be seen without associated symptomatology in up to 30% of cases.[3]

With regard to the herniated disc causing an abnormal extrinsic pressure on a lumbosacral nerve root, the primary signs and symptoms involve radiculopathy, weakness, pain, and sensory changes. Symptoms will vary depending on the size of the disc fragment, its location, and acuity of development. Herniations can be classified based on location within the spinal canal including, posterolateral or paracentral, central, and foraminal or far lateral (▶ Fig. 6.2). Posterolateral or paracentral herniations are the most common variant that occur along the lateral border of the posterior longitudinal ligament and compress the traversing nerve root of a given level. Central herniations can be asymptomatic, especially if the volume of herniated material is small, or, in case of very large discs, can cause claudication or rarely cauda

equine syndrome. Foraminal disc herniations will typically cause compressive symptoms of the exiting nerve root at the level in question.

Both back pain and radicular pain are often positional. Discogenic back pain is typically worse with sitting upright without any rear support or with forward flexion; these activities increase intradiskal pressure up to an estimated 1,000 N.[32] Peterson et al. performed a systematic review focused on diagnostic criteria for various etiologies of lower back pain and recommend screening for presence of a motor weakness, abnormal reflexes, and dermatomal pain with an associated sensory deficit.[33] Having three out of these four findings, commonly referred to as the Hancock rules, coupled with presence of a positive crossed straight leg raise (SLR), is associated with favorable positive likelihood ratios of the patient having a herniated disc with specificities ranging from 0.83 to 0.94 depending on level involved.[33,34]

Central compression concentrated at the termination of the spinal cord or distally along the cauda equina may bring a constellation of emergent findings of varying acuity, most notably conus medullaris syndrome or cauda equina syndrome (CES). These syndromes must be managed expeditiously in order to limit neurologic compromise.

While variable or partial presentations can occur, a large central herniation at L1–L2 will cause conus medullaris syndrome, which is typically characterized as lower extremity weakness, variable hyperreflexia, symmetric saddle paresthesias, and early bowel/bladder incontinence.[35] Central compression distal to L2 may elicit a CES, with common presentations involving severe radicular pain, saddle/perineal anesthesia, urinary/fecal incontinence, and areflexic paraplegia.[36]

6.5 Imaging

First-line imaging for lower back pain with or without associated radicular symptoms typically begins with orthogonal plain radiographs. Dynamic flexion and extension views should be obtained to investigate presence of instability. In the absence of significant osseous abnormality, absence of red flag signs or symptoms, including neurologic compromise, and absence of symptoms of infection or tumor, a course of nonoperative treatment is usually recommended prior to obtaining further imaging. If these initial treatment modalities fail, advanced imaging, ideally in the form of an MRI, should be obtained to evaluate the soft tissues and neural elements of the spine.

Disc degeneration will typically manifest as progressive loss of T2-weighted signal intensity within the NP, loss of a distinct contrast between the NP and AF, and eventual loss of disc height. Herniated disc material typically appears with intermediate signal intensity on T1 W and high signal intensity on T2 W imaging, though more chronic herniations appear to have low–intermediate T2 W signal. Care should be taken to evaluate the prevertebral soft tissue structures and the aorta with T1 W MRI for pathology which may present with lumbar spine type symptoms. A linear area of high T2 W signal along the posterior AF, known as a high-intensity zone (HIZ), can be associated with disc degeneration. The signal is distinctly brighter than that of the associated NP.[37] Though an HIZ was initially thought to indicate a radial tear in the posterior anulus, conflicting studies have made its interpretation controversial and it is not thought to be a specific sign for disc pathology.[38,39,40]

High signal intensity on T1- or T2-weighted images may also be appreciated in the CEP and vertebral bone marrow. These findings were classified by Modic et al based on their relative signal strengths on T1 W and T2 W imaging.[41] So-called MCs are classified into three categories: MC type 1

appear hypointense on T1 W and hyperintense on T2 W, MC type 2 are hyperintense on T1 W and may appear either isointense or hypointense on T2 W, and MC type 3 are hypointense on both T1 W and T2 W imaging.[41] These changes may be indicative of chronic inflammatory changes within the affected disc and adjacent CEP with bone marrow changes suggestive of inflammatory factor outflow; however, the correlation with clinical presentation is tenuous.[42,43]

6.6 Treatment of DDD

In the absence of red flag findings, initial treatments of degenerative disease in the lumbar spine are typically nonoperative and multimodal in nature. Patient education regarding basic spinal mechanics, anatomy, proper posture, and accessible ways of minimizing discomfort are first-line and have been shown in recent systematic reviews to be effective in achieving short-term improvement in symptoms.[44] Activity modification and rest can be helpful in the acute setting; however, the clinician should encourage the patient to avoid prolonged bedrest as deconditioning can exacerbate symptoms.[45] Core strengthening, trunk stabilization exercises, and physical therapy have also become mainstays of nonoperative treatment. While these modalities have not been convincingly shown to be helpful in reducing pain compared to no treatment in patients with acute back pain, those patients with chronic pain may indeed benefit.[46,47] Furthermore, the benefits of exercise in improving mood and overall health cannot be overstated.

The most readily available treatment for lower back pain remains pharmacological with the most common medications being NSAIDs, antidepressants, and opioids.[48] A meta-analysis of existing Cochrane reviews regarding the efficacy of opioids for chronic degenerative lower back pain concluded that compared to placebo opioids do indeed help decrease pain in the acute setting, though this clinical improvement is significantly marred by a large side-effect profile and risk of addiction; opioids are therefore not recommended in the management of degenerative lumbar disease.[48,49] Furthermore this benefit can also be seemingly achieved by prescribing NSAIDs, though these medications also have a non-negligible side-effect profile that should not be overlooked.[48] Antidepressants are also a common treatment; however, these have not been shown to be superior to placebo.[48]

Surgical management is generally considered for patients who experience no clinical improvement in 6 months despite active, conservative treatment. Lumbar interbody fusion can take many forms depending on the desired surgical approach (anterior, posterior, transforaminal, lateral lumbar); however, the goal remains to induce a union of adjacent vertebral bodies across the degenerated segment via instrumentation and/or bone graft. A recent meta-analysis focused on comparing the various interbody fusion techniques found that fusion rates were statistically similar among the approaches though anterior lumbar interbody fusion allowed for better ability to restore lumbar lordosis of the desired segment as well as achieve the greatest postoperative restoration of disc height.[50] They additionally noted a statistically greater blood loss in posterior approaches; however, they caution that anterior approaches risk major vascular injury, which would dramatically alter intraoperative blood loss and operative time, were it to occur.[50] Cage migration is also a concern and appeared to occur with the greatest frequency in patients treated with anterior fusion.[50]

With regard to concerns with fusion, such as pseudoarthrosis, hardware failure, and adjacent segment disease, total lumbar disc replacement (TDR) represents an alternative surgical strategy aimed at restoring disc height and physiologic load across the degenerative segment while theoretically not sacrificing additional motion segments. Originally implanted in the 1950s in the form of a steel sphere designed to mimic the NP, TDR has undergone many iterations and currently can be implanted in constrained or unconstrained designs, each with varying benefits and drawbacks.[51] In a meta-analysis of randomized controlled trials investigating the clinical efficacy of TDR versus lumbar fusion at 5-year follow-up, Zigler et al. report statistically and clinically significant improvements in the Oswestry Disability Index in 68 to 79% of patients and in satisfaction in 70 to 79% of patients that underwent TDR for degenerative disease.[52] This compared to significant improvement in ODI in 64 to 76% of patients and in satisfaction in 63 to 72% of patient who underwent fusion surgery. Improvement in pain scores was found to be clinically significant in both treatment groups, though TDR offered a lower risk of reoperation.[52] A meta-analysis by Mu et al. also reports an increased safety profile in TDR compared with anterior lumbar interbody fusion, though the authors cautiously note that heterogeneity in artificial disc

implants and lack of blinding may have been sources of bias.[53]

Regardless of the approach chosen, surgical intervention involves increased risks, costs, and rehabilitation times compared to nonoperative treatment. Patients must be carefully selected, including a thorough psychosocial evaluation, and counseled to increase chances of a successful clinical outcome.

6.7 Treatments of Lumbar HNP

In the absence of red flags such as CES, functional neurological deficits or intractable pain, treatment for HNP first starts with a conservative approach of rest, activity modification, nonsteroidal anti-inflammatory medication, and physical therapy. Epidural steroid injections are also typically considered, though treatment success is historically variable and can be practitioner dependent.[23] Size of the disc may also determine efficacy of injections with larger discs favoring surgical intervention; Kim et al. reported that transforaminal injections showed substantial clinical improvement in patients with disc herniations of 6.2 mm and smaller.[54]

For those patients whose radiculopathy persists for at least 6 to 8 weeks, operative intervention is generally considered, and depending on the patient's body habitus, disc level, and fragment location, minimally invasive surgery (MIS) may be an option. There are several described endoscopic approaches including transforaminal, interlaminar, posterolateral, and transiliac.[23,55,56] While discussion of these approaches in detail is beyond the scope of this chapter, a recent systematic review and pooled meta-analysis of available literature comparing endoscopic outcomes with that of traditional open approaches found shorter hospital stays and reduced blood loss in the endoscopic cohort but did not detect any statistically significant clinical improvements favoring the endoscopic group nor any decrease in rates of complications.[56]

In a large, multicenter, prospective observational study known as the Spine Patient Outcomes Research Trial (SPORT), outcomes of 503 open discectomy patients were compared with those of 216 patients treated nonoperatively and found that for patients with at least 6 weeks of persistent radiculopathy surgical intervention showed statistically significant clinical improvements in their Medical Outcomes Study Short-Form Health Survey (SF-36) and their Oswestry Disability Index (ODI) in as early as 3 months post-intervention compared with those of the nonoperative group.[57,58,59] Although the nonoperative group did show persistent improvement during the study's time course and difference in outcome magnitude lessened between 3 months and 2 years postintervention, those patients who underwent surgical intervention enjoyed statistically significant improvement throughout the study's timeline.[57] These findings were similarly found in the randomized component of the SPORT trial, though the authors mention that nonadherence was a major limitation in interpreting the results of that treatment arm.[60]

Pearls

- Many herniated discs are asymptomatic and the differential diagnosis for radiculopathy is broad. Must carefully correlate clinical presentation and imaging findings.
- Most patients with symptomatic herniated discs without neurologic compromise will have resolution of symptoms within 6 to 12 weeks.
- Absolute indications for surgery are rare but include cauda equina syndrome, acute disabling motor deficit, progressive neurologic compromise, and disabling intractable pain not responding to other treatment modalities.
- Most patient should have at least a 4 to 8 week trial of nonoperative care. Duration of nonoperative treatment depends on patient preference, severity of symptoms, and/or presence or absence of neurologic deficit.
- A limited discectomy, removing only free/extruded fragment of disc material is the current standard of care. Care should be taken to preserve bony and soft tissue elements to the extent possible without compromising decompression of neural elements, to avoid iatrogenic instability.
- There is an approximate 15% symptomatic disc herniation recurrence rate after discectomy surgery. Fusion of the involved motion segment should be considered after multiple recurrences at the same level.

6.8 Case Examples

6.8.1 Case 1

A 56-year-old, otherwise healthy, female presented with a 3-week history of back pain radiating down her right leg. She described numbness in an S1 distribution and had 4+/5 plantar flexion strength on the right side. Imaging (below) revealed a large right-sided L5–S1 posterolateral disc herniation. She had already been prescribed an oral steroid taper and physical therapy, both of which provided only mild relief. Treatment options were discussed and the patient elected to have an L5–S1 transforaminal epidural injection. The injection provided 5 days of pain relief followed by the pain returning. At follow-up 7 weeks after initial onset of symptoms, the patient remained debilitated due to her symptoms and elected to undergo a microdiscectomy. Tubular microdiscectomy was undertaken without complication (see video on L5-S1 Tubular Microdisc). The patient had complete resolution of leg pain immediately postop. Plantar flexion strength returned to normal by 2-week follow-up. Numbness resolved slowly over the following 2 to 3 months. MRI obtained 3 months postop demonstrates successful resection of herniated fragment as preservation of disc height as compared to preop MRI.

Preop MRI:

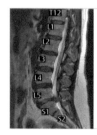 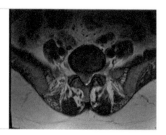

Postop MRI:

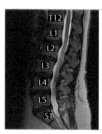 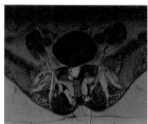

6.8.2 Case 2

A 45-year-old female presented with a 3-month history of back pain radiating down the right leg in an L5 and S1 distribution. She reported undergoing L5–S1 discectomy 5 years earlier with excellent relief of symptoms. Motor and sensory exam were normal. She had not responded to physical therapy or medications including NSAIDs, oral steroids, or gabapentin. Imaging revealed asymmetric disc collapse, right-sided foraminal stenosis, and recurrent disc herniation at L5–S1. The patient elected to undergo a trial of epidural injections. After these failed to provide relief, surgical options were discussed. Given the recurrence of herniation, as well as the significant foraminal stenosis, Anterior lumbar interbody fusion (ALIF) was recommended to resect the herniated disc and provide indirect decompression of the neural foramen. Surgery was successfully carried out with a stand-alone ALIF device with integrated fixation. The patient experienced complete relief of radicular symptoms and a 80% reduction in low back pain. Plain X-rays 1 year postop demonstrate restoration of disc height with bone growth across the disc space indicating successful fusion.

1 year postop:

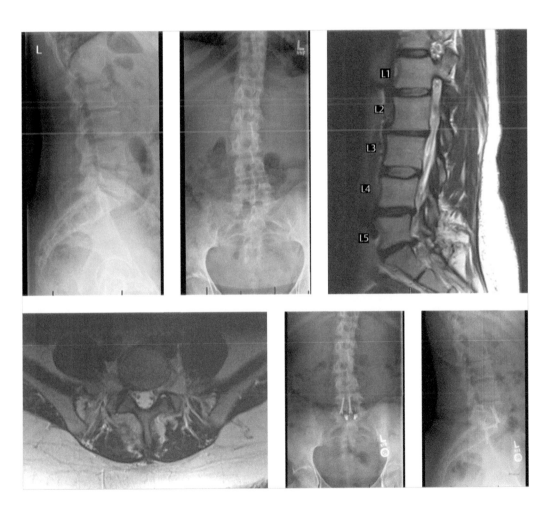

6.9 Board-style Questions

1. A 33-year-old man arrives to the ED complaining of a 24-hour history of severe lower back pain with radiation to his legs after he began a new weightlifting routine. He reports saddle anesthesia and some difficulty with urinating. MRI shows a large central disc herniation at L5–S1. What is the next best step?
   a) Recommend rest, NSAIDs, and a steroid taper
   b) Epidural steroid injection
   c) Determine NPO status and discuss need for surgical intervention today
   d) Recommend PT

2. What is the estimated financial impact of work lost due to lower back pain?
   a) < $5 billion
   b) $5–10 billion
   c) $10–20 billion
   d) $20–50 billion
   e) $50–100 billion

3. For a large foraminal disc herniation at L4–L5, what nerve root would be typically affected and what would be the associated sensory finding?
   a) Traversing, L4, anterolateral leg numbness
   b) Traversing, L5, anterolateral leg numbness
   c) Exiting, L4, anteromedial leg numbness
   d) Exiting, L5, anteromedial leg numbness
   e) Both exiting and traversing roots, mixed anteromedial/anterolateral leg numbness

4. A 60-year-old woman complains of bilateral leg pain that has persisted for 7 months and has failed to improve with rest, physical therapy, or epidural steroid injections. Pain is worsened by ambulation and improved with leaning forward or resting. Physical exam reveals no evidence of neuromotor compromise. MRI reveals no focal disc herniations but multiple areas of disc bulges and a hypertrophied ligamentum flavum at L4–L5. There is no radiographic evidence of instability. What treatment would likely provide the most effective pain relief?
   a) Oral gabapentin
   b) Continued physical therapy with focus on core strengthening
   c) Posterior lumbar decompression at L4–L5
   d) Posterior lumbar decompression and arthrodesis at L4–L5
   e) Bilateral transforaminal epidural steroid injection at L4–L5

5. An MRI is performed on a 40-year-old patient referred to you for management of severe lower back pain that has been present for roughly 12 months and has not been associated with any radiculopathy. Nonoperative care including physical therapy, oral NSAIDs, muscle relaxants, and epidural steroid injections has provided minimal relief. Pain continues to affect her activities of daily living. MRI shows high signal along the L5 and S1 vertebral bodies and end plates on T2 W imaging. There is no history of fevers/chills/malaise. What is the most appropriate treatment?
   a) Continue nonoperative care and add extended-release narcotics
   b) Referral to interventional pain management
   c) Posterior lumbar arthrodesis at L5–S1
   d) Referral for repeat epidural steroid injection

Answers

1. c
2. e
3. c
4. c
5. c

References

[1] Hurwitz EL, Randhawa K, Yu H, Côté P, Haldeman S. The global spine care initiative: a summary of the global burden of low back and neck pain studies. Eur Spine J. 2018; 27 Suppl 6:796–801

[2] Luo X, Pietrobon R, Sun SX, Liu GG, Hey L. Estimates and patterns of direct health care expenditures among individuals with back pain in the United States. Spine. 2004; 29(1):79–86

[3] Luoma K, Riihimäki H, Luukkonen R, Raininko R, Viikari-Juntura E, Lamminen A. Low back pain in relation to lumbar disc degeneration. Spine. 2000; 25(4):487–492

[4] Urban JPG, Roberts S. Degeneration of the intervertebral disc. Arthritis Res Ther. 2003; 5(3):120–130

[5] Daly C, Ghosh P, Jenkin G, Oehme D, Goldschlager T. A review of animal models of intervertebral disc degeneration: pathophysiology, regeneration, and translation to the clinic. BioMed Res Int. 2016; 2016:5952165

[6] Moon SM, Yoder JH, Wright AC, Smith LJ, Vresilovic EJ, Elliott DM. Evaluation of intervertebral disc cartilaginous endplate structure using magnetic resonance imaging. Eur Spine J. 2013; 22(8):1820–1828

[7] Vergroesen PP, Kingma I, Emanuel KS, et al. Mechanics and biology in intervertebral disc degeneration: a vicious circle. Osteoarthritis Cartilage. 2015; 23(7):1057–1070

[8] Buckwalter JA. Aging and degeneration of the human intervertebral disc. Spine. 1995; 20(11):1307–1314

[9] Zhao CQ, Wang LM, Jiang LS, Dai LY. The cell biology of intervertebral disc aging and degeneration. Ageing Res Rev. 2007; 6(3):247–261

[10] Roberts S, Caterson B, Menage J, Evans EH, Jaffray DC, Eisenstein SM. Matrix metalloproteinases and aggrecanase: their role in disorders of the human intervertebral disc. Spine. 2000; 25(23):3005–3013

[11] Iatridis JC, Nicoll SB, Michalek AJ, Walter BA, Gupta MS. Role of biomechanics in intervertebral disc degeneration and regenerative therapies: what needs repairing in the disc and what are promising biomaterials for its repair? Spine J. 2013; 13(3):243–262

[12] Sakai D, Grad S. Advancing the cellular and molecular therapy for intervertebral disc disease. Adv Drug Deliv Rev. 2015; 84:159–171

[13] Kepler CK, Ponnappan RK, Tannoury CA, Risbud MV, Anderson DG. The molecular basis of intervertebral disc degeneration. Spine J. 2013; 13(3):318–330

[14] Wang F, Cai F, Shi R, Wang XH, Wu XT. Aging and age related stresses: a senescence mechanism of intervertebral disc degeneration. Osteoarthritis Cartilage. 2016; 24 (3):398–408

[15] Uchiyama Y, Cheng CC, Danielson KG, et al. Expression of acid-sensing ion channel 3 (ASIC3) in nucleus pulposus cells of the intervertebral disc is regulated by p75NTR and ERK signaling. J Bone Miner Res. 2007; 22(12):1996–2006

[16] van Deursen JM. The role of senescent cells in ageing. Nature. 2014; 509(7501):439–446

[17] Feng C, Liu H, Yang M, Zhang Y, Huang B, Zhou Y. Disc cell senescence in intervertebral disc degeneration: causes and molecular pathways. Cell Cycle. 2016; 15(13):1674–1684

[18] Roberts S, Evans EH, Kletsas D, Jaffray DC, Eisenstein SM. Senescence in human intervertebral discs. Eur Spine J. 2006; 15 Suppl 3:S312–S316

[19] Määttä JH, Kraatari M, Wolber L, et al. Vertebral endplate change as a feature of intervertebral disc degeneration: a heritability study. Eur Spine J. 2014; 23(9):1856–1862

[20] Li Y, Samartzis D, Campbell DD, et al. Two subtypes of intervertebral disc degeneration distinguished by large-scale population-based study. Spine J. 2016; 16(9):1079–1089

[21] Battié MC, Videman T. Lumbar disc degeneration: epidemiology and genetics. J Bone Joint Surg Am. 2006; 88 Suppl 2: 3–9

[22] Fardon DF, Williams AL, Dohring EJ, Murtagh FR, Gabriel Rothman SL, Sze GK. Lumbar disc nomenclature: version 2.0: recommendations of the combined task forces of the North American Spine Society, the American Society of Spine Radiology and the American Society of Neuroradiology. Spine J. 2014; 14(11):2525–2545

[23] Amin RM, Andrade NS, Neuman BJ. Lumbar disc herniation. Curr Rev Musculoskelet Med. 2017; 10(4):507–516

[24] Cunha C, Silva AJ, Pereira P, Vaz R, Gonçalves RM, Barbosa MA. The inflammatory response in the regression of lumbar disc herniation. Arthritis Res Ther. 2018; 20(1):251

[25] Rao R. Neck pain, cervical radiculopathy, and cervical myelopathy: pathophysiology, natural history, and clinical evaluation. J Bone Joint Surg Am. 2002; 84(10): 1872–1881

[26] Cooper RG, Freemont AJ, Hoyland JA, et al. Herniated intervertebral disc-associated periradicular fibrosis and vascular abnormalities occur without inflammatory cell infiltration. Spine. 1995; 20(5):591–598

[27] Todd AG. Cervical spine: degenerative conditions. Curr Rev Musculoskelet Med. 2011; 4(4):168–174

[28] Kalichman L, Hunter DJ. The genetics of intervertebral disc degeneration: familial predisposition and heritability estimation. Joint Bone Spine. 2008; 75(4):383–387

[29] Teichtahl AJ, Urquhart DM, Wang Y, et al. Lumbar disc degeneration is associated with modic change and high paraspinal fat content: a 3.0 T magnetic resonance imaging study. BMC Musculoskelet Disord. 2016; 17(1):439

[30] Pfirrmann CW, Metzdorf A, Zanetti M, Hodler J, Boos N. Magnetic resonance classification of lumbar intervertebral disc degeneration. Spine. 2001; 26(17):1873–1878

[31] Hicks GE, Morone N, Weiner DK. Degenerative lumbar disc and facet disease in older adults: prevalence and clinical correlates. Spine. 2009; 34(12):1301–1306

[32] Nachemson AL. Disc pressure measurements. Spine. 1981; 6 (1):93–97

[33] Petersen T, Laslett M, Juhl C. Clinical classification in low back pain: best-evidence diagnostic rules based on systematic reviews. BMC Musculoskelet Disord. 2017; 18(1):188

[34] Hancock MJ, Maher CG, Latimer J, et al. Systematic review of tests to identify the disc, SIJ or facet joint as the source of low back pain. Eur Spine J. 2007; 16(10):1539–1550

[35] Ropper AE, Ropper AH. Acute spinal cord compression. N Engl J Med. 2017; 376(14):1358–1369

[36] Todd NV. Guidelines for cauda equina syndrome. Red flags and white flags. Systematic review and implications for triage. Br J Neurosurg. 2017; 31(3):336–339

[37] Park KW, Song KS, Chung JY, et al. High-intensity zone on L-spine MRI: clinical relevance and association with trauma history. Asian Spine J. 2007; 1(1):38–42

[38] Ricketson R, Simmons JW, Hauser BO. The prolapsed intervertebral disc: the high-intensity zone with discography correlation. Spine. 1996; 21(23):2758–2762

[39] Carragee EJ, Paragioudakis SJ, Khurana S. 2000 Volvo Award winner in clinical studies: lumbar high-intensity zone and discography in subjects without low back problems. Spine. 2000; 25(23):2987–2992

[40] Schellhas KP, Pollei SR, Gundry CR, Heithoff KB. Lumbar disc high-intensity zone: correlation of magnetic resonance imaging and discography. Spine. 1996; 21(1):79–86

[41] Modic MT, Steinberg PM, Ross JS, Masaryk TJ, Carter JR. Degenerative disk disease: assessment of changes in vertebral body marrow with MR imaging. Radiology. 1988; 166(1 Pt 1):193–199

[42] Dudli S, Fields AJ, Samartzis D, Karppinen J, Lotz JC. Pathobiology of Modic changes. Eur Spine J. 2016; 25(11):3723–3734

[43] Zhang Y-H, Zhao C-Q, Jiang L-S, Chen X-D, Dai L-Y. Modic changes: a systematic review of the literature. Eur Spine J. 2008; 17(10):1289–1299

[44] Heymans M, Van Tulder M, Esmail R, Bombardier C, Koes B. Pharmacologic management of chronic low back pain: synthesis of the evidence. Spine. 2005; 30:2153–2163

[45] Waddell G, Feder G, Lewis M. Systematic reviews of bed rest and advice to stay active for acute low back pain. Br J Gen Pract. 1997; 47(423):647–652

[46] Anshel MH, Russell KG. Effect of aerobic and strength training on pain tolerance, pain appraisal and mood of unfit males as a function of pain location. J Sports Sci. 1994; 12 (6):535–547

[47] Chou R, Huffman LH, American Pain Society, American College of Physicians. Nonpharmacologic therapies for acute and chronic low back pain: a review of the evidence for an American Pain Society/American College of Physicians clinical practice guideline. Ann Intern Med. 2007; 147(7):492–504

[48] White AP, Arnold PM, Norvell DC, Ecker E, Fehlings MG. Pharmacologic management of chronic low back pain: synthesis of the evidence. Spine. 2011; 36(21) Suppl: S131–S143

[49] Deyo RA, Smith DH, Johnson ES, et al. Opioids for back pain patients: primary care prescribing patterns and use of services. J Am Board Fam Med. 2011; 24(6):717–727

[50] Teng I, Han J, Phan K, Mobbs R. A meta-analysis comparing ALIF, PLIF, TLIF and LLIF. J Clin Neurosci. 2017; 44: 11–17

[51] Salzmann SN, Plais N, Shue J, Girardi FP. Lumbar disc replacement surgery: successes and obstacles to widespread adoption. Curr Rev Musculoskelet Med. 2017; 10 (2):153–159

[52] Zigler J, Gornet MF, Ferko N, Cameron C, Schranck FW, Patel L. Comparison of lumbar total disc replacement with surgical spinal fusion for the treatment of single-level degenerative disc disease: a meta-analysis of 5-year outcomes from randomized controlled trials. Global Spine J. 2018; 8(4):413–423

[53] Mu X, Wei J, A J, Li Z, Ou Y. The short-term efficacy and safety of artificial total disc replacement for selected patients with lumbar degenerative disc disease compared with anterior lumbar interbody fusion: a systematic review and meta-analysis. PLoS One. 2018; 13(12): e0209660

[54] Kim J, Hur JW, Lee J-B, Park JY. Surgery versus nerve blocks for lumbar disc herniation : quantitative analysis of radiological factors as a predictor for successful outcomes. J Korean Neurosurg Soc. 2016; 59(5):478–484

[55] Millhouse PW, Schroeder GD, Kurd MF, Kepler CK, Vaccaro AR, Savage JW. Microdiscectomy for a paracentral lumbar herniated disk. Clin Spine Surg. 2016; 29(1):17–20

[56] Phan K, Xu J, Schultz K, et al. Full-endoscopic versus micro-endoscopic and open discectomy: a systematic review and meta-analysis of outcomes and complications. Clin Neurol Neurosurg. 2017; 154:1–12

[57] Weinstein JN, Lurie JD, Tosteson TD, et al. Surgical vs nonoperative treatment for lumbar disk herniation: the Spine Patient Outcomes Research Trial (SPORT) observational cohort. JAMA. 2006; 296(20):2451–2459

[58] McHorney CA, Ware JE, Jr, Lu JF, Sherbourne CD. The MOS 36-item Short-Form Health Survey (SF-36): III. Tests of data quality, scaling assumptions, and reliability across diverse patient groups. Med Care. 1994; 32(1):40–66

[59] Daltroy LH, Cats-Baril WL, Katz JN, Fossel AH, Liang MH. The North American spine society lumbar spine outcome assessment instrument: reliability and validity tests. Spine. 1996; 21(6):741–749

[60] Weinstein JN, Tosteson TD, Lurie JD, et al. Surgical vs nonoperative treatment for lumbar disk herniation: the Spine Patient Outcomes Research Trial (SPORT): a randomized trial. JAMA. 2006; 296(20):2441–2450

7 Lumbar Spinal Stenosis

Patrick K. Cronin and Thomas D. Cha

Abstract

Lumbar spinal stenosis (LSS) is a common condition of the spine. With an increasing segment of the population reaching advanced ages and expecting higher level functionality into later life, effective management of LSS will be a common problem facing spine surgeons. Neurogenic claudication, often present with LSS, is caused by impingement on the neural elements due to a combination of anatomic considerations including the intervertebral disc, hypertrophic facet capsule, ligamentum flavum, impinging osteophytes, and vertebral body instability. While nonoperative treatments can be effective in providing temporary symptom relief, LSS is a progressive disease and definitive treatment generally requires surgical decompression once conservative measures fail. There are multiple options for effective surgical decompression including open and minimally invasive techniques, each with its own risk profile and specific set of indications.

Keywords: lumbar stenosis, neurogenic claudication, laminectomy, minimally invasive decompression

7.1 Introduction

Since 1900, the percentage of Americans over the age of 65 has increased from 4.1 to 14.9%, representing approximately 47.8 million people.[1] By 2040, an estimated 21.7% of Americans will be over the age of 65.[1] This aging demographic is associated with an increased incidence in degenerative orthopaedic conditions. Of those conditions, lumbar spinal stenosis (LSS) is the most common relating to the spine, with up to 75% of elderly individuals displaying moderate-to-severe stenosis on MRI.[2,3] Furthermore, changing expectations toward a higher level of function into the later years has led to an increasing demand for interventions to remedy symptoms and preserve active lifestyles. In fact, LSS is the most common indication for spinal surgery in patients over the age of 65,[4] and the most likely diagnosis for elderly patients undergoing spinal fusion.[5] Although LSS often presents as a degenerative condition, some patients present with symptoms from lifelong narrowing of the spinal canal. These patients have congenital stenosis (CS) and present with symptoms of stenosis at a younger age. CS patients often have a distinct pathophysiology with fewer degenerative changes but present with multilevel involvement.[6,7,8]

Commonly, spinal stenosis is not symptomatic until patients reach late into middle age.[9,10] Across a lifetime there is no difference in the prevalence of symptomatic LSS between men and women,[9] although from age 60 to 69 years, there is a higher prevalence in men (12 vs. 9%), and beyond age 70 (10–12% vs. 12–13%),[11] a higher prevalence in women.[2] Although nonoperative care can alleviate symptoms,[12] there is good evidence that patients with symptomatic spinal stenosis, who are addressed surgically, have higher functional outcomes than those who receive nonoperative treatment.[13,14]

7.2 Pathogenesis

Spinal stenosis refers to narrowing of the spinal canal causing a constellation of clinical symptoms resulting from impingement upon the conus medullaris or descending neural elements. The etiology of this narrowing includes degenerative conditions, traumatic injury, metabolic disorders, infection, and rheumatologic disease. For the purposes of this chapter we will focus on the former and most common etiology, degenerative LSS.[15] The degenerative pathogenesis of stenosis is often related to one or a combination of disc degeneration, facet osteoarthritis and hypertrophy, ligamentum flavum hypertrophy, instability, or scoliosis.

The earliest changes associated with degenerative LSS involve desiccation and flattening of the intervertebral disc spaces.[16] This loss of structural stability stresses the ligamentum flavum and facet joints, which act as posterior stabilizers of the spine. Subsequent compensatory hypertrophy of these posterior elements and the development of osteophytes occur. A combination of impingement via the intervertebral disc anteriorly and posterior/foraminal impingement by the hypertrophic facet capsule, ligamentum flavum, and osteophytes leads to diminished space for the neural elements. Due to compression of the neural elements, the characteristic neurogenic claudication often begins to manifest.[17] In some cases, the hypertrophic facet joints and ligamentum flavum are unable to control motion between segments. In this scenario, dynamic impingement on the neural elements occurs, depending on body positioning.[18] There is also a vascular component to claudication. As mechanical deformation of the neural elements occurs, venous congestion leads to diminished blood flow and ischemia that can impair nerve conduction.[19,20] Additionally, a scoliosis deformity can also develop, as the cross-sectional area of the central canal becomes narrowed due to lateral shift or angulation of vertebral body motion segments.[21] This narrowing, compounded by posterior element hypertrophy, osteophyte formation and/or spinal instability can result in worsened neural element compression.[21]

7.3 Clinical Presentation

LSS has an insidious manifestation, which usually does not present until late in middle-age.[13,15] Initial symptoms include back pain as well as radiculitis with pain and paresthesias radiating from the buttock to the lower extremities. Symptoms can progress to neurogenic claudication with diminished ambulatory endurance. It is important to differentiate neurogenically derived claudication from vascular sources of claudication.[15] Claudication of neurologic origin tends to start proximally and radiate distally.[15] Patients experience relief after sitting, whereas vascular claudication patients will often have relief with rest regardless of position. This differentiation is due to the lumbar kyphosis that occurs when in the seated position, which creates a relative increase in the amount of central cord space. For the same reason, it is frequently more difficult for patients with LSS to ambulate downstairs as opposed to upstairs. Chronic LSS may present with dense numbness, weakness, or a foot drop without a history of antecedent back pain. The symptoms of patients presenting with CS may be somewhat different than the degenerative condition, in that LBP may be prominent with or without claudication symptoms.[6,7,8]

Even with characteristic history, abnormal neurologic exam findings are observed in fewer than 50% of patients with LSS.[22,23,24] The most common finding is exacerbated pain and radicular symptoms with spine extension. Despite this, a full neurologic exam is indicated for all patients who present with a clinical constellation that raises suspicion for LSS. To further differentiate vascular from neurogenic claudication, a motorized treadmill test (MTT) or self-paced walking test (SPWT) can be used as an effective provocative evaluation of stenosis, as studies have also shown pathologic test results to be directly correlated to the dural sac cross-sectional area.[25,26]

7.4 Imaging Findings

Imaging evaluation for patients presenting with LSS includes multiple modalities. Standing plain radiographs of the lumbosacral spine with flexion and extension views are often the initial imaging study of choice. The gold standard for diagnosis of lumbar stenosis is MRI without contrast.[23,24,27] T2-weighted sequences provide high imaging resolution with the ability to contrast neural elements against the hyperintense signal of the cerebral spinal fluid (CSF) centrally or perineural fat in the neural foramen. Structures frequently complicit in spinal stenosis include the intervertebral disc, ligamentum flavum, facet capsule, and osteophytes. The extent to which stenosis can be classified by MRI alone is somewhat limited because of the dynamic nature of this condition.[23] Additionally, there is a high degree of radiographic stenosis that may be asymptomatic.[10,15,22,27] Some researchers have advocated the use of upright MRI scans to evaluate how weightbearing affects stenosis.[23,27] If the patient is unable to tolerate an MRI study, computed tomography (CT) with and without myelography is a second-line modality.[24,28] With contrast, one can evaluate the perineural space in the foramen and throughout the spinal column, in addition to the bony anatomy. CT myelography provides comparatively low-resolution analysis of the neural elements compared to modern MRI, which can allow distinct visualization of structures as discrete as the dorsal root ganglion or similar size structures. While myelography is not a first-line choice, CT itself is frequently helpful in a preoperative setting due to its superior ability to image bone architecture, particularly the bony stenosis in the foramen. Sagittal reconstruction images can assess bony spikes that impinge the nerve roots in the foramen better than MRI. Some surgeons consider a CT alongside standing radiographs with flexion and extension views to be an essential part of the preoperative imaging workup.[29]

The severity of LSS is not easily defined by imaging measurements alone. Generally, in cross-sectional images, mild stenosis represents a compromise of the area in the dural sac by 1/3 of its normal size, moderate represents compromise between 1/3 and 2/3 of normal size, and severe represents compromise of more than 2/3 its normal size.[30] The SPORT cohort was used to determine the reliability of this method, indicating substantial interobserver reliability for central stenosis, moderate reliability for foraminal stenosis, and fair reliability for far lateral recess stenosis.[30] The overall cross-sectional area of the dural sac is another method to measure the severity of LSS on imaging. When area is less than 75 mm^2, the stenosis is considered severe, and when it is less than 100 mm^2, stenosis is deemed moderate.[31] A more nuanced approach to severity was proposed by Lee et al, who evaluated 61 lumbar spine MRIs and graded stenosis 0 to 3 based upon effacement of the neural elements. Grade 0 stenosis has no effacement of CSF; Grade 1 has no CSF anterior to the nerve rootlets; Grade 2, moderate stenosis, leads to some bunching of the nerve rootlets; and Grade 3, severe stenosis, occurs when there is complete effacement of the nerve rootlets.[32,33]

In cases where LSS affects the cord or conus medullaris, relative signal intensity on variable weighted imaging series can provide information on the duration of compression and likelihood of recovery. In general, hyperintensity on T2-weighted imaging may be indicative of the presence of compression and inflammation, but provides less specific information regarding the presence of demyelination and myelopathy.[34,35] Conversely, hypointensity on preoperative T1-weighted images correlates with longer disease duration and poorer outcomes as measured by the Japanese Orthopaedic Association (JOA) scoring system, when compared to patients who display hyperintense T2-weighted lesions.[36]

In 1975, Verbiest recommended defining absolute measurement of less than 10 mm in sagittal canal diameter.[37] The first modern classification system of LSS categorized stenosis into degenerative/acquired stenosis or CS. While this definition subdivided narrowing of the spinal canal into dysplastic or nondisplastic etiologies, no threshold value of narrowing had been adopted at the time.[38] Today, a common way of classifying stenosis is according to the location of the compression, which can occur centrally or laterally.[39] Central stenosis is stenosis that narrows the central canal compressing the dural sac, which can cause neurogenic claudication. In lateral recess stenosis, also termed subarticular stenosis, the traversing nerve root is impinged under the superior articular facet to the

medial aspect of the pedicle. Foraminal stenosis occurs from the medial aspect of the pedicle to the lateral aspect of the pedicle, and extraforaminal zone stenosis is self-explanatory. For example, L4–L5 lateral recess stenosis could cause radiculopathy compressing the L5 traversing nerve root, while foraminal stenosis impinges the L4 exiting root.

7.5 Treatment

While conservative treatment remains the standard of care in the initial management of patients with LSS, the data is conflicting regarding the long-term benefit of nonoperative management. Some medication options for symptomatic control are commonly used including: nonsteroidal anti-inflammatory drugs (NSAIDs), acetaminophen, gabapentin, calcitonin, and prostaglandins. These modalities in combination with physical therapy can be successful in the short term for symptom alleviation, but recurrence and secondary need for surgical management is common.[40] A lumbosacral corset may aid ambulatory endurance at the time of use, but it is impractical for long-term use given the incidence of skin breakdown and inconvenience.[41] Approximately 45% of patients who undergo attempted nonoperative management also undergo at least one epidural or foraminal steroid injection; the data behind these interventions is of fairly low quality.[42,43,44]

Care should be taken to rule out vascular claudication, hip arthritis, or upper motor neuron dysfunction due to cervical-associated myelopathy. Once LSS is clarified by physical exam and radiographic evaluation, patients should undergo at least 6 to 12 weeks of nonsurgical treatment before any operative intervention is initiated. Common nonsurgical treatment options include physical therapy (44%), use of NSAIDs (49%), analgesics, and anti-inflammatory steroid injection (45%).[42,44,45]

When symptoms persist following a trial of conservative treatments, surgical decompression of LSS is an effective means of altering the natural history of stenosis. The absolute and urgent indications are cauda equina syndrome or progressive motor weakness.

Direct decompression through removal of the offending bone or soft tissue remains a common effective method of reducing encroachment on the involved neural elements. The key to an adequate decompression while preserving the stability of the motion segment is by undercutting the facet joint and preserving the pars interarticularis. The most frequent approach utilizes a direct posterior incision with dissection through a subperiosteal or para-midline plane.[46] While first described in the 7th century by Paulus of Aegina, the midline posterior approach remains the most common method utilizing meticulous subperiosteal dissection of all muscle and tissue from the spinous process down to the lamina then extending laterally to the pars interarticularis and facet joints.[47,48] If a multilevel decompression is necessary, care must be taken to preserve the pars interarticularis in the upper lumbar spine, because the pars are more medial. Therefore, the lateral borders of the laminectomy need to get narrower cephalad and less lateral at the pars. A laminoplasty is another option for stability-preservation, where a unilateral approach is utilized to perform a central and/or bilateral decompression.[49,50,51] These procedures allow for the maintenance of the posterior bony arch and stability. A fenestration technique can also be applied in which a laminotomy and lateral recess decompression is performed at places or nerve root compression, preserving midline structures.[52,53]

For anatomic reasons, foraminal stenosis can be difficult to address. The constraint of the pedicles and the dural sac restricts movement and increases technical difficulty. Foraminal decompression requires more facet removal; thus, every effort should be made to preserve the facet joint as much as possible by undercutting and using special instruments, such as a curved foraminotomy rongeur or rasp. Decompression of the length of the nerve root from canal to extraforaminal zone frequently requires removal of the facet joint and thereby destabilization of the posterior elements.[54] In some cases, a combined central and paramedical approach can be used to perform foraminotomy to preserve the facet joint. New techniques that use a minimally invasive approach or tubular retractor coupled with microendoscopic visualization utilizing the removal of the inferior pedicle have been shown to be potential sources for a non-destabilizing decompression.[54] Similarly, microsurgical techniques have successfully been used to safely decompress compression in the setting of intraspinal juxta facet joint cyst.[55,56] If the nerve root remains tight after laminectomy and facet undercutting, there may be additional sites causing nerve compression. These compression sites include the superior facet against the posterior vertebral body, the superior facet against the pedicle, the superior facet or pedicle against a bulging lateral anulus, the inferior facet and vertebral body (if instability is present), or the transverse processes of L5 and the sacral ala ("far-out syndrome").

Minimally invasive approaches focus attention on muscle-splitting approaches that preserve innervation. These have been shown to preserve as much as 28% more functional muscle when compared with a direct midline posterior approach.[57] The muscle-preserving benefit of minimally invasive surgery was quantified by postoperative measurement of muscle necrosis and inflammatory markers by Kim et al.[58] Minimally invasive approaches can be especially effective in unilateral radicular symptoms where an approach on the ipsilateral side may allow undercutting of the facet joints. This procedure may be employed to achieve decompression in far lateral, foraminal, and central stenosis.[59,60] Complex patients or those with prior surgery at the involved level should be approached with caution when utilizing a minimally invasive technique.[60] Revision cases are especially susceptible to complications such as durotomy or nerve root injury secondary to surgical adhesions and absence of normal anatomic localizing markers.[59] While the paramedian, muscle-splitting approach is among the most common minimally invasive approach, Hatta et al recently demonstrated that a midline muscle-sparing approach, utilizing judicious spinous process resection with a burr, can allow safe access to the interlaminar space.[61]

Interspinous process devices (IPDs) were developed as a minimally invasive method for treating poor surgical candidates with LSS, especially in the setting of instability (low-grade "stable" spondylolisthesis). These devices capitalize on the increased canal diameter that is produced by the kyphosis that occurs during forward flexion.[62,63] Distraction of the spinous processes leads to an increased space available for the neural elements and coincident symptom relief. Some IPDs such as Coflex allow direct decompression of the nerve roots as well as interlaminar or interspinous dynamic stabilization. Careful patient selection is important for the success of outcome. A biomechanical study evaluating proof of concept showed that on review of postinstrumentation radiographs the space available centrally was minimally changed; however, the foramen height and width were significantly increased.[64] While this project indicated these devices seem to have endurance with regard to cyclic loading and proof of concept for foramina stenosis, the overall indication for IPD is still being refined.

In the setting of revision surgery, careful preoperative planning is necessary to assess the thecal sac. During the approach, the surgeon should leave some, but not an excessive amount of midline scar tissue for protection. Careful dissection between the previous laminectomy edges and scar and meticulous mobilization of the scar tissue before using the Kerrison rongeur can help prevent a durotomy. The mobilization of scar tissue should begin at the pars region first, then at the level of the facet joint, as the scar tissue is often more adherent at the facet joint. To mobilize the nerve at the lateral recess, expose the nerve roots at the pedicle and into the foramen first.

7.6 Expected Outcomes

Direct open decompression has been established to be effective for treatment of LSS in several retrospective and prospective trials. Malmivaara et al prospectively evaluated direct surgical decompression compared with nonoperative usual care including physiotherapy and nonsteroidal anti-inflammatory medications among 94 patients with spinal stenosis, and found improvement in both groups with a larger improvement in Oswestry Disability Index (ODI) at 1 year in the surgical group and a slight loss in gains at 2-year follow-up.[14] A long-term prospective observational cohort study reflected these findings and found that outcomes early on (at 1- and 4-year follow-up) favored initial surgical treatment. At 8- to 10-year follow-up, patients reported similar improvement in pain, relief of primary presenting symptom, and treatment satisfaction. However, there was a greater functional status benefit that persisted in patients who initially received surgical treatment.[11] Herkowitz and Kurz evaluated outcomes of the setting of spinal stenosis in 50 patients with concomitant spondylolisthesis and found that approximately one-third of patients experienced subjective improvement in back pain and 55% described improved radicular leg at 3-year follow-up with significantly better results in patients in whom arthrodesis was performed.[65] Among 76 patients with LSS and spondylolisthesis, Fischgrund et al found similar results with regard to subjectively reported pain relief and physical function among patients who underwent decompression with instrumented and noninstrumented fusion. In a recent *New England Journal of Medicine* article, Ghogawala et al evaluated laminectomy versus laminectomy with arthrodesis in patients with grade 1 spondylolisthesis and found meaningful improvement in overall physical health-related quality of life and lower reoperation rates than laminectomy alone at the expense of increased blood loss and longer hospitalization rates.[66]

The largest prospective study, the Spine Outcomes Research Trial (SPORT) has solidly established open direct decompression to be an effective treatment method with superior outcomes to nonoperative usual care in both the short- and mid-term follow-up, with results currently established out to 4 years.[13] The SPORT trials additionally showed a relatively low complication profile with a reoperation rate of 8% at 2 years and 13% at 4 years.[13] Perioperative mortality from open decompression was approximately 0.2%,[13] which is similar to other previously reported rates.[67]

Both patients with congenital and degenerative stenosis respond well to decompression-alone, without a supplemental fusion, despite differences in pain experience and presentation.[6] The degenerative patients were more susceptible to require another operation resulting in a fusion, which supports the theory that micro-instability can progress in degenerative stenosis, but is likely not part of the disease process in CS.[6] Laminoplasty in the setting of LSS has shown promising results, similar to that in the cervical spine.[49,50,51] Fenestration has similarly shown excellent results for LSS patients with operation rates of 0.8% at 1 year, 2.9% at 5 years, 5.2% at 10 years, 7.5% at 15 years, and 8.6% at > 17.7 years.[52]

The burgeoning field of minimally invasive surgery (MIS) for lumbar stenosis lacks the high volume level I studies that have been possible for standard direct open decompression. Currently, the literature evaluating MIS depends on patient cohorts that are frequently heterogeneous. Furthermore, while standard open decompressive laminectomy is generally the standard to which minimally invasive techniques are compared, there is gradation in the individual open techniques such as the degree of facetectomy or foraminotomy. A function of the novelty and innovation within the minimally invasive field is an inability to obtain long-term results.

In 1988 Young et al described decompression of both sides of the thecal sac from a unilateral approach.[53] Although this approach was minimally invasive in its preservation of the spinous processes, interspinous ligament, and the lateral two-thirds of the facet joints, it still called for bilateral dissection of paraspinous muscles.[53] Furthermore, the complication profile was substantial with a 28% complication rate overall, including a 9% durotomy incidence.[53] Still, patients responded well and none of the 32 patients required conversion to a standard laminectomy or required fusion.[53] Subsequent attempts at minimally invasive endoscopic decompressions have experienced similarly high rates of durotomy.[68] Despite this, with the advent of managed care and the importance of early functional recovery, patient satisfaction, and enthusiasm for minimized duration of hospitalization, interest for endoscopic spine surgery persisted among orthopaedic surgeons.[68] The addition of the operating microscope and tubular retractor systems in the early 2000s provided tools to speed the safety and development of minimally invasive techniques.[69,70,71]

Early use of tubular retractors for LSS was reported by Palmer et al, who prospectively evaluated 17 consecutive patients who underwent bilateral decompression from a unilateral approach with a tubular retractor system.[72] Patients were assessed with MRI and a VAS pain questionnaire administered preoperatively and again at 4 to 7 months after decompression which showed significant improvements in VAS scores.[72] Although promising, Palmer's data was not randomized and was not compared to a control group. However, it was an important step in establishing the feasibility of bilateral decompression from a unilateral approach in patients. Over a decade later, Mobbs et al performed a prospective, randomized trial comparing unilateral laminectomy for bilateral decompression with standard open laminectomy in 54 consecutively enrolled randomized patients.[73] Both groups experienced a substantial decrease in VAS and ODI scores. However, the minimally invasive group was observed to have significantly better mean improvement in the VAS scores compared to the standard open group. Additionally, the minimally invasive group achieved shorter lengths of postoperative hospitalization (55 vs. 100 hours) and time to mobilization (16 vs. 33 hours), while displaying a 37% lower postoperative opiate requirement. Additionally, the durotomy profile was more than halved from the 9% durotomy rate reported by Young et al[53] to approximately

3%, without an observed difference between the two groups.[73] A retrospective review of 48 patients with mid-term follow-up compared to a historical control showed patients with minimally invasive laminectomy had shorter length of hospitalization (36 vs. 94 hours) and similar functional improvements as measured via ODI and SF-36.[59] These findings were replicated by Yagi et al in a prospective study that compared microendoscopic decompression with open laminectomy at 18-month follow-up.[74] Patients experienced symptomatic relief with over half the average length of hospital stay and nearly half the amount of blood loss for minimally invasive decompression when compared to open laminectomy.[74]

For patients who are at excessive risk for perioperative complication, Chopko recently published a technique to attempt percutaneous remodeling of ligamentum flavum and lamina (PRLL). This method utilizes contrast injected into an involved segment to delineate the dura mater from the lamina and ligamentum flavum and allow percutaneous decompression with fluoroscopic assistance.[75] In his initial publication describing the study, Chopko evaluated 14 patients treated via this method and reported improvements in VAS scores at short-term follow-up. However, subsequent attempts to validate this method revealed unacceptably high failure rates of this procedure.[56,76]

7.7 Complications

The most common complications of a lumbar decompression surgery for LSS include nerve root damage, dural tear, infection, bleeding, and postoperative instability at the operative levels.

A review of 10,329 patients treated surgically for LSS compiled by the Scoliosis Research Society (SRS) revealed that complication rates did not differ based on patient age or whether fusion was performed.[77] Additionally, MIS procedures were associated with fewer complications and new neurological deficits.[77] An added benefit of minimally invasive procedures is the more favorable risk profile associated to BMI.[78] While standard open and minimally invasive procedures generally have similar risk profiles, the increased dependence of minimally invasive surgery does add an increased opportunity for disorientation.[79]

Pearls

- To clinically distinguish vascular from neurogenic claudication, it may be helpful to ask if the patient must sit down to experience relief or if relief will occur while resting standing up. Similarly, patients with vascular claudication will frequently feel relief if they dangle their feet over the edge of the bed to increase blood flow.
- If a patient has a T2-weighted hyperintensity on MRI in the cord, look for concomitant T1-weighted hypointensity, which has been shown to be more correlated with prognostic outcome.
- Facet diastasis on a supine MRI can be an indication, but not definitive, that instability is present; in scenarios when this is observed flexion and extension radiographs may be helpful in the determination of spinal stenosis.
- The key to an adequate decompression while preserving the stability of the motion segment is by undercutting the facet joint and preserving the pars interarticularis. The lateral margin of the laminectomy is the lateral edge of the thecal sac, and the nerve roots in the lateral recess are decompressed by undercutting the facet joints and are only visible with medial retraction. Every decompressed nerve root should be "free and mobile" except in revision cases as the nerve root is free but necessarily mobile due to adhesion. "Free" means that a Woodson can be passed into the foramen, and "mobile" means that the nerve root can be retracted about 1 cm medially without tension at the lateral recess or intervertebral disc region.
- If a multilevel decompression is necessary, care must be taken to preserve the pars interarticularis in the upper lumbar spine, because the pars are more medial. Therefore, the lateral borders of the laminectomy need to get narrower cephalad and less lateral at the pars.
- Foraminal decompression requires more facet removal; thus, every effort should be made to preserve the facet joint as much as possible by undercutting and using special instruments, such as a curved foraminotomy rongeur or rasp.
- If the nerve root does not appear free and mobile following a laminectomy, check the following locations for regions of compression: superior facet against the pedicle or posterior vertebral body, superior facet or pedicle against a bulging lateral anulus, inferior facet and vertebral body (spondylolisthesis), or between the transverse processes of L5 and sacral ala.
- In the setting of revision surgery, careful preoperative planning is necessary to assess the thecal sac. During the approach, the surgeon should leave some, but not an excessive amount of midline scar tissue for protection. Careful dissection between the previous laminectomy edges and scar and meticulous mobilization of the scar tissue before using the Kerrison rongeur can help prevent a durotomy.

7.8 Case Examples

7.8.1 Case 1

A 63-year-old woman presents with a two-year history of pain radiating down her posterior thigh, lateral leg to the dorsum of her foot. She reports difficulty with ambulation or when standing for a long period of time. To relieve her symptoms she must sit down. Multiple epidural steroid injections have provided short lived relief with diminishing improvement. Physical therapy was attempted with insufficient relief. The patient is otherwise healthy with a normal sensory and motor exam (▶ Fig. 7.1, ▶ Fig. 7.2, ▶ Fig. 7.3, ▶ Fig. 7.4).

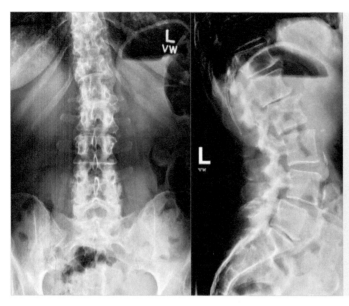

Fig. 7.1 Anteroposterior (AP) and lateral standing radiographs of lumbar spine.

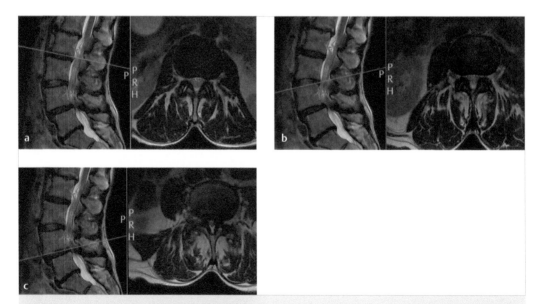

Fig. 7.2 (a–c) Sagittal and axial T2-weighted MRI of the lumbar spine. Lumbar spinal stenosis (LSS) at L2–L3, L3–L4, and L4–L5 with degenerative spondylolisthesis of L4–L5.

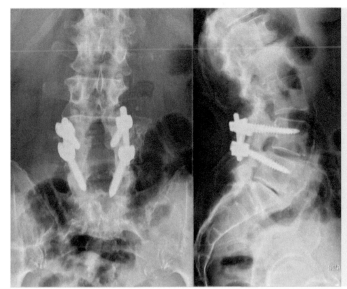

Fig. 7.3 Postoperative anteroposterior (AP) and lateral radiographs following L2–L3, L3–L4, and L4–L5 decompression via open laminectomy with pedicle screw instrumentation and fusion of L4–L5. Postoperatively the patient regained ambulatory endurance and right leg pain resolved.

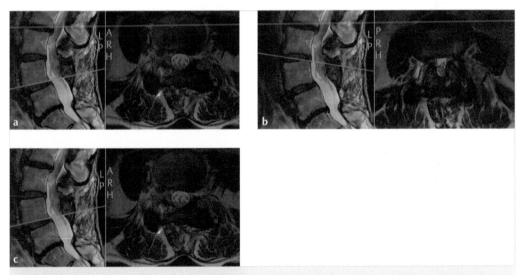

Fig. 7.4 (a–c) Postoperative sagittal and axial MRI following L2–L3, L3–L4, and L4–L5 decompression via open laminectomy with pedicle screw instrumentation and fusion of L4–L5.

7.8.2 Case 2

A 79-year-old male with multiple medical comorbidities and an 18-month history of bilateral buttock pain radiating down the posterior thigh and lower leg. Patient reported pain and heaviness in his legs, which became prevalent with standing and worsened with walking. Steroid injections have provided short-term relief. Physical therapy provided insufficient improvements in symptoms. On examination the patient stands with a forward station. Sensation and motor exam was intact with normal reflexes and without long track signs (▶ Fig. 7.5, ▶ Fig. 7.6, ▶ Fig. 7.7).

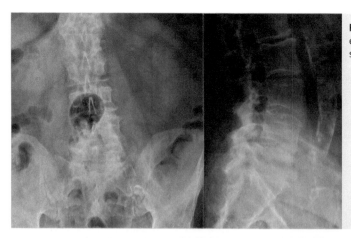

Fig. 7.5 Anteroposterior (AP) and lateral standing radiographs of lumbar spine.

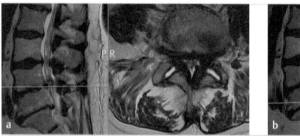
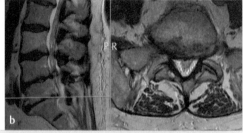

Fig. 7.6 (a, b) Sagittal and axial T2-weighted MRI of the lumbar spine. Lumbar spinal stenosis (LSS) L4–L5 and L5–S1.

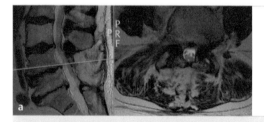
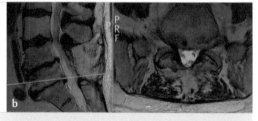

Fig. 7.7 (a, b) Sagittal and axial MRI following L4 and L5 laminectomy. Postoperatively the patient regained ambulatory endurance and forward station improved while claudication symptoms resolved completely.

7.9 Board-style Questions

1. A 75-year-old woman presents with leg pain that is worse with prolonged standing and relieved with sitting. She reports she is only able to walk 50 feet but can walk slightly longer if she leans over a shopping cart or walker. Physical therapy, NSAIDs, and an epidural steroid injection provided temporary relief but her symptoms are returning. Flexion and extension radiographs show no instability. MRI shows complete effacement of the neural rootlets without any visible CSF at the effected level. What is the next step in management?

a) Referral for evaluation by vascular surgery to rule out coincident vascular claudication
b) Continuation of physical therapy
c) Decompressive laminectomy with instrumented fusion
d) Repeat corticosteroid injection
e) Decompressive laminectomy without fusion

2. Which of the following describes a patient who would most benefit from an IPD for treatment of single-level LSS?

a) A 70-year-old male with single-level LSS who has significant cardiac comorbidities and who must sit down after 100 ft of walking to experience relief from his symptoms

b) A 65-year-old female with symptomatic single-level LSS who recently sustained a ground-level fall with resultant distal radius fracture

c) A 69 year-old male with multiple medical comorbidities who has spondylolisthesis with concomitant spinal stenosis

d) A 75-year-old female who is otherwise healthy with severe two-level spinal stenosis that is not relieved with forward flexion

3. A 68-year-old male with severe bilateral buttock and leg claudication which has not improved with physical therapy or several corticosteroid injections. Patient has normal ABIs. MRI shows severe two-level central LSS. You discuss the option of going forward with a surgical decompression. What is the most notable prognostic factor for clinical outcome?

a) History of depression

b) Active tobacco use

c) Multilevel stenosis

d) Medical comorbidities

4. Select option(s) that are known outcomes of minimally invasive surgery.

a) Diminished denervation of the paraspinal musculature

b) Less blood loss

c) Lower durotomy rate

d) Shorter hospital stay

5. Which minimally invasive implants have been shown to be motion preserving, while adequately stabilizing the spinal segment?

a) Segmental pedicular stabilization

b) X-STOP Interspinous Process Devices (X-STOP)

c) Segmental pars screw stabilization

d) Interlaminar stabilizing system (Coflex)

Answers

1. e
2. a
3. d
4. a, b, d
5. d

References

[1] Administration on Aging. A Profile of Older Americans: 2015. US Department of Health and Human Services; 2015

[2] Ishimoto Y, Yoshimura N, Muraki S, et al. Prevalence of symptomatic lumbar spinal stenosis and its association with physical performance in a population-based cohort in Japan: The Wakayama Spine Study. Osteoarthr Cartil. 2012. doi:10.1016/j.joca.2012.06.018

[3] Sasaki K. Magnetic resonance imaging findings of the lumbar root pathway in patients over 50 years old. Eur Spine J. 1995; 4(2):71–76

[4] Jansson KÅ, Blomqvist P, Granath F, Németh G. Spinal stenosis surgery in Sweden 1987–1999. Eur Spine J. 2003; 12(5): 535–541

[5] Deyo RA, Gray DT, Kreuter W, Mirza S, Martin BI. United States trends in lumbar fusion surgery for degenerative conditions. Spine(Phila Pa 1976). 2005; 30(12):1441–1445, discussion 1446–1447

[6] Louie PK, Paul JC, Markowitz J, et al. Stability-preserving decompression in degenerative versus congenital spinal stenosis: demographic patterns and patient outcomes. Spine J. 2017; 17(10):1420–1425

[7] Singh K, Samartzis D, Vaccaro AR, et al. Congenital lumbar spinal stenosis: a prospective, control-matched, cohort radiographic analysis. Spine J. 2005; 5(6):615–622

[8] Kitab SA, Alsulaiman AM, Benzel EC. Anatomic radiological variations in developmental lumbar spinal stenosis: a prospective, control-matched comparative analysis. Spine J. 2014; 14(5):808–815

[9] Kalichman L, Cole R, Kim DH, et al. Spinal stenosis prevalence and association with symptoms: the Framingham Study. Spine J. 2009; 9(7):545–550

[10] Boden SD, Davis DO, Dina TS, Patronas NJ, Wiesel SW. Abnormal magnetic-resonance scans of the lumbar spine in asymptomatic subjects: a prospective investigation. J Bone Joint Surg Am. 1990; 72(3):403–408

[11] Atlas SJ, Deyo RA, Keller RB, et al. The Maine Lumbar Spine Study, Part II. 1-year outcomes of surgical and nonsurgical management of sciatica. Spine. 1996; 21(15): 1777–1786

[12] Simotas AC, Dorey FJ, Hansraj KK, Cammisa F, Jr. Nonoperative treatment for lumbar spinal stenosis: clinical and outcome results and a 3-year survivorship analysis. Spine. 2000; 25(2):197–203, 203–204

[13] Weinstein JN, Tosteson TD, Lurie JD, et al. Surgical versus nonoperative treatment for lumbar spinal stenosis four-year results of the Spine Patient Outcomes Research Trial. Spine. 2010; 35(14):1329–1338

[14] Malmivaara A, Slätis P, Heliövaara M, et al. Finnish Lumbar Spinal Research Group. Surgical or nonoperative treatment for lumbar spinal stenosis? A randomized controlled trial. Spine. 2007; 32(1):1–8

[15] Melancia JL, Francisco AF, Antunes JL. Spinal stenosis. In: Neurologic Aspects of Systemic Disease Part I; 2014

[16] Djurasovic M, Glassman SD, Carreon LY, Dimar JR, II. Contemporary management of symptomatic lumbar spinal stenosis. Orthop Clin North Am. 2010; 41(2):183–191

[17] Butler D, Trafimow JH, Andersson GBJ, McNeill TW, Huckman MS. Discs degenerate before facets. Spine. 1990; 15(2): 111–113

[18] Fischgrund JS, Mackay M, Herkowitz HN, Brower R, Montgomery DM, Kurz LT. 1997 Volvo Award winner in clinical studies. Degenerative lumbar spondylolisthesis with spinal stenosis: a prospective, randomized study comparing decompressive laminectomy and arthrodesis with and without spinal instrumentation. Spine. 1997; 22(24): 2807–2812

[19] Dommisse GF, Grobler L. Arteries and veins of the lumbar nerve roots and cauda equina. Clin Orthop Relat Res. 1976 (115):22–29

[20] Akuthota V, Lento P, Sowa G. Pathogenesis of lumbar spinal stenosis pain: why does an asymptomatic stenotic patient flare? In: Physical Medicine and Rehabilitation Clinics of North America.; 2003. doi:10.1016/S1047-9651(02)00078-5

[21] Yamada K, Matsuda H, Nabeta M, Habunaga H, Suzuki A, Nakamura H. Clinical outcomes of microscopic decompression for degenerative lumbar foraminal stenosis: a comparison between patients with and without degenerative lumbar scoliosis. Eur Spine J. 2011; 20(6):947–953

[22] Alsaleh K, Ho D, Rosas-Arellano MP, Stewart TC, Gurr KR, Bailey CS. Radiographic assessment of degenerative lumbar spinal stenosis: is MRI superior to CT? Eur Spine J. 2017; 26 (2):362–367

[23] Alyas F, Connell D, Saifuddin A. Upright positional MRI of the lumbar spine. Clin Radiol. 2008; 63(9):1035–1048

[24] Cowley P. Neuroimaging of spinal canal stenosis. Magn Reson Imaging Clin N Am. 2016; 24(3):523–539

[25] Barz T, Melloh M, Staub L, et al. The diagnostic value of a treadmill test in predicting lumbar spinal stenosis. Eur Spine J. 2008; 17(5):686–690

[26] Rainville J, Childs LA, Peña EB, et al. Quantification of walking ability in subjects with neurogenic claudication from lumbar spinal stenosis: a comparative study. Spine J. 2012; 12(2):101–109

[27] Kinder A, Filho FP, Ribeiro E, et al. Magnetic resonance imaging of the lumbar spine with axial loading: a review of 120 cases. Eur J Radiol. 2012; 81(4):e561–e564

[28] Harrop JS, Hilibrand A, Mihalovich KE, Dettori JR, Chapman J. Cost-effectiveness of surgical treatment for degenerative spondylolisthesis and spinal stenosis. Spine. 2014; 39(22) Suppl 1:S75–S85

[29] Eun SS, Lee HY, Lee SH, Kim KH, Liu WC. MRI versus CT for the diagnosis of lumbar spinal stenosis. J Neuroradiol. 2012; 39(2):104–109

[30] Lurie JD, Tosteson AN, Tosteson TD, et al. Reliability of readings of magnetic resonance imaging features of lumbar spinal stenosis. Spine. 2008; 33(14):1605–1610

[31] Schönström N, Lindahl S, Willén J, Hansson T. Dynamic changes in the dimensions of the lumbar spinal canal: an experimental study in vitro. J Orthop Res. 1989; 7(1):115–121

[32] Lee GY, Lee JW, Choi HS, Oh KJ, Kang HS. A new grading system of lumbar central canal stenosis on MRI: an easy and reliable method. Skeletal Radiol. 2011; 40(8):1033–1039

[33] Park HJ, Kim SS, Lee YJ, et al. Clinical correlation of a new practical MRI method for assessing central lumbar spinal stenosis. Br J Radiol. 2013; 86(1025):20120180

[34] Avadhani A, Rajasekaran S, Shetty AP. Comparison of prognostic value of different MRI classifications of signal intensity change in cervical spondylotic myelopathy. Spine J. 2010; 10(6):475–485

[35] Fernández de Rota JJ, Meschian S, Fernández de Rota A, Urbano V, Baron M. Cervical spondylotic myelopathy due to chronic compression: the role of signal intensity changes in magnetic resonance images. J Neurosurg Spine. 2007; 6(1):17–22

[36] Mastronardi L, Elsawaf A, Roperto R, et al. Prognostic relevance of the postoperative evolution of intramedullary spinal cord changes in signal intensity on magnetic resonance imaging after anterior decompression for cervical spondylotic myelopathy. J Neurosurg Spine. 2007; 7(6):615–622

[37] Verbiest H. Pathomorphologic aspects of developmental lumbar stenosis. Orthop Clin North Am. 1975; 6(1):177–196

[38] Arnoldi CC, Brodsky AE, Cauchoix J, et al. Lumbar spinal stenosis and nerve root entrapment syndromes: definition and classification. Clin Orthop Relat Res. 1976(115):4–5

[39] Schroeder GD, Kurd MF, Vaccaro AR. Lumbar spinal stenosis: how is it classified? J Am Acad Orthop Surg. 2016; 24(12): 843–852

[40] Albert HB, Manniche C. The efficacy of systematic active conservative treatment for patients with severe sciatica: a single-blind, randomized, clinical, controlled trial. Spine. 2012; 37(7):531–542

[41] Prateepavanich P, Thanapipatsiri S, Santisatisakul P, Somshevita P, Charoensak T. The effectiveness of lumbosacral corset in symptomatic degenerative lumbar spinal stenosis. J Med Assoc Thai. 2001; 84(4):572–576

[42] Botwin KP, Gruber RD, Bouchlas CG, et al. Fluoroscopically guided lumbar transformational epidural steroid injections in degenerative lumbar stenosis: an outcome study. Am J Phys Med Rehabil. 2002; 81(12):898–905

[43] Ng L, Chaudhary N, Sell P. The efficacy of corticosteroids in periradicular infiltration for chronic radicular pain: a randomized, double-blind, controlled trial. Spine. 2005; 30 (8):857–862

[44] Peul WC, van den Hout WB, Brand R, Thomeer RTWM, Koes BW, Leiden-The Hague Spine Intervention Prognostic Study Group. Prolonged conservative care versus early surgery in patients with sciatica caused by lumbar disc herniation: two year results of a randomised controlled trial. BMJ. 2008; 336 (7657):1355–1358

[45] Atlas SJ, Keller RB, Wu YA, Deyo RA, Singer DE. Long-term outcomes of surgical and nonsurgical management of lumbar spinal stenosis: 8 to 10 year results from the Maine Lumbar Spine Study. Spine (03622436). 2005; 30(8): 936–943

[46] Moghimi MH, Leonard DA, Cho CH, et al. Virtually bloodless posterior midline exposure of the lumbar spine using the "para-midline" fatty plane. Eur Spine J. 2016; 25(3): 956–962

[47] Hoppenfeld S, DeBoer P, Buckley R. Surgical Exposures in Orthopaedics: The Anatomic Approach. 4th ed. Philadelphia: Walters Kluwer/Lippincott Williams & Wilkins Health; 2009

[48] Rothman, Richard H, Frederick A. Simeone, Harry N. In: Posterior and Lateral Approaches. Herkowitz. Rothman-Simeone, the Spine: Vol. 1. Philadelphia, PA: Saunders Elsevier; 2006

[49] O'Leary PF, McCance SE. Distraction laminoplasty for decompression of lumbar spinal stenosis. Clin Orthop Relat Res. 2001(384):26–34

[50] Kakiuchi M, Fukushima W. Impact of spinous process integrity on ten to twelve-year outcomes after posterior decompression for lumbar spinal stenosis: study of open-door laminoplasty using a spinous process-splitting approach. J Bone Joint Surg Am. 2015; 97(20):1667–1677

[51] Matsui H, Tsuji H, Sekido H, Hirano N, Katoh Y, Makiyama N. Results of expansive laminoplasty for lumbar spinal stenosis in active manual workers. Spine (Philadelphia, PA: 1976). 1992 Mar;17(3 Suppl): S37–40

[52] Aizawa T, Ozawa H, Kusakabe T, et al. Reoperation rates after fenestration for lumbar spinal canal stenosis: a 20-year period survival function method analysis. Eur Spine J. 2015; 24 (2):381–387

[53] Young S, Veerapen R, O'Laoire SA. Relief of lumbar canal stenosis using multilevel subarticular fenestrations as an alternative to wide laminectomy: preliminary report. Neurosurgery. 1988; 23(5):628–633

[54] Yoshimoto M, Takebayashi T, Kawaguchi S, et al. Minimally invasive technique for decompression of lumbar foraminal

stenosis using a spinal microendoscope: technical note. Minim Invasive Neurosurg. 2011; 54(3):142–146

[55] Deinsberger R, Kinn E, Ungersböck K. Microsurgical treatment of juxta facet cysts of the lumbar spine. J Spinal Disord Tech. 2006; 19(3):155–160

[56] Chopko B, Caraway DL. MiDAS I (mild Decompression Alternative to Open Surgery): a preliminary report of a prospective, multi-center clinical study. Pain Physician. 2010; 13(4): 369–378

[57] Junhui L, Zhengbao P, Wenbin X, et al. Comparison of pedicle fixation by the Wiltse approach and the conventional posterior open approach for thoracolumbar fractures, using MRI, histological and electrophysiological analyses of the multifidus muscle. Eur Spine J. 2017; 26(5):1506–1514

[58] Kim K-T, Lee S-H, Suk K-S, Bae S-C. The quantitative analysis of tissue injury markers after mini-open lumbar fusion. Spine. 2006; 31(6):712–716

[59] Asgarzadie F, Khoo LT. Minimally invasive operative management for lumbar spinal stenosis: overview of early and long-term outcomes. Orthop Clin North Am. 2007; 38(3): 387–399, abstract vi–vii

[60] Komp M, Hahn P, Merk H, Godolias G, Ruetten S. Bilateral operation of lumbar degenerative central spinal stenosis in full-endoscopic interlaminar technique with unilateral approach: prospective 2-year results of 74 patients. J Spinal Disord Tech. 2011; 24(5):281–287

[61] Hatta Y, Shiraishi T, Sakamoto A, et al. Muscle-preserving interlaminar decompression for the lumbar spine: a minimally invasive new procedure for the lumbar spinal canal stenosis. Spine. 2009; 34(8):E276–E280

[62] Chiu JC. Interspinous process decompression (IPD) system (X-STOP) for the treatment of lumbar spinal stenosis. Surg Technol Int. 2006; 15:265–275

[63] Lauryssen C. Appropriate selection of patients with lumbar spinal stenosis for interspinous process decompression with the X STOP device. Neurosurg Focus. 2007; 22(1):E5

[64] Goyal A, Goel VK, Mehta A, Dick D, Chinthakunta SR, Ferrara L. Cyclic loads do not compromise functionality of the interspinous spacer or cause damage to the spinal segment: an in vitro analysis. J Long Term Eff Med Implants. 2008; 18(4): 289–302

[65] Herkowitz HN, Kurz LT. Degenerative lumbar spondylolisthesis with spinal stenosis: a prospective study comparing decompression with decompression and intertransverse process arthrodesis. J Bone Joint Surg Am. 1991; 73(6): 802–808

[66] Ghogawala Z, Dziura J, Butler WE, et al. Laminectomy plus fusion versus laminectomy alone for lumbar spondylolisthesis. N Engl J Med. 2016; 374(15):1424–1434

[67] Deyo RA, Cherkin DC, Ciol MA. Adapting a clinical comorbidity index for use with ICD-9-CM administrative databases. J Clin Epidemiol. 1992; 45(6):613–619

[68] Oppenheimer JH, DeCastro I, McDonnell DE. Minimally invasive spine technology and minimally invasive spine surgery: a historical review. Neurosurg Focus. 2009; 27(3):E9

[69] Guiot BH, Khoo LT, Fessler RG. A minimally invasive technique for decompression of the lumbar spine. Spine. 2002; 27 (4):432–438

[70] Palmer S. Use of a tubular retractor system in microscopic lumbar discectomy: 1 year prospective results in 135 patients. Neurosurg Focus. 2002; 13(2):E5

[71] Parker SL, Adogwa O, Davis BJ, et al. Cost-utility analysis of minimally invasive versus open multilevel hemilaminectomy for lumbar stenosis. J Spinal Disord Tech. 2013; 26(1):42–47

[72] Palmer S, Turner R, Palmer R. Bilateral decompression of lumbar spinal stenosis involving a unilateral approach with microscope and tubular retractor system. J Neurosurg. 2002; 97(2) Suppl:213–217

[73] Mobbs RJ, Li J, Sivabalan P, Raley D, Rao PJ. Outcomes after decompressive laminectomy for lumbar spinal stenosis: comparison between minimally invasive unilateral laminectomy for bilateral decompression and open laminectomy: clinical article. J Neurosurg Spine. 2014; 21(2): 179–186

[74] Yagi M, Okada E, Ninomiya K, Kihara M. Postoperative outcome after modified unilateral-approach microendoscopic midline decompression for degenerative spinal stenosis. J Neurosurg Spine. 2009; 10(4):293–299

[75] Chopko BW. A novel method for treatment of lumbar spinal stenosis in high-risk surgical candidates: pilot study experience with percutaneous remodeling of ligamentum flavum and lamina. J Neurosurg Spine. 2011; 14(1):46–50

[76] Wilkinson JS, Fourney DR. Failure of percutaneous remodeling of the ligamentum flavum and lamina for neurogenic claudication. Neurosurgery. 2012; 71(1):86–92

[77] Fu K-MG, Smith JS, Polly DW, Jr, et al. Morbidity and mortality in the surgical treatment of 10,329 adults with degenerative lumbar stenosis. J Neurosurg Spine. 2010; 12 (5):443–446

[78] Senker W, Meznik C, Avian A, Berghold A. Perioperative morbidity and complications in minimal access surgery techniques in obese patients with degenerative lumbar disease. Eur Spine J. 2011; 20(7):1182–1187

[79] Pao J-L, Chen W-C, Chen P-Q. Clinical outcomes of microendoscopic decompressive laminotomy for degenerative lumbar spinal stenosis. Eur Spine J. 2009; 18(5):672–678

Suggested Readings

Boden SD, Davis DO, Dina TS, Patronas NJ, Wiesel SW. Abnormal magnetic-resonance scans of the lumbar spine in asymptomatic subjects. A prospective investigation. J Bone Joint Surg Am. 1990; 72(3):403–408

Fairbank JC, Pynsent PB. The Oswestry Disability Index. Spine. 2000; 25(22):2940–2952, discussion 2952 Review

Fischgrund JS, Mackay M, Herkowitz HN, Brower R, Montgomery DM, Kurz LT. 1997 Volvo Award winner in clinical studies. Degenerative lumbar spondylolisthesis with spinal stenosis: a prospective, randomized study comparing decompressive laminectomy and arthrodesis with and without spinal instrumentation. Spine. 1997; 22(24):2807–2812

Herkowitz HN, Kurz LT. Degenerative lumbar spondylolisthesis with spinal stenosis. A prospective study comparing decompression with decompression and intertransverse process arthrodesis. J Bone Joint Surg Am. 1991; 73(6):802–808

Jensen MC, Brant-Zawadzki MN, Obuchowski N, Modic MT, Malkasian D, Ross JS. Magnetic resonance imaging of the lumbar spine in people without back pain. N Engl J Med. 1994; 331(2):69–73

Verbiest H. A radicular syndrome from developmental narrowing of the lumbar vertebral canal. J Bone Joint Surg Br. 1954; 36-B (2):230–237

Weinstein JN, Tosteson TD, Lurie JD, et al. Surgical versus nonoperative treatment for lumbar spinal stenosis four-year results of the spine patient outcomes research trial. Spine (Phila Pa 1976).

Zdeblick TA. A prospective, randomized study of lumbar fusion. Preliminary results. Spine. 1993; 18(8):983–991

8 Degenerative Spondylolisthesis

Craig Forsthoefel and Kris Siemionow

Abstract

Degenerative spondylolisthesis is the result of arthritic changes in the lumbar spine, usually L4–L5, and can lead to debilitating axial back pain and neurogenic claudication due to spinal stenosis. Canal stenosis results from encroachment by the subluxating posterior elements of the unstable vertebral body. Neuroforaminal stenosis results from the narrowing of the foramina by loss of disc height and arthrosis of the facet joints. Patients will frequently report leg and buttock pain with back extension due to spinal stenosis and lower back pain when leaning forward due to vertebral instability. Evaluation involves standing AP, lateral, flexion, and extension radiographs as well as lumbar spine magnetic resonance imaging. Initial treatment involves conservative measures including physical therapy, NSAIDs, and activity modification. Surgical treatment is recommended if conservative measures fail after 3 months. Lumbar laminectomy with instrumented posterolateral fusion remains the gold standard of treatment. Other techniques, such as interbody fusion, have been described with similar outcomes, but with the added benefit of indirect decompression by increasing the neuroforaminal area. Minimally invasive techniques have the added benefit of reduced blood loss, pain scores, and faster recovery time. Surgical outcomes are favorable to nonoperative treatment with regard to functional outcome scores, back pain, and leg pain.

Keywords: spondylolisthesis, interbody fusion, posterolateral fusion, spinal stenosis, instrumentation

8.1 Introduction

Degenerative spondylolisthesis (DS) is a condition where one vertebral body slips on the other that can lead to spinal symptoms, which most commonly involves the L4–L5 segment. When visualized on the lateral radiographs, the L4 vertebral body will be positioned anteriorly compared to the inferior L5 vertebral body. However, this can occur in nearly any spinal segment or can involve retrolisthesis, with posterior subluxation of the superior vertebral body. The pathology that is seen in this condition occurs in the presence of degenerative disc disease, which leads to instability of the spinal segment and thus radiographic slippage (▶ Fig. 8.1). In comparison to isthmic spondylolisthesis that occurs in young athletes who participate in hyperextension activities of the lumbar spine, there is preservation of the link to the posterior elements and the vertebral body. This can subsequently lead to spinal stenosis in higher grade slippages. Because of this difference, DS has been termed pseudospondylolisthesis.

8.1.1 Demographics

The incidence for DS is approximately 4.1%, but only a small percentage of these patients will ever require surgical intervention.[1] Patients under the age of 50 years are rarely affected, as the condition occurs in the context of degenerative disc disease. Females are more commonly affected with an observed 4:1 incidence,[2] which is believed to be the result of ligamentous laxity from hormonal

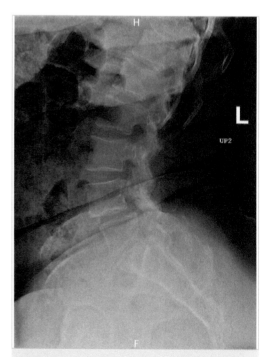

Fig. 8.1 Lateral radiograph of the lumbar spine demonstrating L4–L5 spondylolisthesis.

changes related to the menstrual cycle. Additionally, African-Americans tend to be more affected which is believed to be secondary to decreased lumbar lordosis, and increased sacralization of the L5 vertebral body, leading to greater force transmission to the L4–L5 segment.[3]

8.2 Pathogenesis

As previously mentioned, the pathology begins with degeneration of the lumbar spine leading to instability. Radiographically these manifest from loss of disc height and then arthritis of the facet joints which further becomes unstable. This leads to the superior vertebral body settling anteriorly in reference to the inferior body, which occurs approximately 70% of the time.[2] Otherwise there can be retrolisthesis where the opposite occurs, but is less common. Furthermore, degenerative scoliosis can occur as the unstable segments settle in a coronally deformed fashion, which can lead to worsening foraminal stenosis.

Sagittally oriented facets can potentiate instability as the morphology reduces the efficacy of the "boney hook" against shear forces (▶ Fig. 8.2). This aberrancy is thought to be secondary to degenerative changes rather than a congenital anomaly. Beyond coronally oriented facets, sacralized L5 (▶ Fig. 8.3), vertebral body and coronally oriented facets at L5–S1 have been associated with the DS. These variations produce greater force transmission to the L4–L5 segment, leading to a greater slippage force, which combined with degenerative changes at that segment can lead to overall anterolisthesis of the L4–L5 segment.

Symptoms of L4–L5 anterolisthesis can be related to diskogenic pain, facet pain, or neurologic pain. The neurologic symptoms are related to the specific nerve root compressed and the location in the spinal canal or foramen. If there is lateral recess stenosis due to hypertrophic arthritic changes at the L4–L5 facet joint, the L5 nerve root is compressed. This can lead to pain in the dorsum of the foot and weakness of the extensor hallucis longus. Furthermore, if foraminal stenosis exists from the subluxation of the L4 vertebral body and concomitant bulging and buckling of the L4–L5 disc then the L4 nerve root will be affected. This can lead to pain in the shin region as well as weakness of the tibialis anterior, possibly leading to foot drop. If there is a high-grade slip of the L4–L5 segment, the hypertrophic ligamentum flavum and the bulging intervertebral discs can encroach the spinal canal leading to spinal stenosis and presenting with classic neurogenic claudication.

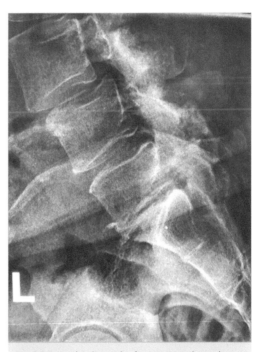

Fig. 8.3 Lateral radiograph of a transitional vertebra.

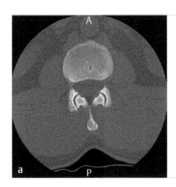
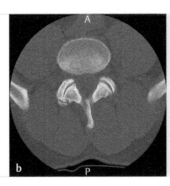

Fig. 8.2 (a) Axial CT of sagittally oriented facets. (b) Axial CT of more coronally oriented facets.

8.3 Clinical Presentation

The most common complaint of patients affected by DS is lower back pain. Pain is typically exacerbated by rising up from a forward bent position, which originates from the instability of the spinal segment leading to abnormal loading of the vertebral end plates, termed mechanical back pain. Many patients will use their hands to walk themselves up their thighs to avoid exacerbating their pain. Additionally, from the degenerative process of the arthritic facet joint lower back extension may cause increased pain.

When there are higher grade Meyerding slips, the posterior elements can cause narrowing of the spinal canal leading to spinal stenosis and neurogenic claudication. The compression on the nerves leads to a hypoxia event of the affected nerve roots that worsens when the lower back extends and improves with forward bending, which increases the surface area of the neuroforamina. Pain usually radiates down the patient's buttock and sometimes into their thighs. The common clinical sign discussed is the shopping cart sign, which describes improvement in pain while leaning over a shopping cart rather than walking up straight. Frequently, this must be contrasted with vascular claudication where there is similar pain in the legs with activity but improves with rest while standing upright. Correspondingly, riding a bicycle would cause less pain with neurogenic compared to vascular claudication.

Patients may also experience radicular symptoms as a result of compression on nerve roots. Depending on the affected nerve root, there will be different motor and sensory manifestations. When the L4–L5 segment is involved, stenosis in the lateral recess will affect the traversing nerve root, which would involve the L5 root. A far buckling of the disc and hypertrophic facet joints results in foraminal stenosis affecting the exiting nerve root, which would be L4. When the L4 root is involved there will be pain over the shin with associated tibialis anterior weakness. In the same way, L5 compression will cause pain in the dorsum of the foot as well as weakness of the extensor hallucis longus and hip abductors.

8.3.1 Clinical Findings

Patients may ambulate with a stooped over posture, also termed a lumbar lurch, characterized by flexed hips, flexed knees, and lumbar hypolordosis. The slipped segment in conjunction with other degenerative disc changes in spine results in lumbar hypolordosis and subsequent sagittal imbalance. Likewise, this is further initiated by the patient assuming a stooped over posture to reduce stenosis symptoms. In an effort to correct the imbalance and increase muscle efficiency with weightbearing, the patient will extend the hips followed by flexing the knees to increase pelvic retroversion.[4] Physical examination will reveal hip flexion contractures and tight hamstring muscles. Palpation of the lumbar spine may reveal a boney step-off in higher grade slips, but this remains rare in DS. Most patients will demonstrate normal motor and sensory examinations, but there may be deficits depending on the severity of radiculopathy. However, lateral recess stenosis will have more profound motor deficits compared to central stenosis. Pain can further be provoked by having the patient stand up erect, which decreases the surface area for the exiting nerve root in the neuroforamina.

Since many of these patients will complain of leg or hip pain and may have coexisting knee or hip arthritis, a full hip and knee exam should be performed. Most often, patients with arthritic pain in their hip will complain of groin pain, whereas patients with spinal stenosis and diskogenic back pain will present with buttock pain. It is crucial to differentiate these locations in order to obtain the appropriate workup and diagnosis. Similarly, knee osteoarthritis can present with knee pain and radiating pain proximally and distally in severe cases, which can be confused for radiculopathy. In this case, pain would be elicited by manipulating the knee versus pain elicited with straight leg raise. In equivocal cases, a diagnostic and therapeutic corticosteroid injection can help elucidate the primary pain generator.

8.4 Imaging Findings

Radiographs consisting of flexion and extension views will demonstrate if there is any underlying instability in patients with DS. A dynamically unstable segment will have greater than 4 mm of translation or 10° angulation compared to the adjacent segment.[5] The presence of vacuum disc phenomenon and facet joint fusions on magnetic resonance imaging (MRI) has been correlated with instability of the segment as well.[6] Plain lateral X-ray views will reveal the presence of spondylolisthesis.

When there are associated signs and symptoms of radiculopathy or spinal stenosis, MRI is indicated to identify the source of the pathology. Nerve compression can best be identified on the axial and sagittal T2 slices. Additionally, axial T2 slices can demonstrate effusions in the facet joints, which is a reported finding of segment instability. Computed tomography can also be used to gather greater boney detail, especially for surgical planning. Patients with suspected osteoporosis should undergo DEXA scanning to determine if they need bone health optimization prior to surgery or if they are candidates for certain interbody fusion procedures.

8.5 Classification Systems

8.5.1 Wiltse Classification

The Wiltse classification groups spondylolisthesis based on the etiology of the finding. Under this classification scheme DS is type III. The following briefly describes the classification system:
1. Type I—dysplastic
2. Type II—isthmic (subdivided into three groups)
   a) A—Pars fatigue fracture
   b) B—Pars elongation due to multiple healed stress fractures
   c) C—Acute pars fracture
3. Type III—Degenerative
4. Type IV—Traumatic
5. Type V—Neoplastic

8.5.2 Meyerding Classification

The Meyerding classification grades the degree of the anterolisthesis based on the percentage of vertebral body length of the unstable vertebral body compared to the inferior vertebral body.
1. Grade I: 0–25%
2. Grade II: 26–50%
3. Grade III: 51–75%
4. Grade IV: 76–100%
5. Grade V: > 100%, also known as spondyloptosis

Unlike isthmic spondylolisthesis, DS slips greater than grade II are rare given that the posterior arch remains intact. Additionally, with the degenerative process, the unstable segment tends to become stabilized adaptive changes which include osteophytes, ligament hypertrophy, and subchondral sclerosis.

8.6 Treatment

8.6.1 Nonoperative Treatment

Nonoperative measures are typically employed first unless in severe circumstances. A course of physical therapy focusing on core strengthening and flexibility of the hamstrings, activity modifications, and NSAIDs is effective in most symptomatic patients. If these initial conservative options fail, epidural steroid injections are a secondary fall back treatment option. If there are signs and symptoms of radiculopathy with dermatomal pain, gabapentin can be utilized in addition to the above regimen.

8.6.2 Indications for Surgery

Conservative treatment tends to be very effective in treating DS, with only 10 to 15% of patients requiring surgical intervention.[3] The typical cutoff for failed conservative treatment is 6 months of adequate physical therapy and anti-pain regimen. However, if the patient is presenting with progressive neurological deficit, bowel or bladder symptoms, or a surgical emergency such as cauda equina, surgical decompression should be performed without delay.

8.6.3 Surgical Options

The objective of surgical intervention is to decompress the neurological elements and stabilize the segment. In cases where the segment is relatively stable, a decompressive laminectomy alone can be performed. Relative stability is defined with the absence of mechanical lower back pain, facet angles < 50°, spondylolisthesis motion < 1.25 mm, disc height < 6.5 mm, as well as extensive osteophytes and facet hypertrophy with sclerosis.[7] This can be especially attractive in medically high-risk patients as it results in a shorter operative time and less blood loss, attributed to limited exposure and the lack of instrumentation. Additionally, it comes with a lower cost of the procedure and higher QALYs, but comes at the expense of not addressing the inherent instability. Several studies examining outcomes of decompressions alone compared to decompression with posterolateral fusion have demonstrated a higher reoperation rate for slip progression with continued spinal stenosis symptoms at the index level. These cases are successfully treated with posterolateral fusion and instrumentation.

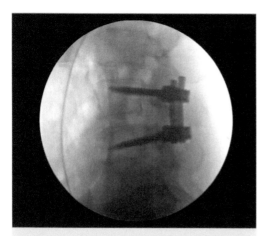

Fig. 8.4 Lateral fluoroscopic image of posterior spinal instrumentation with posterolateral fusion. Spondylolisthesis reduction was achieved with posterior spinal instrumentation.

Decompression with posterolateral fusion remains the gold standard for treatment of DS (▶ Fig. 8.4). The surgical procedure consists of a standard laminectomy of the involved segment followed by fusion between the transverse processes of the affected vertebra and the inferior vertebra, most commonly L4–L5. This can be performed instrumented and uninstrumented, with there being no difference between the two in regard to short-term outcomes. Studies have reported a higher fusion rate with instrumentation and higher long-term complications secondary to pseudoarthrosis in uninstrumented fusions. For this reason, most surgeons opt for instrumented over uninstrumented fusions. In order to gain enough surface area for fusion, posterolateral fusion requires exposure of the transverse processes compared to a decompressive laminectomy alone. Compared to laminectomy alone, there is a significantly lower reoperation rate, with revision cases addressing degeneration at the adjacent segment. Furthermore, fusions have been reported to have a higher improvement in SF-36 scores compared to laminectomy alone.[8]

The adjacent segment degeneration with lumbar fusion is believed to occur as a result of increased motion at the adjacent segments in response to the fused segment. Newer techniques, consisting of a decompressive laminectomy and insertion of interlaminar device that stabilizes the segment, but permits motion, are available.[9,10] There are reportedly high success rates and equivalent outcomes compared to lumbar spine fusion in select patients, with the benefit of preserved lumbar spine motion. Cases that have failed this approach are subsequently revised to a lumbar fusion with a high success rate. Spinous process fractures are possible complications, occurring in approximately 14% of cases, but this has not been proven to affect outcomes.

Instead of fusing the unstable segment between the transverse processes, fusion between the vertebral bodies has been reported with a high degree of success. There are various approaches to perform this technique, but the success stems from the increased surface area for fusion compared to posterolateral fusion. Some surgeons suggest that interbody fusion be reserved for revision cases. Given that an interbody device is inserted in the disc space, there is the advantage of potential reconstitution of the original disc height, reduction of the spondylolisthesis, and restoration of lumbar lordosis, which all can further decompress the segment. The extent to which these goals are accomplished is often technique-dependent. This process further stabilizes the anterior column and can correct kyphosis. However, the increased stiffness of the interbody device can lead to adjacent segment disease. When there is osteoporotic bone, the weakened vertebral end plates can lead to implant subsidence and compression fractures.

Transforaminal lumbar interbody fusion (TLIF) is very similar to the surgical approach of a posterolateral fusion; however, a more unilateral approach to the spine is pursued. The disc space is prepped allowing for insertion of an interbody device and simultaneously direct decompression of the affected nerve root via foraminotomy and partial facetectomy. Additionally, a circumferential fusion can be achieved from this single approach, given that posterior instrumentation can be performed adjunctively. This method does provide some benefits compared to the posterior lumbar interbody fusion (PLIF) counterpart. Since the interbody device and graft are inserted into the disc space from a lateral approach, there is less retraction of the dura and thus less potential neurological complications. Additionally, there is the opportunity for both direct and indirect decompression of the segment. However, there are some challenges with this approach, given that it places the nerve root directly into the surgical field and the subsequent narrow corridor for interbody device insertion.

Using a similar approach, PLIF places an interbody device with bone graft using a direct posterior approach. Much like the TLIF it allows for correct kyphosis of the affected segment, direct

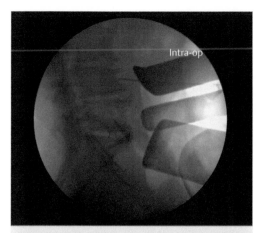

Fig. 8.5 Lateral intraop fluoroscopic image of an ALIF approach with interbody device present between L5 and S1.

decompression of the neurologic elements, and circumferential fusion. This necessitates a wide laminectomy and partial facetectomies in order to permit interbody device placement, which allows for direct decompression of the neural elements. Additionally, this approach requires retraction of the dura for effective placement of the device, often to a greater extent than the TLIF, which potentially can cause a durotomy and nerve root injuries. This method takes advantage of a well-known posterior surgical approach compared to the paramedian approach of the TLIF.

Utilizing an isolated anterior approach to the affected segment and anterior lumbar interbody fusion (ALIF) avoids any posterior dissection and disruption of the paraspinal musculature (▶ Fig. 8.5). This approach utilizes the exposure through the retroperitoneal space, often with the assistance of a general or vascular approach surgeon. Because of the presence of the great vessels, typically L4–L5 and L5–S1 are the levels most easily accessible using the anterior approach. However, the anterior to psoas approach utilizes the natural plane between the psoas and the great vessels and can allow for access to L2–L5. There are some risks with this method that are inherent to the approach: specifically, retrograde ejaculation if there is damage to the parasympathetic plexus, with higher rates associated with BMP compared to autograft (7.2 vs. 0.6%).[11] Additionally, given the proximity of the structures there are risks of visceral and vascular injury as well as damage to the sympathetic chain.

A lateral lumbar interbody fusion (LLIF or XLIF) is another technique that can be used to access the intervertebral disc space anteriorly. This method is advantageous compared to the ALIF approach, in that it preserves the anterior longitudinal ligament. This aids in reduction of spondylolisthesis once the disc height is reconstituted with the interbody device and bone graft. This additionally provides more anterior stability to the construct overall. Much like the ALIF procedure, there is preservation of the posterior elements and the paraspinal musculature remains intact. However, given the presence of the iliac wing, there can be difficulty accessing L4–L5. The approach requires retraction of the psoas muscle or passage through the muscle belly, which may result in postoperative groin and thigh pain. Furthermore, there may be damage to the lumbar plexus, and in an unlikely event if a vascular or visceral injury does occur, there will be extreme difficulty to manage due to the surgical corridor.

Minimally invasive techniques have become increasingly attractive in spine surgery. Perioperative metrics including blood loss, hospital stay, and return to activity are statistically improved compared to traditional open techniques.[12] There have been concerns about increased radiation exposure in these procedures with the increased reliance on fluoroscopic guidance. Additionally, there is a learning curve with the approaches compared to the universal posterior approach.

8.6.4 Postoperative Care

Patients should be instructed to limit any lifting of more than 10 pounds for 3 months postop, as to protect the fusion. Most regimens begin physical therapy at 6 weeks postop, when boney union becomes apparent. Follow-up should continue until 2 years postop if there has been an uneventful recovery. Complications should be followed for a long period and may require increased follow-up studies including CT scans and MRI.

8.6.5 Expected Outcomes

Regardless of fusion method and approach, all patients undergoing surgery will have significantly improved functional outcome scores, back pain, and leg pain compared to nonoperative modalities. These findings were reported in the landmark

SPORT study.[13] Other studies have reported slightly better short-term outcome with interbody fusion (IBF), but long-term follow-up IBF and PLF are comparable.[14,15] Meta-analyses comparing the two fusion methods have concluded that there are no differences with regard to outcomes.[15] One reported advantage of PLF is shorter hospital stays.[15]

Pearls   i

- DS almost always occurs at L4–L5.
- Neural arch is intact (vs. isthmic spondylolisthesis) which can cause spinal canal stenosis.
- Patients are almost never younger than 50-year-old.
- Instability on flex-ex films is defined at greater than 4 mm of translation or 10 degrees angulation.
- DS typically does not exceed slip percentage greater than 30% due to the stabilizing degenerative changes that occur with the pathogenesis.
- Conservative treatment consisting of NSAIDs, physical therapy, and activity modification should be pursued for a minimum of 3 months before surgical options are considered.
- Gold standard of surgical treatment of DS is decompressive laminectomy with posterolateral fusion.
- IBF provides added benefit of increasing the fusion area, indirect decompression, restoring disc height, and correcting sagittal balance.
- LLIF has the added benefit of preserving the anterior longitudinal ligament compared to ALIF.
- Minimally invasive procedures have been associated with faster recoveries and less tissue trauma, but comes with steeper learning curves.

8.7 Case Examples

8.7.1 Case 1

The patient is a 59-year-old female who had been a patient in the clinic for 2 years prior to undergoing surgery. Her initial complaint was lower back pain with bilateral radicular pain in the L5–S1 distribution. Her motor and sensory examine was unremarkable. Lumbar spine X-rays were obtained at her first visit and demonstrated mild grade I spondylolisthesis of L4–L5 (▶ Fig. 8.6a). Her symptoms were initially managed with physical therapy, steroid injections, Medrol dosepak, and anti-inflammatories. However, she achieved no relief from these measures. She opted for surgical management, which consisted of an L4 laminectomy and decompression, L5 hemilaminectomy, L4–L5 posterolateral fusion, with posterior spinal instrumentation. At 10 weeks follow-up the patient reported complete resolution of her bilateral radicular pain, but with residual lower back pain that was lower in quality preoperatively. Her 10-week postop radiographs are shown in ▶ Fig. 8.6b.

8.7.2 Case 2

The patient is a 52-year-old female who presented to the clinic with several years of back pain with occasional right leg pain. An extensive nonoperative management regimen was attempted for several years, which included several epidural steroid

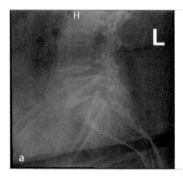
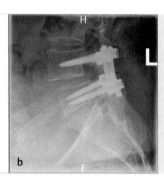

Fig. 8.6 (a) Preop radiographs with L4–L5 spondylolisthesis. (b) Postop radiograph with instrumentation.

injections, multiple courses of physical therapy, and anti-inflammatory medications. The patient did not obtain any relief with these measures and in fact experienced worsening of her symptoms. She opted for surgical management which included an L4 laminectomy and decompression, posterolateral spinal fusion L4–L5, and posterior spinal instrumentation L4–L5. Her preoperative radiographs are shown in ▶ Fig. 8.7a. Bilateral Wiltse posterolateral approaches were used. At 1-year follow-up, the patient reported complete resolution of her radicular symptoms, but mild intermittent lower back pain. She was given physical therapy and responded well. Her postoperative radiographs are shown in ▶ Fig. 8.7b.

8.7.3 Case 3

The patient is a 57-year-old female presenting with a several year history of lower back pain and right leg pain. She had a previous microdiscectomy at L4–L5 performed 10 years prior to presentation. Her back pain and right leg pain have gradually worsened over the past several years. Her current radiographs are shown in ▶ Fig. 8.8a. She has attempted steroid injections, physical therapy, gabapentin, and anti-inflammatories. Radiographs at the time of presentation demonstrated grade II L4–L5 spondylolisthesis. She also presented with multiple cervical spine issues, of which she underwent operative management prior to undergoing surgery for her lumbar spine afflictions. After she had recovered from her cervical spine procedure, she proceeded with an L4–L5 laminectomy and decompression, S1 hemilaminectomy, L4–L5 posterolateral fusion, with posterior spinal instrumentation. At 4-month follow-up she reported resolution of her radicular symptoms, although had persistent low-quality back pain. Follow-up radiographs are shown in ▶ Fig. 8.8b.

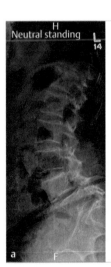
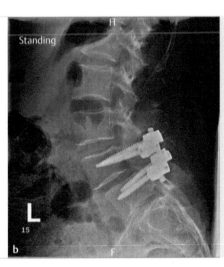

Fig. 8.7 (a) Preop demonstrating Grade I L4–L5 spondylolisthesis and facet arthrosis. (b) Postop demonstrating positioned posterior spinal instrumentation.

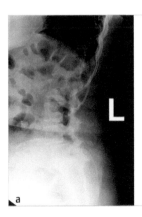
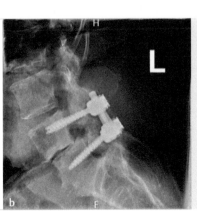

Fig. 8.8 (a) Preop radiograph demonstrating grade II L4–L5 spondylolisthesis. (b) Postop radiographs.

8.8 Board-style Questions

1. A 65-year-old African-American female is presenting with lower back pain. Neurovascular exam demonstrates 5/5 motor strength in her iliopsoas, quadriceps, hamstrings, tibialis anterior, extensor hallucis longus, and gastrocsoleus complex muscles. Patellar and Achilles reflexes are 2/4. Radiographs taken demonstrate anterolisthesis at L4–L5 with diffuse degenerative disc changes. What would be the next step in treatment?
   a) ALIF
   b) Posterolateral fusion without instrumentation
   c) Posterolateral fusion with instrumentation
   d) Physical therapy, NSAIDs, and activity modification
   e) Decompression without fusion

2. A radiograph of a 73-year-old male demonstrates grade II anterolisthesis at L4–L5. What findings would suggest instability in the motion segment?
   a) MRI with hypertrophy of the ligamentum flavum and buckling of the intervertebral disc
   b) Sagittally oriented facets on CT scan
   c) Greater than 4 mm of subluxation on lateral flexion-extension radiographs of the lumbar spine
   d) Increased pelvic incidence on lateral radiographs of the lumbar spine
   e) Loss of disc height on lateral radiographs

3. A 59-year-old male patient is found to have left-side radicular symptoms due to L4–L5 spondylolisthesis. What would be the most likely finding of his physical exam?
   a) Pain, numbness, and tingling in the L5 dermatome
   b) Palpable boney step-off in the lumbar spine
   c) 4/5 motor strength in the extensor hallucis longus
   d) 4/5 motor strength in the tibialis anterior
   e) Babinski sign bilaterally

4. LLIF has the added benefit in treating DS compared to ALIF?
   a) Direct decompression of the neuroforamina
   b) Better exposure to the L4–L5 segment
   c) Preservation of the posterior elements
   d) Restoring disc height
   e) Retaining the anterior longitudinal ligament

5. A 77-year-old female with L4–L5 DS has been undergoing 2 months of conservative treatment for lower back pain and left leg radicular symptoms consisting of physical therapy, activity modification, and NSAIDs. Despite these measures, she is still experiencing consistent pain in her L4 dermatome. What is the next step in treatment?
   a) Epidural steroid injections and gabapentin
   b) Laminectomy without fusion
   c) Posterolateral fusion without instrumentation
   d) Posterolateral fusion with instrumentation
   e) Interbody fusion

6. Which one of the following is not generally accepted as a risk factor for the development of DS?
   a) Age over 50 years old
   b) Sagittally oriented facets
   c) Sacralized L5
   d) Caucasian male
   e) Ligamentous laxity

7. A 62-year-old African-American female presents with lower back and right leg pain 6 months ago. She was diagnosed with L4–L5 DS with flexion-extension radiographs that was graded Meyerding II and subsequently treated with conservative measures including epidural steroid injections. Recent flexion-extension radiographs demonstrate 7 mm of subluxation of the L4 vertebral body. Despite these efforts she continues to experience 6/10 pain that limits her daily functional capacity. What is the next step in treatment?
   a) Additional 3 months of conservative measures and reassess
   b) MRI lumbar spine
   c) CT lumbar spine
   d) Laminectomy without fusion
   e) Laminectomy with instrumented posterolateral fusion

8. Which of the following is the biggest complication between PLF without versus with instrumentation?
   a) Pseudoarthrosis
   b) Infection
   c) Increased risk of injury to the neural elements
   d) Increased blood loss intraoperatively
   e) Loss of the posterior longitudinal ligament

9. Which of the following is an absolute indication for surgery in DS?
   a) Radicular symptoms
   b) Persistent back pain for 3 months despite conservative measures
   c) Instability on flexion-extension radiographs
   d) Cauda equina syndrome
   e) Meyerding grade II anterolisthesis

10. What are the outcomes of PLF compared to IBF techniques in the treatment of DS?
    a) Improved SF-36 scores
    b) Statistically significant increased fusion rates
    c) Reduced pain scores
    d) Increased blood loss intraoperatively
    e) No difference in outcomes

Answers

1. d: Newly diagnosed DS should always be treated with conservative treatment initially. If symptoms persist for 6 months in the presence of adequate conservative measures, then surgical options can be pursued. All other choices are surgical options.

2. c: Instability of the motion segment of L4–L5 would be the presence of greater than 4 mm of translation or greater than 10 degrees in angulation on flexion-extension radiographs. Other signs that have been described are vacuum phenomenon. All other choices are parameters associated with DS but are not consistent with instability.

3. a: The L5 nerve root is the most commonly involved nerve root in DS. This is due to lateral recess stenosis which compresses the L5 nerve root. The most common finding with L5 compression is radicular pain followed by L5 myotome weakness. The other choices are not reflective of this.

4. e: The added benefit of the LLIF is the preservation of the anterior longitudinal ligament. This may give added stability to an unstable motion segment in DS. All of the other choices are shared benefits between the two techniques.

5. a: The patient is experiencing symptoms related to DS despite 2 months of conservative treatment. However, she has not attempted epidural steroid injections, which is a second-line treatment in the conservative realm. If she continues to have symptoms after 3 to 6 months of exhaustive conservative measures, surgery can be considered.

6. d: All of the choices except "d" are believed to be risk factors for the development of DS. Instead of Caucasian males, African-American females are at higher risk of developing DS.

7. e: The patient in this stem has symptoms of nerve compression that have persisted despite 6 months of adequate conservative treatment. Additionally, the patient has instability on recent radiographs which makes fusion necessary in the surgical management.

8. a: Pseudoarthrosis is the biggest complication with uninstrumented PLF compared to PLF with instrumentation. Instrumentation increases the rigidity of the segment to facilitate fusion. Some studies have demonstrated no differences between the two despite the increased pseudoarthrosis rate; however, long-term results demonstrate that pseudoarthrosis lead to poor outcomes.

9. d: Cauda equina syndrome is an absolute indication for emergent surgery. All of the other choices are relative and strong indications for surgery, but not as strong as cauda equina syndrome.

10. e: IBF has been established to have increased fusion compared to PLF. However, many studies have not established statistical significance between the two techniques. Additionally, blood loss is typically increased with IBF compared to PLF due to the increased exposure needed. Overall, there has not been any established benefit of one over the other.

References

[1] Steiger F, Becker HJ, Standaert CJ, et al. Surgery in lumbar degenerative spondylolisthesis: indications, outcomes and complications. A systematic review. Eur Spine J. 2014; 23 (5):945–973

[2] Sengupta DK, Herkowitz HN. Degenerative spondylolisthesis: review of current trends and controversies. Spine. 2005; 30(6) Suppl:S71–S81

[3] Vibert BT, Sliva CD, Herkowitz HN. Treatment of instability and spondylolisthesis: surgical versus nonsurgical treatment. Clin Orthop Relat Res. 2006; 443(443):222–227

[4] Lamartina C, Berjano P, Petruzzi M, et al. Criteria to restore the sagittal balance in deformity and degenerative spondylolisthesis. Eur Spine J. 2012; 21 Suppl 1:S27–S31

[5] Simmonds AM, Rampersaud YR, Dvorak MF, Dea N, Melnyk AD, Fisher CG. Defining the inherent stability of degenerative spondylolisthesis: a systematic review. J Neurosurg Spine. 2015; 23(2):178–189

[6] Lattig F, Fekete TF, Grob D, Kleinstück FS, Jeszenszky D, Mannion AF. Lumbar facet joint effusion in MRI: a sign of instability in degenerative spondylolisthesis? Eur Spine J. 2012; 21(2):276–281

[7] Blumenthal C, Curran J, Benzel EC, et al. Radiographic predictors of delayed instability following decompression without fusion for degenerative grade I lumbar spondylolisthesis. J Neurosurg Spine. 2013; 18(4):340–346

[8] Ghogawala Z, Dziura J, Butler WE, et al. Laminectomy plus fusion versus laminectomy alone for lumbar spondylolisthesis. N Engl J Med. 2016; 374(15):1424–1434

[9] Davis RJ, Errico TJ, Bae H, Auerbach JD. Decompression and Coflex interlaminar stabilization compared with decompression and instrumented spinal fusion for spinal stenosis and low-grade degenerative spondylolisthesis: two-year results from the prospective, randomized, multicenter, Food and Drug Administration Investigational Device Exemption trial. Spine. 2013; 38(18):1529–1539

[10] Davis R, Auerbach JD, Bae H, Errico TJ. Can low-grade spondylolisthesis be effectively treated by either coflex interlaminar stabilization or laminectomy and posterior spinal fusion? Two-year clinical and radiographic results from the randomized, prospective, multicenter US investigational device exemption trial: clinical article. J Neurosurg Spine. 2013; 19(2):174–184

[11] Lindley EM, McBeth ZL, Henry SE, et al. Retrograde ejaculation after anterior lumbar spine surgery. Spine. 2012; 37 (20):1785–1789

[12] Wu A-M, Hu Z-C, Li X-B, et al. Comparison of minimally invasive and open transforaminal lumbar interbody fusion in the treatment of single segmental lumbar spondylolisthesis: minimum two-year follow up. Ann Transl Med. 2018; 6(6):105–105

[13] Weinstein JN, Lurie JD, Tosteson TD, et al. Surgical compared with nonoperative treatment for lumbar degenerative spondylolisthesis: four-year results in the Spine Patient Outcomes Research Trial (SPORT) randomized and observational cohorts. J Bone Joint Surg Am - Ser A. 2009; 91(6):1295–1304

[14] Campbell RC, Mobbs RJ, Lu VM, Xu J, Rao PJ, Phan K. Posterolateral fusion versus interbody fusion for degenerative spondylolisthesis: systematic review and meta-analysis. Global Spine J. 2017; 7(5):482–490

[15] McAnany SJ, Baird EO, Qureshi SA, Hecht AC, Heller JG, Anderson PA. Posterolateral fusion versus interbody fusion for degenerative spondylolisthesis: a systematic review and meta-analysis. Spine. 2016; 41(23):E1408–E1414

9 Spinal Cord Injury

Jakub Sikora-Klak, Ryan O'Leary, and R. Todd Allen

Abstract

Spinal cord injuries (SCIs) comprise a heterogeneous group of potentially devastating events. Spinal cord anatomy is essential in order to provide a foundation for understanding the types of SCIs and the expected deficits. SCIs can be classified by the location of disruption and the associated phenotype, both of which help guide the prognosis. Regardless of the specific injury, every traumatic SCI patient should be resuscitated following advanced trauma life support (ATLS) protocol, with care taken to maintain adequate blood pressure to prevent further insult to the cord. This can be followed by a thorough physical exam and the appropriate imaging studies. The decision for surgical intervention is largely based on findings of instability and progressive neurologic deficits, and the specific surgical approach is dictated by the injury pattern. The current literature is reviewed, showing a trend toward support of early intervention.

The chapter concludes with a discussion of current controversies and future directions. There is a slackening enthusiasm for the use of high-dose steroids in SCI; however, there are a lot of exciting new treatment options being explored.

Keywords: spinal cord injury, spinal cord anatomy, SCI intervention

9.1 Introduction

Spinal cord injuries (SCIs) are devastating events that have significant impact on a patient's independence, function, and quality of life. There are an estimated 17,700 new SCIs in the United States each year, an incidence of 54 cases per one million people. SCI is the second most expensive medical condition to treat, behind only respiratory distress in preterm infants (▶ Table 9.1).[1] Presentations and outcomes vary, depending on level, location of injury, and highly heterogenous baseline patient factors. Mechanisms of injury include high-energy accidents, falls from standing, and athletic participation and pathology can range from contusions to complete spinal cord transections.

9.2 Spinal Cord Anatomy

Ascending and descending tracts of the spinal cord are contained in the white matter (▶ Fig. 9.1). It is through these tracts that motor and sensory information is conveyed. Descending tracts carry information from the cortex to the periphery via the lateral and anterior corticospinal tracts, rubrospinal, reticulospinal, and vestibulospinal spinal tract. The lateral corticospinal and rubrospinal tracts mediate voluntary movement of large muscles and fine motor control. The anterior corticospinal, reticulospinal, and vestibulospinal tracts mediate balance and postural movements. Important ascending tracts include the dorsal columns and both the lateral and ventral spinothalamic tract. The ascending tracts carry information from the peripheries to the central nervous system. The dorsal columns transmit information regarding deep touch, vibration, and proprioception. The lateral spinothalamic tract carries pain and temperature from the contralateral side. The ventral spinothalamic tract is responsible for light touch.

Table 9.1 National SCI cost to treat.

Severity of injury	Average yearly expenses (in 2017 dollars)		Estimated lifetime costs by age at injury (discounted at 2%)	
	First year	Each subsequent year	25 years old	50 years old
High Tetraplegia (C1–C4) AIS ABC	$1,102,403	$191,436	$4,891,398	$2,688,229
Low Tetraplegia (C5–C8) AIS ABC	$796,583	$117,437	$3,573,960	$2,198,305
Paraplegia AIS ABC	$537,271	$71,172	$2,391,872	$1,569,714
Motor Functional at Any Level AIS D	$359,783	$43,700	$1,634,139	$1,153,420

Data source: Economic Impact of SCI published in the journal Topics in Spinal Cord Injury Rehabilitation, Volume 16, Number 4, in 2011.
Note: ASIA Impairment Scale (AIS) is used to grade the severity of a person's neurological impairment following spinal cord injury.

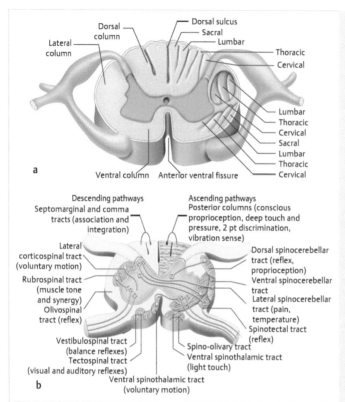

Fig. 9.1 (a,b) Spinal cord tracts. (Reproduced with permission from An HS, Singh K. Synopsis of Spine Surgery. 3rd Edition. Thieme; 2016.)

9.3 Presentation

Initial evaluation and resuscitation must be performed per the advanced trauma life support (ATLS) protocol. During initial evaluation, providers should assume that an unstable traumatic SCI is present and proper precautions must be undertaken, which include cervical collars and maintaining spinal precautions.

Injuries at the C3 vertebral body or cephalad may present with respiratory arrest; thus, intubation should be managed emergently. If intubation is necessary, the spine should be maintained in neutral alignment. Excessive flexion or extension during airway management and positioning (especially prone positioning) can compromise the spinal cord.[2] Lower level injuries can decrease respiratory function via impaired diaphragm and accessory muscles.

Hypotension is a common finding on initial presentation of trauma patients. After hemorrhage has been ruled out, neurogenic shock should be considered as a cause of hypotension. Hypotension must be aggressively resuscitated and systolic pressure less than 90 mmHg should be avoided.[3] A mean arterial pressure between 85 and 90 mmHg for the first 7 days after an acute SCI has been shown to result in improved outcomes.[4] However, one must be careful to avoid fluid overload in SCI patients, as they are at high risk for pulmonary edema.

Systemic hypothermia induction via a central venous catheter has shown modest improvement in motor function at the expense of respiratory complications and urinary tract infections,[5] but future studies are needed to establish its role.

Assessment of voluntary movement of all four extremities, palpation of the entirety of the spine, perianal sensation, digital rectal exam, and bulbocavernosus reflex should be performed. The bulbocavernosus reflex responds to squeezing the glans of the penis or clitoris. Through the local S2–S4 spinal reflex arc it initiates contraction of the bulbocavernosus arc. The bulbocavernosus reflex is generally the first reflex to appear following SCI.[6] Therefore, an absent bulbocavernosus reflex reveals that spinal shock is present, and a definitive diagnosis of SCI level cannot be made. The presence of the reflex in the setting of a complete SCI signifies an upper motor neuron lesion through loss of supraspinal inhibition.

9.4 Injury Types

The level and extent of SCI determines the injury and its classification. The American Spinal Injury Association (ASIA) created the International Standards for Neurological Classification of SCI (ISNCSCSI) examination to classify the level of neurologic injury and extent of function (▶ Fig. 9.2). Injuries are deemed complete when there is no sensory or motor function at S4–S5 after spinal shock has resolved.[7,8] Complete neurological deficits (classification ASIA A) are most prevalent in thoracic spine injuries, likely due to the smaller central canal in the thoracic spine when compared to the cervical or lumbar spine.[9]

Incomplete injuries are highly variable. They can be grouped using the ASIA classification or by identifying the associated syndrome. The incomplete SCI syndromes include: central cord, Brown-Sequard, anterior cord, and posterior cord syndromes. Classification by syndrome can aid in communication with other caretakers,

improve diagnostic ability, help predict prognosis, and guide treatment decisions.[10]

Central cord syndrome presents as motor weakness in the extremities, with more significant motor deficits in the upper extremities as compared to the lower extremities. There is variable associated sensory loss. The classic presentation is a hyperflexion/extension injury in elderly patients with pre-existing stenosis. Other common causes include acute disc herniation, fracture, or dislocation.

Central cord syndrome had traditionally been treated nonoperatively. Contemporary literature now supports operative intervention within one week to promote earlier recovery, decreased length of stay, and lower hospital costs.[11] Decompression is an effective treatment in patients with pre-existing cervical spondylosis and canal narrowing.[12] For associated injuries, fractures are generally treated with ACCF and disc herniations with ACDF. While early operative management with decompression and stabilization has not been shown

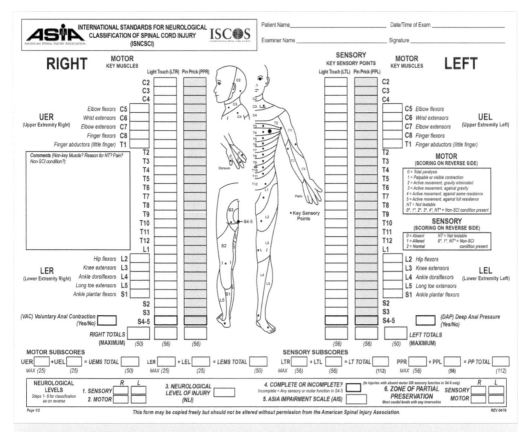

Fig. 9.2 ASIA classification. © 2019 American Spinal Injury Association. Reproduced with permission.

to impact final ASIA score, younger age was positively correlated with motor recovery and therefore a higher score.[13]

Brown-Sequard syndrome (BSS) occurs with spinal hemisection, typically from a penetrating source. Hemorrhage, disc herniation, and edema are other potential causes. Classically, these patients experience ipsilateral loss of motor and proprioception and contralateral loss of pain and temperature. The "plus" variation of BSS is more common and refers to a relative hemiplegia and contralateral relative hemianalgesia as opposed to a complete loss.[14] Management varies based on the etiology and any associated spinal injuries. Penetrating BSS is often treated nonoperatively (see the Penetrating Injury section), while BSS due to disc herniation has been successfully treated with ACDF with return of normal neurologic function.[15] The prognosis with BSS is generally the most favorable of all the incomplete syndromes, with up to 75% of patients recovering independent ambulation.[14]

Anterior cord syndrome (ACS) occurs with damage to the anterior two-thirds of the spinal cord via ischemia from anterior spinal artery injury or trauma to the anterior cord. Patients present with loss of motor function and pain and temperature sensation, but maintain proprioception and light touch sensation. This syndrome has a poor prognosis for functional recovery and a high mortality rate.[16] Given the rarity of ACS, there is limited data to guide treatment. Current treatment strategies are designed to minimize further insult to the spinal cord. With vascular etiologies it is important to maintain spinal cord perfusion to prevent additional ischemia.[17] ACS associated with trauma is treated with decompression and stabilization as necessary.[18] Rehabilitation and strengthening also play an important role after the acute insult has been managed.

Posterior cord syndrome is a rare injury representing less than one percent of SCI.[19] Patients present with a loss of vibration and proprioception sensation after an injury to the dorsal columns. They have preserved motor function and pain, temperature, and light touch sensation.

Finally, injury to lumbar and sacral nerve roots via fracture, disc herniation, or tumor can present with bowel/bladder dysfunction, variable leg function, and variable bulbocavernosus reflex depending on level of injury. In general, cauda equina syndrome, progressive neurologic deficit, and an unstable spine are indications for surgical management.

9.5 Surgical Intervention and Timing

The indications and approach for surgical intervention are based on the mechanism of injury and associated pathology. Decompression and stabilization are required for all patients with SCI and evidence of compression. There has been a recent movement toward early operative intervention for patients with acute SCI. Benefits include earlier mobilization and rehabilitation, with data to suggest improved neurologic outcomes.

In cervical spine trauma with SCI, early decompression and stabilization (within 24 hours) are associated with greater improvement in ASIA score when compared to later intervention.[20] This study included all ASIA classification levels and incomplete syndromes with imaging evidence of compression and excluded patients with penetrating trauma.

The data on early decompression is less conclusive in thoracolumbar trauma. It has been shown that early operation on thoracolumbar fractures can increase morbidity. However, in a population of *medically stable* patients, decompression and stabilization within 8 hours led to improved postoperative ASIA scores and shorter length of stay.[21]

For thoracolumbar trauma, the thoracolumbar injury severity score (TLICS)[22] can be used to determine when intervention is necessary on thoracolumbar injuries and which approach to take. The patient's neurologic status, integrity of the posterior ligamentous complex, and fracture morphology are the three major determinants guiding operative intervention.

When determining operative approach, there are general principles to consider. For example, canal compression from anterior structures usually requires an anterior approach, while posterior approaches are required for posterior ligamentous complex disruption.[22]

In summary, early decompression and stabilization within 24 hours has shown clear benefit in the cervical spine and is favored for both cervical and thoracolumbar SCI at many centers.

9.6 Penetrating Injury

Gunshot wounds are the most common type of penetrating trauma, with the thoracolumbar region being the most commonly area affected. These injuries typically result in a complete SCI from a combination of direct trauma, blast effect, ischemia, and hemorrhage.[23] Wounds should be treated with local irrigation and debridement as needed, with antibiotic coverage depending on penetration of other structures, with up to 2 weeks of antibiotics if the integumentary system was involved. Incomplete SCI with instability, cauda equina, or worsening neurologic examination benefit from surgical intervention, but otherwise penetrating injuries are managed conservatively with equivocal or better outcomes.[24]

9.7 Imaging

A thorough neurologic exam is the key to diagnostic imaging. Slow recognition of injuries can further delay appropriate studies and care. Plain radiographs are often the first imaging modality for areas of concern. Cervical imaging must include the C7–T1 junction. Typically flexion-extension lateral plain radiographs of the cervical spine are not helpful as most patients will self-protect, thus hiding ligamentous injury.[2] Thoracolumbar radiographs should include anteroposterior (AP) and lateral radiographs, ensuring that the C7–T1 junction is visualized. A swimmer's view can be obtained if the standard lateral image does not capture T1. However, as computer tomography (CT) scans become cheaper and more readily available, they are now supplanting radiographs as the standard C-spine imaging modality in many trauma centers. CT scans offer increased resolution and ability to diagnose skeletal injury as compared to X-rays. In centers relying on plain radiographs for initial screening, CT is recommended with positive radiographic findings, areas of suspicion, or with any high-energy injury. Many trauma centers have protocols regarding abdomen/pelvic imaging, and these should be reviewed in concert to avoid repetitive exposure to radiation. The role of magnetic resonance imaging (MRI) is controversial, given resource limitations and the long scan times in critically ill patients.[25] In those with unexplained neurological deficits, evolving compressive pathologies, and unexaminable patients, we recommend an urgent MRI. MRI can also be used to clarify the presence of posterior ligamentous injury, which can assist operative planning, including when to operate and what approach to use.[22] Recent advances in imaging have been used for developing prognostic scores and outcomes[26,27] based on hemorrhage and cord edema. For example, in the cited studies, patients with single-level cord edema on initial MRI were shown to have improved neurologic function as opposed to patients with diffuse cord edema.

9.8 Steroids

Animal models have shown methylprednisolone to be neuroprotective against inflammation and oxidative stresses.[28,29] The series of prospective National Acute Spinal Cord Injury Studies (NASCIS) trials[30,31,32] queried doses and timing of methylprednisolone administration. The third trial found improved neurological outcomes in those who received methylprednisolone for 48 hours when given within 3 to 8 hours of injury compared with those who received the 24-hour dose, but the 48-hour cohort showed higher rates of severe sepsis and pneumonia. The 2013 AANS/CNS[33] recommended against the use of methylprednisolone, contrarily the 2017 AOSpine guidelines[34] recommend 24 hours of treatment in a nonpenetrating SCI with no significant contraindications.

A survey of the Cervical Spine Research Society members highlights a trend of decreasing steroid use in acute SCI, with only approximately half of the members providing steroids to these patients.[35] Until further data is produced to clarify the issue, it seems reasonable to discontinue use in high risk, elderly patients, while continuing to dose steroids in young, otherwise healthy, trauma patients.

9.9 Venous Thromboembolism

Venous thromboembolism (VTE) events after SCI show an incidence of 3 to 5%, but can be as high as 20% in patients older than 70 years, and occur more often with upper thoracic SCI.[36,37,38] Low-molecular-weight heparin has been shown superior to subcutaneous heparin,[39,40] and offers greater protection with concomitant lower extremity compression devices.[41] Barring contraindication to prophylaxis, authors recommend withholding prophylactic anticoagulation until POD3 and any therapeutic anticoagulation until at least POD7, given the risk of epidural hematoma.

9.10 Future Directions

The next generation of care may incorporate advances in imaging and biomarkers to improve prognosis and outcomes. Studies underway are looking at interleukins, inflammatory proteins, cytokines,[42,43] micro RNAs, astrogliosis,[44] with evaluation of microstructures and insults via MRI sequencing.[45]

9.11 Case Examples

9.11.1 Case 1

An 82-year-old female presented with a T4 burst fracture with posterior ligamentous disruption, associated pelvic fractures, after a fall down multiple steps. On physical exam, her strength was 4/5 bilaterally in her lower extremities, limited

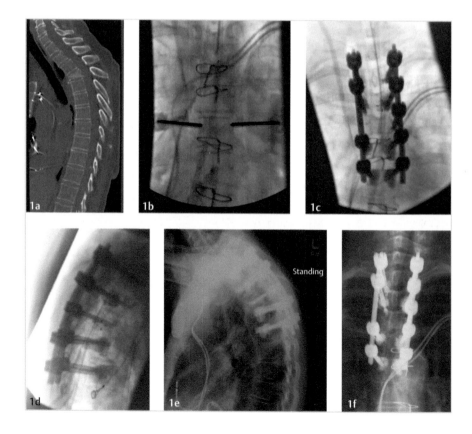

by pain from her pelvis. The decision was made to stabilize her with percutaneous pedicle screws with cement augmentation from T2 to T6. Due to fracture, pedicle size, and mobility, it was deemed unsafe to place a screw at the right T4 pedicle. Image 1a shows the osteoporotic patient with a burst fracture at T4 with posterior ligament disruption. Intraoperative fluoroscopy shows the Jamshidi needle lateral to the medial pedicle wall (Image 1b). Images 1c, 1d show final intraoperative constructs. At 9 months postoperatively, her construct was found to be stable (Images 1e, 1f) and her only complaint was improving soreness after gardening.

9.11.2 Case 2

A 62-year-old female presented to the trauma bay after a pedestrian versus motor vehicle accident. On exam she was localizing cervical neck pain but no neurologic symptoms. On imaging, she was found to have C6–C7, C7–T1 diskoligamentous injuries, an anteroinferior tear drop fracture at C7, along with C4–C6 spinous process fractures (Image 2a). MR imaging (Image 2b) showed tears throughout the posterior ligamentous complex. Two-level anterior cervical discectomy and interbody fusions were done at C6–C7 and C7–T1 without complication (Images 2c–e). At 1-year postoperatively, she is doing well and pain free (Images 2f, g).

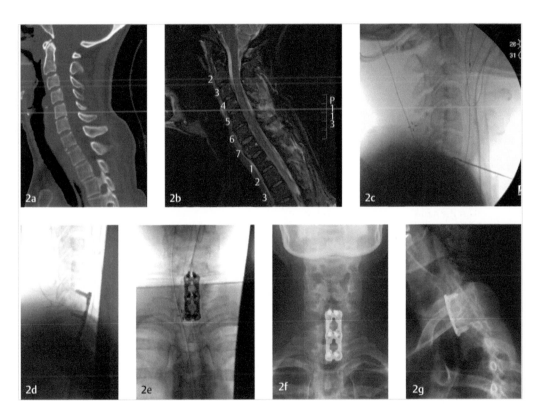

9.12 Board-style Questions

1. A 24-year-old male with a blood alcohol content of 0.12 presents with bilateral cervical facet dislocations at C6–C7 evident on radiographs. Patient has 5/5 strength in bilateral upper and lower extremities and no focal sensory deficits on exam. What is the next step in management?
   a) Computed tomography of the cervical spine
   b) Immediate mobilization of the patient to the operating room for open versus closed reduction and stabilization
   c) Immediate closed reduction, then MRI, then surgical stabilization
   d) MRI of the cervical spine, then surgical stabilization

2. A 74-year-old female on dialysis and significant cardiac history was involved in a motor vehicle accident. She is neurologically intact, with no focal motor or sensory deficits. A CT scan reveals a minimally displaced type-II odontoid fracture. What is the best definitive treatment?
   a) Cervical immobilization in a hard orthosis
   b) Anterior odontoid screw fixation
   c) Posterior C1–C2 fusion
   d) Halo vest immobilization

3. A 47-year-old male was surfing when his head hit the ocean floor and sustained an axial-load through his cervical spine. He complains of neck pain, and an inability to ambulate or to pull himself on the hand rails in the bed. He has grade 2 strength in most muscles of the upper and lower extremity. His bulbocavernosus reflex is intact and he is sensate in all four extremities. Imaging shows a burst fracture of C5. Using the ASIA classification, what severity of injury does the patient have?
   a) Grade 1
   b) Grade 2
   c) Grade 3
   d) Grade 4
   e) Grade 5

4. A 24-year-old male presents after a penetrating stab in his back at approximately T12 level. Patient has advanced imaging showing a hemitransection of the spinal cord. What symptoms is the patient expected to exhibit?
   a) Ipsilateral motor deficit, contralateral temperature, and pain sensation loss
   b) Loss of proprioception alone
   c) Burning in legs, equal bilateral motor deficit
   d) Loss of vibration and motor ipsilaterally
   e) Loss of motor in both feet and ipsilateral proprioception

Answers

1. d
2. a
3. c
4. a

References

[1] Winslow C, Bode RK, Felton D, Chen D, Meyer PR, Jr. Impact of respiratory complications on length of stay and hospital costs in acute cervical spine injury. Chest. 2002; 121(5): 1548–1554. Accessed February 3, 2019

[2] Wang JC, Hatch JD, Sandhu HS, Delamarter RB. Cervical flexion and extension radiographs in acutely injured patients. Clin Orthop Relat Res. 1999(365):111–116. Accessed February 3, 2019

[3] Vale FL, Burns J, Jackson AB, Hadley MN. Combined medical and surgical treatment after acute spinal cord injury: results of a prospective pilot study to assess the merits of aggressive medical resuscitation and blood pressure management. J Neurosurg. 1997; 87(2):239–246

[4] Ryken TC, Hurlbert RJ, Hadley MN, et al. The acute cardiopulmonary management of patients with cervical spinal cord injuries. Neurosurgery. 2013; 72 Suppl 2:84–92

[5] Dididze M, Green BA, Dietrich WD, Vanni S, Wang MY, Levi AD. Systemic hypothermia in acute cervical spinal cord injury: a case-controlled study. Spinal Cord. 2013; 51(5): 395–400

[6] Ko H-Y, Ditunno JF, Jr, Graziani V, Little JW. The pattern of reflex recovery during spinal shock. Spinal Cord. 1999; 37 (6):402–409

[7] Austin N, Krishnamoorthy V, Dagal A. Airway management in cervical spine injury. Int J Crit Illn Inj Sci. 2014; 4(1):50–56

[8] Kirshblum SC, Burns SP, Biering-Sorensen F, et al. International standards for neurological classification of spinal cord injury (revised 2011). J Spinal Cord Med. 2011; 34(6):535–546

[9] Wang H, Zhang Y, Xiang Q, et al. Epidemiology of traumatic spinal fractures: experience from medical university-affiliated hospitals in Chongqing, China, 2001–2010. J Neurosurg Spine. 2012; 17(5):459–468

[10] Eckert MJ, Martin MJ. Trauma: spinal cord injury. Surg Clin North Am. 2017; 97(5):1031–1045

[11] Guest J, Eleraky MA, Apostolides PJ, Dickman CA, Sonntag VKH. Traumatic central cord syndrome: results of surgical management. J Neurosurg. 2002; 97(1) Suppl:25–32. Accessed February 3, 2019

[12] Chen TY, Dickman CA, Eleraky M, Sonntag VK. The role of decompression for acute incomplete cervical spinal cord injury in cervical spondylosis. Spine. 1998; 23(22):2398–2403. Accessed February 3, 2019

[13] Chen L, Yang H, Yang T, Xu Y, Bao Z, Tang T. Effectiveness of surgical treatment for traumatic central cord syndrome. J Neurosurg Spine. 2009; 10(1):3–8

[14] Roth EJ, Park T, Pang T, Yarkony GM, Lee MY. Traumatic cervical Brown-Sequard and Brown-Sequard-plus syndromes: the spectrum of presentations and outcomes. Paraplegia. 1991; 29(9):582–589

[15] Kobayashi N, Asamoto S, Doi H, Sugiyama H. Brown-Sèquard syndrome produced by cervical disc herniation: report of

two cases and review of the literature. Spine J. 2003; 3(6): 530–533

[16] Matos JR, George RM, Wilson SH. It is not always the epidural: a case report of anterior spinal artery ischemia in a trauma patient. A A Pract. 2018; 11(6)

[17] Nasr DM, Rabinstein A. Spinal cord infarcts: risk factors, management, and prognosis. Curr Treat Options Neurol. 2017; 19(8):28

[18] Foo D, Subrahmanyan TS, Rossier AB. Post-traumatic acute anterior spinal cord syndrome. Paraplegia. 1981; 19(4):201–205

[19] McKinley W, Santos K, Meade M, Brooke K. Incidence and outcomes of spinal cord injury clinical syndromes. J Spinal Cord Med. 2007; 30(3):215–224

[20] Fehlings MG, Vaccaro A, Wilson JR, et al. Early versus delayed decompression for traumatic cervical spinal cord injury: results of the Surgical Timing in Acute Spinal Cord Injury Study (STASCIS). PLoS One. 2012; 7(2):e32037

[21] Cengiz ŞL, Kalkan E, Bayir A, Ilik K, Basefer A. Timing of thoracolumbar spine stabilization in trauma patients; impact on neurological outcome and clinical course: a real prospective (rct) randomized controlled study. Arch Orthop Trauma Surg. 2008; 128(9):959–966

[22] Vaccaro AR, Lehman RA, Jr, Hurlbert RJ, et al. A new classification of thoracolumbar injuries: the importance of injury morphology, the integrity of the posterior ligamentous complex, and neurologic status. Spine. 2005; 30(20): 2325–2333. Accessed February 3, 2019

[23] Rosenfeld JV, Bell RS, Armonda R. Current concepts in penetrating and blast injury to the central nervous system. World J Surg. 2015; 39(6):1352–1362

[24] Sidhu GS, Ghag A, Prokuski V, Vaccaro AR, Radcliff KE. Civilian gunshot injuries of the spinal cord: a systematic review of the current literature. Clin Orthop Relat Res. 2013; 471 (12):3945–3955

[25] Blackham J, Benger J. "Clearing" the cervical spine in the unconscious trauma patient. Trauma. 2011; 13(1):65–79

[26] Bozzo A, Marcoux J, Radhakrishna M, Pelletier J, Goulet B. The role of magnetic resonance imaging in the management of acute spinal cord injury. J Neurotrauma. 2011; 28(8): 1401–1411

[27] Wilson JR, Grossman RG, Frankowski RF, et al. A clinical prediction model for long-term functional outcome after traumatic spinal cord injury based on acute clinical and imaging factors. J Neurotrauma. 2012; 29(13):2263–2271

[28] Hall ED, Braughler JM. Glucocorticoid mechanisms in acute spinal cord injury: a review and therapeutic rationale. Surg Neurol. 1982; 18(5):320–327. Accessed February 3, 2019

[29] Braughler JM, Hall ED. Lactate and pyruvate metabolism in injured cat spinal cord before and after a single large intravenous dose of methylprednisolone. J Neurosurg. 1983; 59 (2):256–261

[30] Bracken MB, Shepard MJ, Hellenbrand KG, et al. Methylprednisolone and neurological function 1 year after spinal cord injury: results of the National Acute Spinal Cord Injury Study. J Neurosurg. 1985; 63(5):704–713

[31] Sparkes ML. Methylprednisolone or naloxone treatment after acute spinal cord injury: 1-year follow-up data. J Emerg Med. 1992; 10(5):656

[32] Bracken MB, Shepard MJ, Holford TR, et al. Administration of methylprednisolone for 24 or 48 hours or tirilazad mesylate for 48 hours in the treatment of acute spinal cord injury: results of the Third National Acute Spinal Cord Injury Randomized Controlled Trial. National Acute Spinal Cord Injury Study. JAMA. 1997; 277(20):1597–1604. Accessed February 3, 2019

[33] Walters BC, Hadley MN, Hurlbert RJ, et al. American Association of Neurological Surgeons, Congress of Neurological Surgeons. Guidelines for the management of acute cervical spine and spinal cord injuries: 2013 update. Neurosurgery. 2013; 60 CN_suppl_1:82–91

[34] Fehlings MG, Kwon BK, Tetreault LA. Guidelines for the management of degenerative cervical myelopathy and spinal cord injury: an introduction to a focus issue. Global Spine J. 2017; 7(3) Suppl:6S–7S

[35] Schroeder GD, Kwon BK, Eck JC, Savage JW, Hsu WK, Patel AA. Survey of Cervical Spine Research Society members on the use of high-dose steroids for acute spinal cord injuries. Spine. 2014; 39(12):971–977

[36] Jain NB, Ayers GD, Peterson EN, et al. Traumatic spinal cord injury in the United States, 1993–2012. JAMA. 2015; 313 (22):2236–2243

[37] Jones T, Ugalde V, Franks P, Zhou H, White RH. Venous thromboembolism after spinal cord injury: incidence, time course, and associated risk factors in 16,240 adults and children. Arch Phys Med Rehabil. 2005; 86(12): 2240–2247

[38] Maung AA, Schuster KM, Kaplan LJ, Maerz LL, Davis KA. Risk of venous thromboembolism after spinal cord injury: not all levels are the same. J Trauma. 2011; 71(5):1241–1245

[39] Spinal Cord Injury Thromboprophylaxis Investigators. Prevention of venous thromboembolism in the acute treatment phase after spinal cord injury: a randomized, multicenter trial comparing low-dose heparin plus intermittent pneumatic compression with enoxaparin. J Trauma. 2003; 54(6): 1116–1124, discussion 1125–1126

[40] Teasell RW, Hsieh JT, Aubut J-AL, Eng JJ, Krassioukov A, Tu L, Spinal Cord Injury Rehabilitation Evidence Review Research Team. Venous thromboembolism after spinal cord injury. Arch Phys Med Rehabil. 2009; 90(2):232–245

[41] Aito S, Pieri A, D'Andrea M, Marcelli F, Cominelli E. Primary prevention of deep venous thrombosis and pulmonary embolism in acute spinal cord injured patients. Spinal Cord. 2002; 40(6):300–303

[42] Kwon BK, Casha S, Hurlbert RJ, Yong VW. Inflammatory and structural biomarkers in acute traumatic spinal cord injury. Clin Chem Lab Med. 2011; 49(3):425–433

[43] Kwon BK, Streijger F, Fallah N, et al. Cerebrospinal fluid biomarkers to stratify injury severity and predict outcome in human traumatic spinal cord injury. J Neurotrauma. 2017; 34(3):567–580

[44] Nieto-Diaz M, Esteban FJ, Reigada D, et al. MicroRNA dysregulation in spinal cord injury: causes, consequences and therapeutics. Front Cell Neurosci. 2014; 8:53

[45] Stroman PW, Wheeler-Kingshott C, Bacon M, et al. The current state-of-the-art of spinal cord imaging: methods. Neuroimage. 2014; 84:1070–1081

10 Cervical Spine Injuries

Azeem Tariq Malik, Nikhil Jain, Jeffery Kim, and Safdar N. Khan

Abstract

Trauma to the cervical spine is a relatively rare occurrence associated with high morbidity and mortality. The current chapter provides a brief overview of the clinical anatomy of the cervical spine, the varying types of presentations, associated emergent and surgical management of these injuries, and their eventual prognosis.

Keywords: trauma, cervical spine, injury, fracture, dislocation, surgical technique

10.1 Introduction to Demographics and Epidemiology/Prevalence

10.1.1 Introduction

Injury to the cervical spine is a relatively rare, yet important, manifestation associated with blunt trauma presentations to emergency departments.[1] Despite the low prevalence of this injury, it has been associated with high costs, spinal cord injury (SCI), and mortality.[2] Globally, studies have reported an overall incidence rate of cervical spine injury to range between 2 and 12 per 100,000 populations.[3,4,5,6,7,8,9] However, the actual incidence may even be higher due to the numerous variants and complex patterns of the injury itself, up to 30% of the cervical spine trauma cases are often missed from inadequate radiological examinations[10,11,12] and immature spine formation in children.[13] A recent large-scale database analysis of over 480,000 patients in the United States Nationwide Inpatient Sample (NIS) database showed that overall incidence of cervical spine fractures had increased from 4.1% in 2005 to 5.4% in 2013.[8] Due to a relative lack of large-scale national studies from the United States (US) on the epidemiology of this topic, it is difficult to derive a confirmative number of the incidence of these injuries as the majority of past reported studies are based off estimates from single-study sample sizes that may not be generalized to a national population. Individual incidences of each type of cervical spine injury, based on classification systems, have been reported in the forthcoming relevant subsections of this chapter.

10.1.2 Demographics and Mechanisms of Injury

The incidence of cervical spine injuries typically increases with age, and these injuries have a bimodal occurrence, with the majority of injuries happening between the age group of 15 and 45 years or in elderly individuals over the age of 60 years.[14] Historically, literature has reported that the majority of the injuries are lower cervical (subaxial) in nature, accounting for two-thirds of all cervical injuries.[6] However, recent US based-literature has reported that nearly 32% of injuries involve closed C2 fractures, followed by 21% diagnosed as C7 closed fractures.[8] Around 1% of the cases have associated SCI.[15] While still rare in occurrence, around 1 to 9% of cervical spine injuries also occur in children.[16,17] One of the large-scale epidemiological investigations on CSIs in children < 18 by the National Emergency X-Radiography Utilization Study (NEXUS) reported that nearly 46% of these injuries occurred in the lower cervical spine (C5–C7).[17] Concurrently, Platzer et al analyzed a small case-series of 56 young patients with varying age groups and found that younger children (< 8 years) were more likely to have an injury of the upper cervical spine, whereas older children (9–16 years) more commonly suffered lower cervical spine injuries.[16] It is important to stress that in the pediatric/young population, these injuries often occur in concurrence with head injuries, which can increase their mortality rate up to 40%.[18] The most common mechanism of injury in the pediatric population is a high-mechanism etiology, such as motor vehicle accidents and/or pedestrians hit by vehicles; whereas in older children, injuries were likely to be sustained by sporting activities.[16] A large proportion of lower cervical injuries take place in the elderly, associated with motor vehicle accidents—however, studies have reported a decreasing trend due to an associated increase in traffic regulations worldwide.

10.2 Clinical Anatomy

The cervical spine consists of seven vertebrae (C1–C7), each having their own set of unique articulating joints that play a major role in functionality and complex movements of the neck. Based on similarities in the clinical anatomy, these vertebrae are divided into two major groups: upper cervical (consisting of C1 and C2) and lower cervical/subaxial (C3–C7).

10.2.1 Anatomy of the Upper Cervical Spine

The upper cervical spine, consisting of the atlas (C1) and axis (C2), forms an intricate three-joint unit with the occiput, through articulations and associated ligamentous attachments, to bring about the vital movements at the craniocervical junction. There are a total of six articulating joints (two pairs of occipitoatlantal, atlantoaxial, and the anterior and posterior median atlanto-odontoid joints) in the upper cervical spine which play a major role in determining the range of motion of the neck.

The atlas is a unique C-shaped bone, lacking a vertebral body and spinous process. Lateral masses on each side of the atlas are formed by a superior articular process (which articulates with the clivus of the occipital condyle), an inferior articular surface (which articulates with the superior articular process of the axis [C2]), and a transverse process, containing the transverse foramen (through which the vertebral artery passes). The occipitoatlantal joints are formed by synovial articulations between the convex occipital condyle of the cranium and concave superior articular surface of the atlas. The occipitoatlantal joints are key contributors to flexion/extension (13–15 degrees) and lateral flexion (3–8 degrees) movements of the cervical spine. No rotation takes place at this joint.

Contrary to the atlas, and similar to the remaining vertebrae of the lower cervical spine, the axis (C2) has a vertebral body and spinous process. The axis is also unique in its structure due to a central cranially projecting odontoid process, which is attached to the C1 (via anterior and posterior atlanto-odontoid joints), and the clivus of the occipital condyle by means of ligamentous attachments to atlantoaxial joints supplying rotatory movements (45–50 degrees), with the intercalating ligamentous attachments bringing about overall stability.

When "picturing" the clinical anatomy of the upper vertebrae, it is necessary to describe the ligamentous structures that are a part of the upper cervical spine. There are three main ligamentous complexes in the upper cervical spine—the ligaments supporting the occipital-atlantoaxial joint (anterior atlanto-occipital membrane, the posterior atlanto-occipital membrane, and the tectorial membrane), the occipital-axis joint (apical ligament, cruciform ligament, and the alar ligament), the atlantoaxial complex (transverse portion of cruciform ligament, ligamentum flavum, and accessory atlantoaxial ligaments), and the nuchal ligament (the elastic ligament that merges with the supraspinous ligament, and provides the stretch during neck flexion)— which interplay with each other and the vertebrae to contribute to the stability.

10.2.2 Anatomy of the Lower Cervical Spine

The lower cervical spine (C3–C7) is largely similar in terms of morphology and functionality, with the exception of the C7 vertebrae. C7 is exposed to large amounts of stresses transmitted from the cranium to the thoracic, due to its important articulation with the first thoracic vertebrae to form the cervicothoracic junction. The sizes of the vertebral bodies increase as one moves caudally, with C7 having a large spinous process for the attachment of the nuchal ligaments on either side. On the superior surface of each vertebral body is a cranially rising uncinate process. This is known to hypertrophy with age, and cause significant foraminal stenosis.

The lower cervical vertebrae articulate with each other by means of the intervertebral disc and paired zygoapophyseal facet joints of the superior and inferior articular facets. Two large ligamentous complexes, the anterior longitudinal ligament (ALL) and posterior longitudinal ligament (PLL), are responsible for maintaining the stability of the lower cervical spine. Contrary to upper cervical spine, ligamentous injury is relatively common in the lower cervical spine. The ALL is a continuation of the ALL from the thoracic spine and ends at the C2. The PLL continues above the C2, as the tectorial membrane complex of the upper cervical spine, to attach to the base of the foramen magnum of the skull.

10.3 Radiology

A number of imaging modalities, such as plain radiography (X-rays), computed tomography (CT), and magnetic resonance imaging (MRI), currently exist to diagnose upper and lower cervical spine injuries. Up to 10% of cervical spine injuries have multiple levels, and therefore imaging should be performed for both upper and cervical spine to prevent any missed injuries. X-rays are usually the first imaging modality. Despite up to 90% of all injuries of the upper cervical spine being easily detected on the true lateral view, it is necessary to ensure that both the anteroposterior (AP) and open-mouth views are also ordered as the sensitivity with all three views is known to rise up to 93% (vs. 82% sensitivity of lateral view alone). When evaluating a true-lateral view for the first time, it helps to read the radiograph using a systemic process. First, one should assess for overall cervical spine alignment by forming imaginary lines at anterior and posterior borders of the vertebrae, the spinolaminar line, and the tips of the spinous process. If abnormality is noted, one should then look at the spinous processes to note any widening, which is indicative of ligamentous injury. Finally, the degree of angulation of the spine needs to be evaluated. An angulation of more than 11 degrees should be suspicious for a ligamentous injury and/or fracture. Since ligamentous injury of the upper cervical spine is rare, and difficult to pick up, it is vital to carefully evaluate the soft-tissue swelling on true lateral views that may be the only indicator of ligamentous disruption/injury. AP views are less clinically useful for picking up fractures, with a nonalignment of the spinous processes to be the only indicator of possible rotational injury/facet dislocation. CT scans still remain the most sensitive modality to evaluate suspected injuries of the cervical spine. The superiority of the CT is established by its ability to accurately predict fracture type/pattern at locations, such as the craniocervical junction and C1, which may be difficult to interpret and visualize on standard X-ray. The utility of the MRI in cervical spine injuries is largely limited to assessing for soft tissue/ligamentous disruption and/or spinal cord damage.

10.4 Clinical Presentation and Initial Management

Prior to hospital admission, first-responders need to bear in mind several concerns when arriving at the setting of a trauma patient with suspected spinal injury. First and foremost, the cervical spine should be immobilized with a cervical collar to prevent additional and possibly catastrophic damage to the spinal cord while transferring. Presence of co-existing superficial injury such as abrasion, laceration, and hemorrhage at the region of the

neck or face should raise suspicion of an underlying injury. The cervical collar needs to be in place until a possible unstable injury is ruled out via confirmatory radiography and examination. Initial assessment should involve assessment of associated injuries, followed by a complete neurological examination using the American Spinal Injury Association (ASIA) criteria.[19] Based on clinical symptoms and signs, providers should do a thorough assessment to clear the cervical spine. Asymptomatic patients can be ruled out, using the NEXUS[20] or Canadian Cervical Spine Rule (CCR) criteria,[21] both of which have very good sensitivity. Patients with impaired cognitive function or concurrent injuries located in other extremities should be cleared after 24 to 48 hours. If immediate clearance is required, as in the case of obtunded patients, then timely CT or MRI are preferred imaging modalities for picking up underlying cervical spine injury. Symptomatic patients can undergo conventional radiography or CT scan to rule out possible injury.

10.5 Classification and Treatment

10.5.1 Upper Cervical Spine Injuries

Occipital Condyle

In general, this type of fracture is caused by accidents involving high-energy trauma, such as motor vehicle accidents and sports-related injuries. Younger males, in the second and third decades of life, are typically affected.[22] The incidence of occipital condyle fractures is reported to range from 3% to 16%.[23,24] Extension of the upper part of the cervical spine is limited mainly by the transverse portion of the alar ligaments. When flexion is added to the head rotation, the alar ligament is maximally stretched, and the cervical spine becomes more vulnerable to injury.[25]

The clinical presentation of these injuries can range from minimal deficits to frank quadriparesis. Symptoms and signs can include high cervical pain, torticollis, headaches, and impaired mobility. The most severe neurologic deficits are often seen with concurrent head injury and up to 31% may have acute lower cranial nerve deficits.

CT scan with reconstruction is the imaging modality of choice in the diagnosis and classification of these fractures. MRI can be used to assess for damage to the alar and tectorial membrane but is less useful than CT from a treatment perspective. The occipitocervical transition should be carefully evaluated, particularly in patients with associated facial and cranial trauma.[22]

In 1988, Anderson and Montesano proposed a classification for fractures of the occipital condyle according to the regional anatomy, biomechanics of the structures involved, and fracture morphology.[26] Three types of occipital condyle fractures have been described (▶ Fig. 10.1).

Type I and type II fractures can be treated with a rigid cervical orthosis. Type III injuries can be treated initially with an orthosis or halo vest. However, posterior occipitocervical fusion may be necessary for chronic pain, neurologic deficit, or instability. Because type I injuries can result in considerable articular incongruity, the outcome often depends on the presence or absence of symptomatic posttraumatic arthritis, which may result in neck pain, occipital headaches, restricted occipitocervical motion, and torticollis. Type II and isolated type III injuries generally pose less risk of posttraumatic arthritis because of the lower likelihood of articular incongruity. However, if these injuries are components of occipitocervical dissociation, the prognosis is worse.

Atlanto-Occipital Injuries

The incidence of atlanto-occipital joint injuries is estimated between 5% and 8% of fatal traffic injuries.[27] Children younger than 12 years of age are predisposed to this injury because their atlanto-occipital joints are flatter and their head weight to body weight ratio is significantly greater than adults.

Radiographically, significant retropharyngeal soft tissue swelling is seen at C3. Multiple anatomic lines mark the normal relationship of occiput to C1. The Wackenheim line, a line drawn down the cranial aspect of the clivus should be tangential to the dens. Distance greater than 10 mm between the basion and the dens is considered abnormal.[28] The Powers ratio (▶ Fig. 10.2), the ratio of the distance from the basion to the posterior arch of the atlas divided by the distance from the opisthion to the anterior arch of the atlas, should be 1.0 or less in the absence of anterior occipitoatlantal dislocation.[29] Another method on plain radiographs is by the Harris lines, a posterior axial line as the cranial extent of the posterior cortex of the axis body. If the distance between the basion and the posterior axial line (the basion-axial interval [BAI]) is greater than 12 mm, or if the basion-dental interval is greater than 12 mm, then occipitocervical instability is present (▶ Fig. 10.3).[30,31]

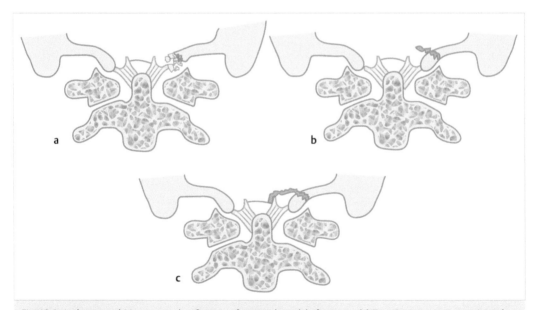

Fig. 10.1 Anderson and Montesano classification of occipital condyle fractures. **(a)** Type I injuries are comminuted, stable impaction fractures caused by axial loading. **(b)** Type II injuries are impaction or shear fractures extending into the base of the skull and are usually stable. **(c)** Type III injuries are alar ligament avulsion fractures and represent unstable distraction injuries of the craniocervical junction. (Source: Smorgick Y, Fischgrund JS. Occipitocervical injuries. Semin Spine Surg 2013;25(1):14–22, ISSN 1040–7383, https://doi.org/10.1053/j.semss.2012.07.004.)

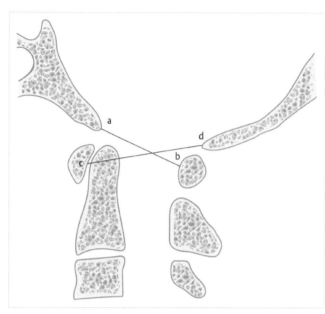

Fig. 10.2 Midsagittal section through the craniocervical junction and demonstration of application of Power's ratio. a, basion; d, opisthion; c, anterior arch of the atlas; b, posterior arch of the atlas. The ratio of ab/cd should always be ≤ 1. If it is > 1, the patient most likely has an anterior occipitocervical subluxation or dislocation. (Source: Smorgick Y, Fischgrund JS. Occipitocervical injuries. Semin Spine Surg 2013;25(1):14–22, ISSN 1040–7383, https://doi.org/10.1053/j.semss.2012.07.004.)

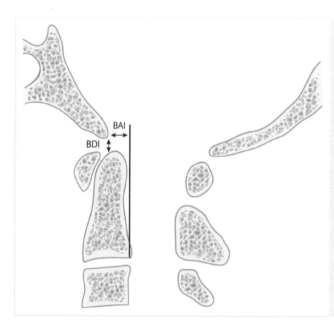

Fig. 10.3 Harris radiographic lines for assessing occipitocervical alignment: If either the basion-dens interval (BDI) or the basion-axial interval (BAI) is greater than 12 mm long on sagittal computed tomography or lateral radiographic measurement, occipitocervical dissociation should be suspected. Because these measurements are more sensitive than they are specific, normal parameters do not exclude the presence of occipitocervical dissociation. PAL, posterior axial line. (Source: Smorgick Y, Fischgrund JS. Occipitocervical injuries. Semin Spine Surg 2013;25(1):14–22, ISSN 1040–7383, https://doi.org/10.1053/j.semss.2012.07.004.)

The most commonly employed classification system for occiput-C1 dislocations was described by Traynelis and colleagues (▶ Fig. 10.4).[32] In type I injuries, there is anterior displacement of the occiput on the atlas. Type II injuries are the result of longitudinal distraction. Any traction applied to a type II injury can result in progression of the existing neurologic deficit. Type III injuries involve a posterior subluxation or dislocation. Very light traction of about 5 pounds applied to type I and type III injuries will help to reduce the dislocation and may improve the neurologic deficit. Radiographs should be taken immediately to ensure that there is no overdistraction.

Signs of instability are translation or distraction of more than 2 mm in any plane,[33] neurologic injury, and concomitant cerebrovascular trauma.[34] There may be less easily recognized unstable occipitocervical dissociative injuries that must be segregated into the following two groups: (1) patients

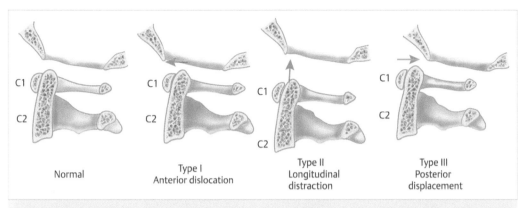

Fig. 10.4 Classification system of Traynelis and coworkers, which describes occipitocervical subluxation and dislocation. (Source: Pneumaticos SG, Triantafyllopoulos GK. Atlantoaxial rotatory fixation. In: Lasanianos N, Kanakaris N, Giannoudis P, eds. Trauma and Orthopaedic Classifications. London: Springer;2015.)

Table 10.1 Harborview classification of craniocervical injuries

Stage	Description
1	Evidence of injury to craniocervical osseoligamentous stabilizers on MRI
	Craniocervical alignment within 2 mm of normal
	Presence of distraction of ≤ 2 mm on provocative traction radiography
2	Evidence of injury to craniocervical osseoligamentous stabilizers on MRI
	Evidence of craniocervical alignment within 2 mm of normal
	Presence of distraction of ≤ 2 mm on provocative traction radiography
3	Presence of craniocervical malalignment of > 2 mm on *static* radiographic studies

with relatively stable injuries who can be treated nonoperatively and (2) patients with highly unstable but partially reduced injuries who require operative stabilization in spite of a misleadingly low degree of displacement. Manual traction testing can be useful in patients with minimally displaced injuries with evidence of extensive occipitocervical injury (ligamentous injury, soft tissue swelling, neurologic or cerebrovascular abnormalities). Surgical stabilization can be reserved for patients with type II and III injuries of the occipitocervical junction, which are defined as dissociations according to the Harborview classification system (▶ Table 10.1).[35]

All occipitocervical dislocations should be treated initially by immediate application of a halo vest. Because the majority of these injuries are unstable, posterior occipitocervical fusion is the procedure of choice.[36,37] This can be done using a variety of techniques, including posterior wiring and structural grafting, Ransford loop fixation with wiring, and plate and rod and screw fixation with structural grafting. The first technique will require the use of postoperative halo immobilization; the latter two techniques will usually only need collar immobilization as external support. Improvements in occipital plate designs allow multiple points of fixation in the occiput, especially in the midline, where the occipital bone is thicker, providing significantly better initial fixation than off-midline plate-rod constructs.[38]

Atlas Fractures

Atlas fractures represent 2% of all vertebral spine fractures and occur when an axial (vertical) compression of the skull on the atlas forces it onto the axis, resulting in a rupture at the weakest points (the anterior and posterior arches) and causing the lateral masses to split; this is known as a Jefferson fracture.[39] Pressure exerted on the atlas may lead not only to fracture of the arches but also to rupture of the transverse ligament, which is the main structure that gives this vertebra its anterior stability and prevents it from slipping on the axis. Thus, in Jefferson fractures, the status of the transverse ligament is essential to the prognosis.[25] Levine and Edwards described a useful four-part classification system: (1) posterior arch fractures, (2) lateral mass fractures, (3) isolated anterior arch fractures, and (4) bursting-type fractures.[39]

Retropharyngeal soft tissue swelling greater than 5 mm at C3 in combination with a fracture of the posterior arch of C1 is highly suggestive

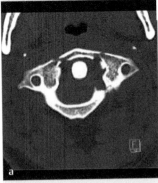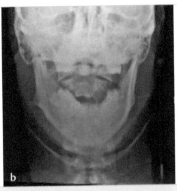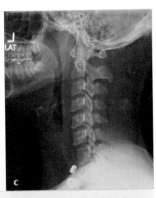

Fig. 10.5 A 28-year-old male involved in altercation sustaining a C1 arch fracture. (**a**) Axial CT image showing bilateral anterior arch fracture and left posterior arch fracture. (**b**) An open mouth odontoid view showing C1 lateral mass displacement. (**c**) It is a lateral X-ray of the cervical spine showing retropharyngeal swelling.

of a burst-type injury. A combined lateral mass displacement on the open-mouth AP view exceeding 6.9 mm is indicative of transverse ligament insufficiency,[40] but this measurement may not be sensitive enough to detect all unstable injuries. MRI can be used to help assess the continuity of the transverse ligament in those cases in which ligament status is unclear.[41] A case example of a C1 arch fracture with radiographic can be seen in ▶ Fig. 10.5.

Most C1 fractures can be treated nonoperatively. Indications for operative management are related mainly to the loss of transverse alar ligament (TAL) integrity, as suggested by combined lateral mass displacement of 6.9 mm or more, which introduces the potential for progressive lateral mass separation, C1–C2 instability, and pseudarthrosis.[42] Halo or rigid cervical collar immobilization alone may be insufficient to maintain acceptable alignment in these patients. If upright radiographs show further lateral mass displacement or an anterior ADI greater than 3 mm, patients must be treated either with prolonged recumbency in cranial tong traction or with operative stabilization, generally with posterior C1–C2 fixation.

Nonoperative treatment, generally in patients without evidence of TAL compromise, consists of either rigid collar or halo vest immobilization, depending on the surgeon's preference. Severe complications are rare. However, with nonoperatively treated fractures, patients have a 17% fracture nonunion rate and an 80% incidence of residual neck pain, possibly because of posttraumatic arthritis. Severe malunion of unstable atlas

fractures may result in painful torticollis, requiring realignment and posterior occipitocervical fusion. Surgical stabilization options consist of C1–C2 transarticular screw fixation or segmental C1–C2 screw and rod fixation. The latter method provides the opportunity to correct the C1 lateral mass widening by approximating the two rods with a cross connector, a procedure that must be performed with a reduction clamp before instrumentation if using the transarticular technique.

Internal fixation of the C1 ring, by simply re-approximating the lateral masses to each other through lateral mass screws connected to a transversely oriented rod, is a useful option that theoretically preserves the C1–C2 motion. A potential problem with direct repair of an unstable C1 fracture is that the associated TAL deficiency may result in persistent C1–C2 instability. However, unlike in shear or distractive injuries, the axial loading mechanism that causes TAL rupture in displaced C1 ring fractures allows secondary restraints to remain intact, thus minimizing any remaining atlantoaxial translational instability once the atlas has been stabilized.[21]

Atlantoaxial Subluxation and Dislocation

Three atlantoaxial instability patterns may manifest either as isolated or combined injuries (▶ Table 10.2).

Traumatic rotatory subluxation or dislocation in adults is most commonly caused by vehicular trauma. Like children, adults will present with a

Table 10.2 Atlantoaxial injuries

Injury type	Characteristics	Treatment
A	Rotation centered on the dens; TAL usually intact	Closed reduction and immobilization; beware of associated fractures
B	Translation between C1 and C2 with TAL disruption	Type 1 (midsubstance TAL tear): C1–C2 arthrodesis Type 2 (TAL avulsion fracture): halo vest versus C1–C2 arthrodesis
C	Distraction injury	Open reduction and posterior instrumented arthrodesis

Abbreviation: TAL, transverse alar ligament.

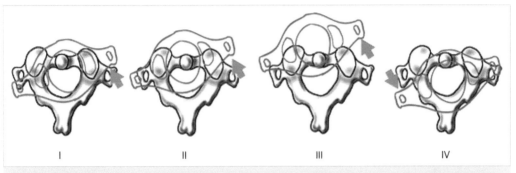

Fig. 10.6 Fielding and Hawkins Classification of Rotatory Atlantoaxial Instability. Type I: rotatory fixation with no anterior displacement and the odontoid acting as the pivot. Type II: rotatory fixation with anterior displacement of 3 to 5 mm, with one lateral articular process acting as the pivot. Type III: rotatory fixation with anterior displacement of > 5 mm. Type IV: rotatory fixation with posterior displacement. (Source: Pneumaticos SG, Triantafyllopoulos GK. Atlantoaxial Rotatory Fixation. In: Lasanianos N, Kanakaris N, Giannoudis P, eds. Trauma and Orthopaedic Classifications. London: Springer; 2015.)

"cock robin" appearance, with the head tilted toward and rotated away from the side of the dislocation. Fielding and Hawkins presented the most commonly used classification scheme for these injuries.[43] Type I dislocations are pure rotational injuries. Type II injuries have both rotatory malalignment with anterior displacement of the atlas less than 3 to 5 mm, suggesting only a mild deficiency of the transverse ligament. Type III injuries combine rotatory subluxation with greater than 5 mm of displacement, suggesting complete deficiency of the transverse ligament. Type IV injuries have both rotational malalignment and posterior displacement (▶ Fig. 10.6).

Rupture of the Transverse Ligament

Insufficiency of the transverse ligament and subsequent C1–C2 instability is suspected if the atlanto-dens interval is greater than 3.5 mm in adults and greater than 5 mm in children on lateral radiographs and in atlas fractures when the combined overhang of the C1 lateral masses on C2 is greater than 6.9 mm on an AP open-mouth view of the upper cervical spine.[40,41] Plain radiographs, however, are often inadequate to assess suspected transverse ligament injuries; a combination of MRI, CT, and dynamic radiographs is often needed to fully assess the type and extent of injury.[41]

Dickman and colleagues classified transverse ligament injuries into two types.[41] Type I injuries encompass intrasubstance ruptures. Type IA injuries occur in the mid-portion of the ligament. Type IB injuries occur at the periosteal insertion of the ligament onto the atlas. Type II injuries occur when there is an avulsion of the tubercular insertion of the transverse ligament from the C1 lateral mass. Type IIA injuries occur if the lateral mass is comminuted, and type IIB injuries occur if the lateral mass is intact.

Type I injuries should be treated surgically with C1–C2 fusion. The most common way to achieve this is posteriorly. Wiring techniques, such as Brooks and Gallie fusions, are effective more than 90% of the time, but are the least biomechanically stable, and a rigid cervical collar is usually used for 3 months postoperatively. Transarticular screw fixation provides sufficient additional stability to allow the immobilization time to be reduced to 6 weeks in a rigid collar or even to allow the patient to be immobilized in a soft cervical collar. There is, however, risk to the vertebral artery when instrumentation is done across the pars interarticularis of C2. C1 lateral mass screw and C2 pedicle screw constructs provide comparable biomechanical rigidity to transarticular screws with less risk to the vertebral artery but with more risk to the internal carotid artery. If necessary, sacrificing the C2 nerve root provides direct visualization of the C1 lateral mass and the C1–C2 joint. The structures can then be instrumented, reduced, and fused under direct visualization. The combination of C1 lateral mass screws connected to C2 translaminar screws is another alternative fixation option that provides the same degree of stability of the C1–C2 complex. C1–C2 fusion can also be achieved by an anterior approach with anteriorly placed C1–C2 screws. Proponents of this technique note that there is less soft tissue dissection involved as compared with posterior approaches. Type II fractures can be treated with external immobilization for 3 months. Up to 74% of these type II injuries will heal with nonoperative care.[44]

Fractures of the Odontoid

Classification of these fractures is based on their location in the odontoid. The most commonly used classification scheme was described by Anderson and D'Alonzo. Type I fractures consist of avulsion injuries at the tip of the dens. Type II fractures occur through the base of the dens at the junction of the dens and the central body of the axis. Type III fractures extend into the body of the axis (▶ Fig. 10.7).[45]

Treatment of type I odontoid fractures relates to their impact on occipitocervical stability. Surgical indications for type II odontoid fractures remain controversial. Fractures for which surgical stabilization can clearly be advocated include fractures with distractive patterns of displacement and those associated with SCI. Relative indications

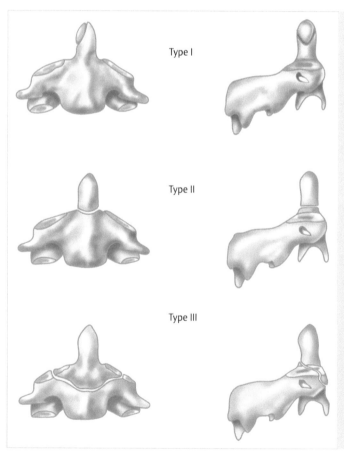

Type I

Type II

Type III

Fig. 10.7 Anderson D'Alonzo odontoid fracture classification. (Source: Kokkino AJ, Lazio BE, Perin NI. Vertical fracture of the odontoid process: case report. Neurosurgery 1996;38(1): 200–203, reproduced from the original "Anderson LD, D'Alonzo RT. Fractures of the odontoid process of the axis. J Bone Joint Surg Am. 1974;56:1663–1674.")

include multiple injuries, associated closed head injury, initial displacement greater than 4 mm, angulation of more than 10 degrees,[46] delayed presentation (> 2 weeks), multiple risk factors for nonunion, the inability to treat with a halo because of advanced age or body habitus,[47] associated cranial or thoracoabdominal injury, other medical comorbidities, and the presence of associated upper cervical fractures.

Operative stabilization of type III injuries is not commonly required, but it is warranted in patients with SCI or distractive instability patterns. Relative indications include highly displaced irreducible fractures, displaced injuries in patients who cannot be treated with a halo, and fractures with initial displacement of 5 mm or more, which have a high potential for nonunion (▶ Table 10.3).[42] A case example can be seen in ▶ Fig. 10.8.

Table 10.3 Odontoid fractures

Injury type	Distinguishing characteristics	Treatment
I	Avulsion at alar ligament insertion	Treated surgically if associated with occipitocervical dissociation
II	Fracture at waist of odontoid process	High risk of nonunion; options include halo vest versus anterior odontoid screw versus posterior C1–C2 arthrodesis, depending on displacement, fracture pattern, and bone quality
III	Fracture extending into cancellous bone within C2 vertebral	Halo versus cervical collar; distraction injuries require posterior C1–C2 arthrodesis

Traumatic Spondylolisthesis of the Axis (Hangman Fractures)

Traumatic spondylolisthesis of the axis, or the hangman fracture, is classified by the modification by Levine and Edwards[48] and by Starr and Eismont[49] of the original classification by Effendi and associates[50] into three primary injury types and two atypical subtypes (▶ Fig. 10.9):

Type I: Minimally displaced (≤ 3 mm), relatively stable fractures of the pars interarticularis that result from hyperextension and axial loading.

Type IA: Atypical unstable lateral bending fractures that are obliquely displaced, with a fracture through one pars and more anteriorly into the body on the contralateral side.

Type II: Displaced injuries (> 3 mm) that occur when a flexion force follows the initial hyperextension and axial loading insult; these may be visible only on upright radiographs if they are spontaneously reduced on supine imaging.

Type IIA: Unstable injury with associated C2–C3 disc and interspinous ligament disruption caused by a flexion-distraction mechanism, in which kyphosis is the prevailing deformity rather than translation.

Type III: Highly unstable injuries in which the pars interarticularis fractures are associated with dislocation of the C2–C3 facet joints.

Most injuries can be treated effectively with a rigid collar or halo immobilization; the pseudarthrosis rate is low, on the order of 5%.[48] Surgical treatment is generally reserved for atypical (type IA), type IIA, and type III fractures, which constitute a greater treatment challenge as a result of their atypical fracture orientation, the amount of displacement, or the associated ligamentous injury. The usefulness of direct osteosynthesis for type II hangman fractures has been questioned

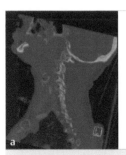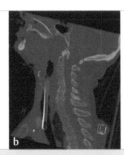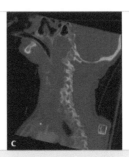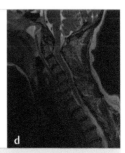

Fig. 10.8 A 55-year-old female who fell, sustaining a C2 dens fracture-dislocation and complete spinal cord injury. **(a–c)** Sagittal images of her cervical spine computed tomography (CT) showing the C2 fracture and bilateral C1–C2 articulations. **(d)** A midsagittal cut of her magnetic resonance imaging (MRI) cervical spine with focal edema/spinal cord signal change.

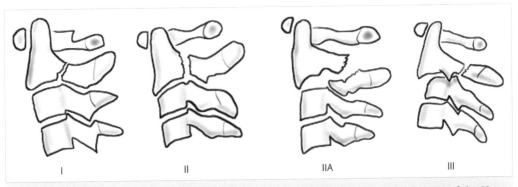

| I | II | IIA | III |

Fig. 10.9 Classification of traumatic spondylolisthesis of the axis. Type I hangman fracture has fractures of the C2 pedicles bilaterally with no angulation and with as much as 3 mm of displacement. Type II fractures have both significant angulation and significant displacement. Type IIA fractures show minimum displacement, but there is severe angulation, apparently hinging from the anterior longitudinal ligament. These fractures have disruption through the disc space and are easily overdistracted with even small amounts of traction. Type III hangman fracture combines bilateral facet dislocations between the second and third cervical vertebra with the fracture of the neural arch. This group of patients will always require surgery to reduce the dislocated facets. (Source: Pneumaticos SG, Triantafyllopoulos GK. Atlantoaxial rotatory fixation. In: Lasanianos N, Kanakaris N, Giannoudis P, eds. Trauma and Orthopaedic Classifications. London: Springer; 2015.)

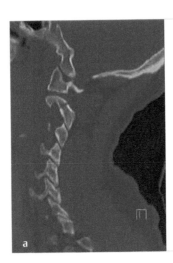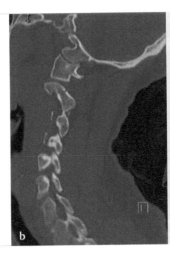

Fig. 10.10 (a) A 24-year-old male involved in ATV accident, sustaining C2 traumatic spondylolisthesis with fractures of his bilateral pars and (b) a left C2–C3 perched facet.

because nonoperative treatment is so effective and because this technique does not address the associated injury to the C2–C3 intervertebral disc.

For the treatment of type IA and IIA fractures, options for minimizing the number of fused levels include C2–C3 anterior cervical discectomy and fusion (ACDF) with plating, as opposed to posterior C2–C3 instrumented fusion, which also requires direct osteosynthesis of the pars interarticularis fracture with C2 pars or pedicle screws. The disadvantage of anterior C2–C3 ACDF is that it compromises the ALL and anterior annulus, the only remaining intact major ligamentous structures at C2–C3. Dysphagia, dysphonia, and swallowing

difficulties are also relatively common with anterior or upper cervical exposures, and access to the C2–C3 level anteriorly can be challenging.[42]

Posterior stabilization is more versatile and stable, but unless adequate purchase can be achieved across the fractured C2 pars interarticularis, loss of atlantoaxial motion results from the need to extend fixation to C1. Stabilization options for type III injuries include posterior C1–C3 fusion, posterior C2–C3 fusion using lag screws across the fracture at C2, and anterior C2–C3 ACDF only in the unusual event that reduction occurs by closed methods.[42] Case examples can be seen in ► Fig. 10.10 and ► Fig. 10.11.

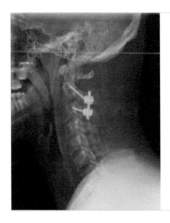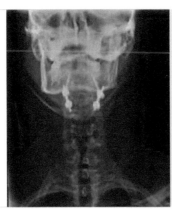

Fig. 10.11 Postoperative images showing C2–C3 posterior cervical fusion with C2 pedicle screws and C3 lateral mass screws.

10.5.2 Subaxial Cervical Spine Injuries

Classification

Many classification systems of lower cervical spine injuries have been described, although none are universally accepted. These systems are based on fracture morphology, presumed mechanism, force vectors of injury, or ratings of severity, such as stable versus unstable.

The subaxial cervical injury classification (SLIC) system was developed to include both severity of injury and the neurologic state to aid in surgical decision making.[51] Three domains are assessed and graded independently: fracture morphology, the osteoligamentous complex, and neurologic function (▶ Table 10.4). The morphology is graded based on a general description of the fracture mechanism: compression, burst, distraction, and translation/rotation. Each of the three domains are scored and summed, giving an SLIC score ranging from 0 to 9. Scores of 3 or less are treated nonoperatively, and scores of greater than 5 are treated surgically. Scores of 4 or 5 may be treated either nonoperatively or operatively. In many cases, an orthosis is attempted and upright serial radiographs are obtained to assess maintenance of alignment. If neurologic symptoms or progressive kyphosis or subluxation develops, then surgery is warranted.

The AO system uses four criteria: injury morphology, facet injury, neurologic status, and case-specific modifiers. When using the system, the user should record level, morphology type, and secondary injuries. In addition, modifiers such as facet injury, neurologic status, and case-specific variants are placed in parentheses. The modified

Table 10.4 Subaxial cervical injury classification (SLIC) system

	Points
Fracture morphology	
Compression	1
Burst	2
Distraction	3
Translation/rotation	4
Discoligamentous complex	
Intact	0
Intermediate	1
Disrupted	2
Neurologic	
Intact	0
Root injury	1
Complete spinal cord injury	2
Incomplete spinal cord injury	3
Ongoing cord compression in setting of neurologic deficit	+ 1
Total SLIC	**0–9**

AO classification system has been updated to simplify its use, promote better direction for treatment, and is based on modern imaging, including MRI. Three basic categories describe the primary injury (▶ Table 10.5).[52] Type A occurs from compressive forces with intact posterior tension band. Type B is distractive injuries of the posterior or anterior tension bands. A type C injury is described as translational displacement in any of the primary axes, including anteroposterior (AP), lateral, rotational, or vertical. If multiple types of injuries are present, then the fracture is graded with its highest score.

Table 10.5 Modified AO classification cervical spine injuries

Type A	A0	No bony or trivial injury
	A1	Compression fracture of only single endplate
	A2	Compression fracture involving two endplates
	A3	Burst fracture with bone retropulsion involving only single endplate
	A4	Burst fracture with bone retropulsion involving both endplates
Type B	B1	Bony injury of either anterior or posterior tension bands
	B2	Posterior ligamentous distractive injury with or without fracture
	B3	Anterior discoligamentous disruption
Type C	C	Translation or rotational injury along any axis
Facet injuries	F1	Nondisplaced facet injury with low potential for subluxation (< 1 cm and < 40% facet)
	F2	Nondisplaced facet injury with low potential for subluxation (> 1 cm and > 40% facet)
	F3	Fracture separation of lateral mass
	F4	Perched facets
Neurologic	N0	Intact
	N1	Transient neurologic deficit
	N2	Root injury or radiculopathy
	N3	Incomplete spinal cord injury
	N4	Complete spinal cord injury
Case-specific modifiers	M1	Possible ligamentous injury
	M2	Traumatic disc herniation
	M3	Fracture in ankylosed spine
	M4	Vertebral artery injury

The fundamental principles of operative intervention are to maximize ultimate neurologic function through neural decompression and to restore spinal alignment and stability while preserving motion segments when possible. In general, the choice of surgical approach, whether anterior or posterior, is based on the location of the pathologic features and the extent of instability. Combined anterior and posterior approaches may be necessary if the extent of the injury warrants them.

Compression and burst injuries to the subaxial spine typically are caused by axial loading. These injuries can result in end plate and vertebral body injury with or without disruption of the discoligamentous complex (DLC). Neurologic status and the presence of residual spinal cord compression typically dictate treatment. In burst-type fractures in which bone is retropulsed into the spinal canal and causes neurologic injury, anterior corpectomy and stabilization comprise the preferred treatment. This treatment allows for direct removal of the impinging bone and realignment and stabilization of the cervical spine. In the presence of intact posterior elements, anterior decompression (corpectomy), fixation, and strut graft provide adequate stability.[53]

Hyperextension distraction injuries typically occur in the stiff spondylotic or ankylosed spine and can be highly unstable. These injuries occur through distraction in the anterior column with sequential propagation through the middle and posterior columns. Radiographically, this injury is typically seen with distraction through the anterior column, usually with a gaped open disc space. The presence of posterior element fractures is typically the result of posterior compression of the lamina or facet joints. These injuries are generally highly unstable and frequently associated with an incomplete central SCI. A widened disc space may be the only apparent radiographic abnormality, and CT may reveal bilateral pedicle fractures. This injury is also observed in patients with near ankylosis secondary to advanced degenerative spondylosis. Surgical management of these lesions should be customized to the patient, the specific injury, and the surgeon's preference. When injuries occur through a spondylotic and ankylosed spine, posterior segmental stabilization may be necessary to achieve adequate fixation points above and below the injury and thus provide adequate spinal stability. Because these injuries act as "long bone fractures," single-level fixation above and below the fracture may not be sufficient.

In patients with a distractive extension injury and a normal, mobile, non-ankylosed spine, consideration of isolated anterior discectomy and fusion with plate fixation alone may be sufficient. In the case of focal or fixed kyphosis, or anterior compression from disc protrusion or a spondylotic bar, anterior surgical decompression and fusion are indicated.[53]

In contrast to distraction injuries, hyperflexion injuries begin with distraction of the posterior elements and propagate anteriorly. In these cases, disruption of the supraspinous and interspinous ligaments with injury to the facet and facet joint can result in injuries ranging from nondisplaced unilateral facet fractures and lateral mass separations to complete bilateral facet fracture-dislocations. The role of closed reduction and traction before operative intervention for facet subluxations or dislocations is controversial. It can dictate the decision whether to perform an anterior or a posterior procedure initially. One of the main controversies focuses on whether MRI is necessary before reducing facet dislocations to assess for the presence of an occult herniated disc. In 1991, Eismont and associates reported on 6 of 86 patients seen between 1980 and 1987 who sustained a fracture or dislocation of a cervical facet with associated disc herniation and spinal cord compression. These investigators recommended MRI to rule out a herniated nucleus pulposus in patients with worsening neurologic symptoms or neurologic deficit after the injury, in patients for whom closed reduction would be difficult, and in patients undergoing operative intervention.[54] In contrast, Vadera and colleagues maintained that baseline MRI in an awake, alert, cooperative patient is unnecessary before closed reduction, provided the patient is closely monitored neurologically during the reduction. These investigators asserted that post-reduction MRI is necessary to determine the presence of a herniated nucleus pulposus and to help define the appropriate operative approach.[55]

Regardless of whether pre-reduction MRI is performed, reduction of dislocated facets is the most effective way to decompress the spinal cord, and it should be done as expeditiously as possible in patients presenting with neurologic deficits. The decision whether to use open or closed reduction depends on the patient's presentation, the institutional resources, and the physician's experience and preference. Closed reduction is contingent on an awake, alert, and cooperative patient. For closed reduction to be successful, the circumstances must be such that the area of interest can be radiographed and serial neurologic examinations can be performed on the patient. In these instances, closed reduction is warranted, and MRI likely is unnecessary. Closed reduction is accomplished by adding sequential weight to skull tongs or a halo ring. Serial radiographs and neurologic examinations are performed as increasing weight is applied.[56,57]

Following closed reduction, surgical treatment by posterior fusion and stabilization with lateral mass screws and rods has been traditionally recommended, but anterior fusion with a rigid plate screw construct is a viable option. It should be remembered that the anterior construct, which leaves the disrupted posterior elements is biomechanically less stable than the posterior tension band construct. However, in the majority of clinical scenarios, the anterior construct is sufficient for good outcome if the rigid construct is used in the nonosteoporotic bone and postoperative bracing.

When MRI reveals a disc fragment dorsal to the posterior cortex of the caudal vertebral body with a facet dislocation or subluxation, an anterior discectomy-decompression procedure is preferred before reduction of the dislocation. This procedure may be followed by anterior reduction of the facet dislocation and placement of an interbody graft and an anterior cervical plate. Because this injury is primarily a posterior ligamentous lesion, complete apposition of the facets, placement of a trapezoidal interbody graft, and contouring of the plate into lordosis optimize the stability of the construct.

Razack and associates conducted a 6-year retrospective study of patients who were treated at a single institution and who had traumatic cervical bilateral facet fracture-dislocations. All fracture-dislocations that could be aligned with traction were later stabilized with ACDF. Twenty-two patients were followed up for an average of 32 months. At final follow-up, all patients had evidence of radiographic fusion.[58] If anterior reduction of the dislocation cannot be safely accomplished, a graft is placed in the disc space after discectomy, and posterior reduction and stabilization are performed. If the graft displaces during the reduction maneuver, repeat placement of the graft anteriorly may be required. The use of an anti-kick plate can be considered and may reduce the risk of graft displacement during the posterior reduction maneuver.

When facet dislocation without a herniated disc is treated surgically, anterior or posterior stabilization is possible. The choice of procedure may be influenced by available equipment and the surgeon's preference. However, consideration of anterior issues, such as the risk of dysphagia and potential injury to visceral structures, should be weighed against the additional muscle dissection and wound infection risk of posterior

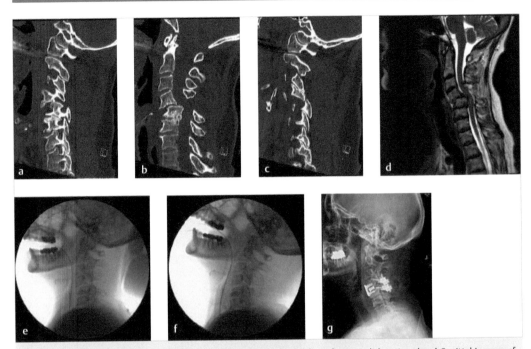

Fig. 10.12 A 66-year-old female who fell, sustaining C4–C5 bilateral facet fracture-dislocation. (a–c) Sagittal images of her computed tomography (CT) scan showing her injury. (d) A pre-reduction magnetic resonance imaging (MRI) of cervical spine with no herniated nucleus pulposus. (e, f) Intraoperative fluoroscopy images showing her injury and reduction. (g) The patient underwent a C4–C5 anterior discectomy and fusion followed by a posterior C4–C5 cervical fusion.

procedures.[53] In addition, performing the surgical procedure anteriorly avoids the need for positioning the patient prone with an unstable cervical spine. One clinical situation in which anterior fixation may be beneficial is fracture of the facet and ipsilateral pedicle, or lateral mass separation. In this injury, only a single-level fusion would be possible anteriorly, whereas posteriorly a multiple-level fusion would be required.[59]

Other specific considerations for anterior fixation for the management of unilateral or bilateral facet injuries include careful preoperative imaging to evaluate for subtle vertebral end plate fractures or displaced fractures of the facet joints, for which consideration of circumferential fixation may be necessary, and consideration given to multiple-level anterior fixation to achieve adequate initial spinal stability. Another potential pitfall of anterior fixation is placement of too large an anterior graft. This situation can cause neurologic injury through a stretch-type mechanism and can distract the facet joints at the level of injury. A case example can be seen in ▶ Fig. 10.12.

10.6 Surgical Techniques

10.6.1 Atlantoaxial fixation

Indications for surgical stabilization of atlantoaxial instability include acute, progressive neurologic compromise from instability at the C1–C2 level. Other indications include an anterior atlantodens interval (AADI) of greater than 3 mm in adults and greater than 5 mm in children. Chronic instability that results in persistent neck pain or occipital headache from C2 nerve root irritation or impingement is another indication for surgical stabilization. Contraindications to use of the C1 lateral mass–C2 pedicle screw technique include bony or vascular anomalies that prohibit safe screw placement. The presence of ponticulus posticus or arcuate foramen at C1, which may be identified by radiographs in approximately 15% of patients is a contraindication. The vertebral artery courses posteriorly through this bony bridge, and can lead to vertebral artery injury if C1 lateral mass screw placement is attempted.

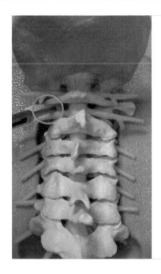

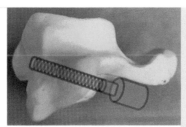

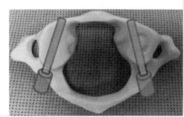

Fig. 10.13 Model representation of the entry point for a C1 lateral mass screw, which is at the midpoint of the mediolateral lateral mass at the junction where it meets the posterior arch of C1.

Technique of C1 Lateral Mass Screw

The patient is positioned prone with the neck held in appropriate alignment with cranial tongs. The atlantoaxial position is confirmed using fluoroscopic imaging. Reduction of any atlantoaxial malalignment may be performed by the cranial tongs. Alternatively, reduction may be performed later in the procedure once instrumentation has been placed. Next, the posterior cervical spine is exposed using sharp dissection and electrocautery from the base of the occiput to approximately the C3 level. The inferior portion of the ring of C1 and lamina of C2 are exposed to their lateral borders. The C1–C2 articulation should be dissected with caution as significant bleeding may arise from the epidural venous plexus and obscure the C1–C2 joint. This bleeding may be effectively controlled with a combination of bipolar electrocautery, absorbable gelatin and thrombin mixture, and cottonoid patties. Identification of the C1–C2 joint is crucial for accurate placement of the C1 lateral mass screw. The C2 nerve must be retracted caudally to expose the entry point for the C1 screw, which is located at the midpoint of the posteroinferior aspect of the C1 lateral mass, where it meets the C1 posterior arch (▶ Fig. 10.13).[60,61] The entry point should be marked with a small, high-speed burr to avoid any slippage of the drill bit. The entry point is classically at the juncture between the lateral mass and C1 ring, in which C2 nerve root sometimes needs to be resected. Another entry point option is 1 mm cephalad at the edge of the inferior C1 ring so that C2 nerve root is out of the

way. Next, the pilot hole is drilled in a straight-ahead or 10-degree convergent trajectory in the mediolateral direction and parallel to the plane of the C1 posterior arch in the craniocaudal direction.[60,61,62,63] The drill tip should be directed toward the anterior arch of C1 on lateral fluoroscopic imaging. Screw violation of the C1–C2 joint caudally or the occipital–C1 joint cranially should be avoided.[64] Intraoperative landmarks and preoperative axial CT images are indispensable aids in safe screw placement. A blunt probe is used to check the integrity of the pilot hole. Then the hole is tapped, and a 3.5-mm polyaxial screw of an appropriate length is inserted bicortically into the lateral mass of C1.

The length of the C1 screw should be determined preoperatively by measurements on fine-cut CT scan. Typically, a 10-mm smooth shank (unthreaded) portion of the C1 screw stays above the lateral mass. This allows the polyaxial portion of the screw to rest above the posterior arch and also decreases irritation to the C2 nerve root.[62] As with placement of all instrumentation, screw position is verified by fluoroscopic imaging.

Next, a small instrument such as a Penfield number 4 dissector can be used to identify the medial border of the C2 pars. This technique helps delineate the entry point for the C2 pedicle screw, which is in the cranial and medial quadrant of the isthmus surface of C2 (▶ Fig. 10.14).[62] After the entry point is marked with a high-speed burr, the pilot hole is drilled bicortically. The trajectory of the drill bit is approximately 20 to 30 degrees

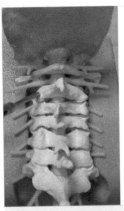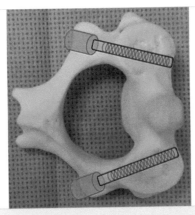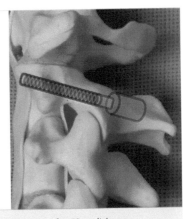

Fig. 10.14 Axial schematic and model views demonstrating the position and trajectory of a C2 pedicle screw.

convergent and cephalad, typically guided by the superior and medial surface of the C2 isthmus.[63] A blunt probe is used to check the integrity of the pilot hole. After the hole is tapped, a 3.5-mm polyaxial screw of an appropriate length is inserted bicortically. At this point, reduction of the C1 ring may be performed by either repositioning of the patient's head using cranial tongs or by direct manipulation of the C1 and C2 vertebrae with the screws. Once adequate alignment is achieved, the screws are then fixed to the rods to maintain the alignment. For definitive fusion, the posterior aspects of C1 and C2 are decorticated, and autograft or allograft bone is placed over the decorticated surfaces. Intra-articular fusion has also been described, involving decortication of the joint surfaces between C1 and C2.[62] However, this step poses an additional risk to neurovascular structures and should be performed only under direct vision.

Posterior C1–C2 Wiring

Surgeons may also prefer the use of posterior C1–C2 wiring, along with the use of adjunct bone-graft placed between the vertebrae, to allow fusion to take place in cases of atlantoaxial instability. While the original technique of posterior/dorsal wiring described by Jenkins et al has been modified, the essentials still remain the same. After insertion of screws and decortication of the inferior surfaces of the posterior C1 arch and superior aspects of the C2 spine process, the inferior aspects of the C2 laminae are bilaterally "notched" to allow the placement of wires. An autologous tricortical bone graft is then obtained from the iliac crest. The graft

is prepared by removing the upper cortical edge using a Lexsell rongeur to create a bicortical curved strut to allow appropriate fitting and restoration of height between the C1 arch and C2 spinous process. The graft is then temporarily placed between the C1–C2 spaces to allow the shape of the structure's curve to approximate the curve of the C1 posterior ring. The graft is also notched in the midline to ensure that the structured is "contoured" substantially to the shape of the C2 spinous process. The graft is then taken out of the C1–C2 space, and wires are placed and secured. The graft is then repositioned and loop of the cable is based over the posterior C1 ring, behind the graft and secured under the C2 spinous process. The knot is tightened so that the graft is compressed between the C1 and C2, and further decortication of posterior C1–C2 arches and bone graft is performed. Further, cancellous bone graft is also packed against the fusion surfaces. Patients are placed in a Philadelphia collar until fusion can be documented radiographically.

10.6.2 C2 Fixation Options

There are several fixation options at C2, including the previously described C1/C2 pedicle screw. Other fixation options include a C2 pars screw and C2 laminar screw.

C2 pars screw: The entry point for a C2 pars screw is approximately 3 to 4 mm cranial to the C2–C3 facet joint and at the midpoint of the pars (▶ Fig. 10.15). After the entry point is marked with a high-speed burr, the pilot hole is drilled. The trajectory is traditionally more dorsal and straight ahead than the pedicle screw similarly to the

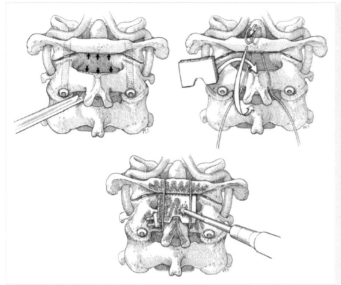

Fig. 10.15 Model views demonstrating the position and trajectory of a C2 pars screw.

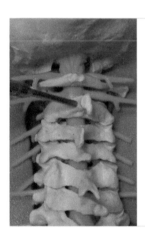
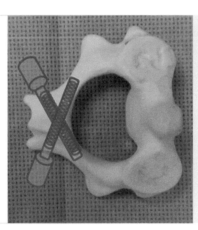

Fig. 10.16 Model views demonstrating the position and trajectory of C2 laminar screw.

trajectory of a transarticular screw.[65] A blunt probe is used to check the integrity of the pilot hole. After the hole is tapped, a screw of an appropriate length is inserted.[66]

C2 laminar screw: The entry point for a C2 laminar screw is at the junction of the spinous process and the lamina (▶ Fig. 10.16). If using bilateral laminar screws, the entry points should be planned accordingly to allow the placement of both screws with one starting point more cranial and the other more caudally. After the entry point is marked with a high-speed burr, the pilot hole is drilled. The trajectory can be aligned with the angle of the expose contralateral laminar surface. To avoid possible cortical breakthrough into the canal, the trajectory can be kept slightly less than the downslope of the lamina. After the hole is tapped, a screw of an appropriate length is inserted.[67]

10.6.3 Lateral Mass Screws

Technique

Several different techniques have been described for placement of lateral mass screws (▶ Fig. 10.17). All the techniques are compromises that attempt to balance anatomic safety and mechanical competence with ease of placement. Nerve roots, the vertebral artery, facet joints, and, to a lesser extent, the spinal cord are at risk during placement of lateral mass screws. Direct anterior trajectories such as the Roy-Camille are technically straightforward,

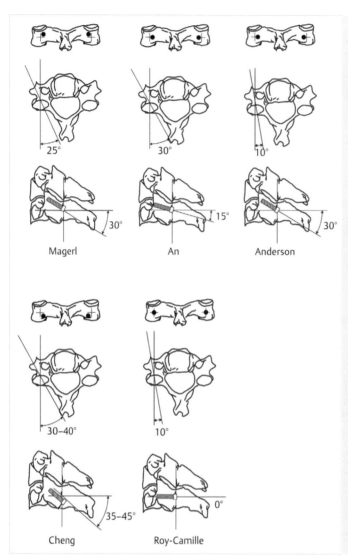

Fig. 10.17 Comparison of the entry points and screw trajectories described by various authors. The *black dots* indicate the entry points for the lateral mass screws. (Source: Wu JC, Huang WC, Chen YC, et al. Stabilization of subaxial cervical spines by lateral mass screw fixation with modified Magerl's technique. Surg Neurol 2008;70(Suppl 1):S25-S33.)

Magerl   An   Anderson

30–40°   10°

Cheng   Roy-Camille

but the screw length is shorter and has a higher chance of violating the inferior facet joint at C6–C7. Screws that angle cranially have a longer, biomechanically stronger screw tract, but they also have a higher chance of damaging the exiting nerve root and of entering the superior facet joint. A more outward (lateral) trajectory, such as used by the An technique, avoids the vertebral artery but has less bone stock available for the screw to traverse (resulting in a shorter screw length) and a higher probability of lateral mass fracture. Trajectory-based methods rely on the surgeon's feel of the angle of screw placement, either freehand or by using a mechanical angle guide or C-arm fluoroscopy.

Safe lateral mass screw placement requires familiarity with the articular pillar anatomy. Exposure should be done till the lateral edge of the pillar. Osteophytes should be removed to better delineate the articular pillar's margins. A Penfield No. 4 dissector can be inserted into the facet to ascertain its angulation. Locate the center of the lateral mass by defining the notch between the lamina and the lateral mass. The Roy-Camille technique describes screw insertion at the apex of convexity of the lateral mass. Aim 10 degrees laterally to decrease the risk of nerve root injury. To decrease facet violation, Magerl recommended an entry point 2 to 3 mm medial and superior to the apex, a 25-degree lateral drill angle, and a superior trajectory parallel to the facet (typically 45 degrees). An and colleagues suggested lateral mass entry 1 mm medial to its center. The drill is angled 30 degrees lateral and 15 degrees cranially.[68,69]

Bicortical penetration improves failure resistance by 20% but increases root injury risk. Consider bicortical screws in the presence of osteoporotic bone, few acceptable anchor points, unstable spines, and, particularly, in those with anterior column collapse and decreased axial load-bearing capability. To place a bicortical screw, gradually increase the drill's set depth. Palpate the opposite cortex. To avoid stripping the threads, be sure to tap the full screw depth.

Pearls ⓘ

- All trauma patients have a cervical spine injury until proven otherwise. Up to 10% of the cases with cervical spine injuries have multiple levels and therefore imaging should be performed for both upper and cervical spine to prevent any missed injuries.
- Patient positioning is critical to prevent iatrogenic injuries and also to obtain an optimal alignment.
- A small instrument such as a Penfield number 4 dissector can be used to identify the medial border of the C2 pars. This technique helps delineate the entry point for the C2 pedicle screw, which is in the cranial and medial quadrant of the isthmus surface of C2.
- The C1–C2 articulation should be dissected with caution, as significant bleeding may arise from the epidural venous plexus and obscure the C1–C2 joint.
- Intraoperative landmarks and preoperative axial CT images are indispensable aids in safe screw placement.
- For C2 laminar screws, if using bilateral laminar screws, the entry points should be planned accordingly to allow the placement of both screws with one starting point more cranial and the other more caudally.
- Safe lateral mass screw placement requires familiarity with the articular pillar anatomy. Exposure should be done till the lateral edge of the pillar. Osteophytes should be removed to better delineate the articular pillar's margins.
- For lateral mass screws, bicortical penetration improves failure resistance by 20% but increases root injury risk. Consider bicortical screws in the presence of osteoporotic bone, few acceptable anchor points, unstable spines, and, particularly, in those with anterior column collapse and decreased axial load-bearing capability.

10.7 Case Examples

10.7.1 Case 1

A 24-year-old right-hand dominant male presented to hospital following an ATV injury. X-rays showed presence of a C2 hangman fracture and subsequently received a C2–C3 fixation.

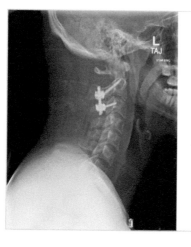
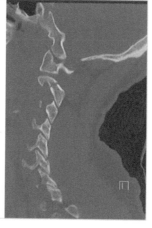

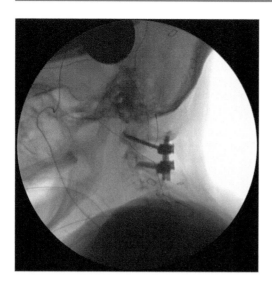

10.7.2 Case 2

A 75-year-old female presenting with a displaced C2 odontoid fracture with bilateral subluxation of her C1–C2 facet joints following a fall. Due to displacement, an operative approach was preferred, which consisted of C1–C2 posterior fusion consisting of C1 lateral mass screws and C2 pars screws. A tricortical iliac crest allograft was retrieved and placed between the posterior arch of C1 and cephalad aspect of C2 pars and lamina, and secured into place using FiberWire sutures. Fibergraft matrix was used to fill in the remaining gaps around the allograft to further supplement fusion.

References

[1] Umana E, Khan K, Baig MN, Binchy J. Epidemiology and characteristics of cervical spine injury in patients presenting to a regional emergency department. Cureus. 2018; 10(2): e2179

[2] Baaj AA, Uribe JS, Nichols TA, et al. Health care burden of cervical spine fractures in the United States: analysis of a nationwide database over a 10-year period. J Neurosurg Spine. 2010; 13(1):61–66

[3] Kamravan HR, Haghnegahdar A, Paydar S, Khalife M, Sedighi M, Ghaffarpasand F. Epidemiological and clinical features of cervical column and cord injuries: a 2-year experience from a large trauma center in Southern Iran. Bull Emerg Trauma. 2014; 2(1):32–37

[4] Clayton JL, Harris MB, Weintraub SL, et al. Risk factors for cervical spine injury. Injury. 2012; 43(4):431–435

[5] Lowery DW, Wald MM, Browne BJ, Tigges S, Hoffman JR, Mower WR, NEXUS Group. Epidemiology of cervical spine injury victims. Ann Emerg Med. 2001; 38(1):12–16

[6] Goldberg W, Mueller C, Panacek E, Tigges S, Hoffman JR, Mower WR, NEXUS Group. Distribution and patterns of blunt traumatic cervical spine injury. Ann Emerg Med. 2001; 38(1):17–21

[7] Hu R, Mustard CA, Burns C. Epidemiology of incident spinal fracture in a complete population. Spine. 1996; 21(4): 492–499

[8] Passias PG, Poorman GW, Segreto FA, et al. Traumatic fractures of the cervical spine: analysis of changes in incidence, cause, concurrent injuries, and complications among 488,262 patients from 2005 to 2013. World Neurosurg. 2018; 110:e427–e437

[9] Fredø HL, Rizvi SA, Lied B, Rønning P, Helseth E. The epidemiology of traumatic cervical spine fractures: a prospective population study from Norway. Scand J Trauma Resusc Emerg Med. 2012; 20:85

[10] Bohlman HH. Acute fractures and dislocations of the cervical spine: an analysis of three hundred hospitalized patients and review of the literature. J Bone Joint Surg Am. 1979; 61 (8):1119–1142

[11] Reid DC, Henderson R, Saboe L, Miller JD. Etiology and clinical course of missed spine fractures. J Trauma. 1987; 27(9): 980–986

[12] Avellino AM, Mann FA, Grady MS, et al. The misdiagnosis of acute cervical spine injuries and fractures in infants and children: the 12-year experience of a level I pediatric and adult trauma center. Childs Nerv Syst. 2005; 21(2): 122–127

[13] Gornet ME, Kelly MP. Fractures of the axis: a review of pediatric, adult, and geriatric injuries. Curr Rev Musculoskelet Med. 2016; 9(4):505–512

[14] Schoenfeld AJ, Sielski B, Rivera KP, Bader JO, Harris MB. Epidemiology of cervical spine fractures in the US military. Spine J. 2012; 12(9):777–783

[15] Tee JW, Chan CH, Fitzgerald MC, Liew SM, Rosenfeld JV. Epidemiological trends of spine trauma: an Australian level 1 trauma centre study. Global Spine J. 2013; 3(2):75–84

[16] Platzer P, Jaindl M, Thalhammer G, et al. Cervical spine injuries in pediatric patients. J Trauma. 2007; 62(2):389–396, discussion 394–396

[17] Viccellio P, Simon H, Pressman BD, Shah MN, Mower WR, Hoffman JR, NEXUS Group. A prospective multicenter study of cervical spine injury in children. Pediatrics. 2001; 108(2):E20

[18] Givens TG, Polley KA, Smith GF, Hardin WD, Jr. Pediatric cervical spine injury: a three-year experience. J Trauma. 1996; 41(2):310–314

[19] Kirshblum SC, Burns SP, Biering-Sorensen F, et al. International standards for neurological classification of spinal cord injury (revised 2011). J Spinal Cord Med. 2011; 34(6): 535–546

[20] Tran J, Jeanmonod D, Agresti D, Hamden K, Jeanmonod RK. Prospective validation of modified NEXUS cervical spine injury criteria in low-risk elderly fall patients. West J Emerg Med. 2016; 17(3):252–257

[21] Saragiotto BT, Michaleff ZA. The Canadian C-spine rule. J Physiother. 2016; 62(3):170

[22] Bolender N, Cromwell LD, Wendling L. Fracture of the occipital condyle. AJR Am J Roentgenol. 1978; 131(4):729–731

[23] Blacksin MF, Lee HJ. Frequency and significance of fractures of the upper cervical spine detected by CT in patients with severe neck trauma. AJR Am J Roentgenol. 1995; 165(5): 1201–1204

[24] Bloom AI, Neeman Z, Slasky BS, et al. Fracture of the occipital condyles and associated craniocervical ligament injury: incidence, CT imaging and implications. Clin Radiol. 1997; 52(3):198–202

[25] Dvorak J, Panjabi MM. Functional anatomy of the alar ligaments. Spine. 1987; 12(2):183–189

[26] Anderson PA, Montesano PX. Morphology and treatment of occipital condyle fractures. Spine. 1988; 13(7):731–736

[27] Bucholz RW, Burkhead WZ, Graham W, Petty C. Occult cervical spine injuries in fatal traffic accidents. J Trauma. 1979; 19(10):768–771

[28] Wholey MH, Bruwer AJ, Baker HL, Jr. The lateral roentgenogram of the neck, with comments on the atlanto-odontoid-basion relationship. Radiology. 1958; 71(3): 350–356

[29] Powers B, Miller MD, Kramer RS, Martinez S, Gehweiler JA, Jr. Traumatic anterior atlanto-occipital dislocation. Neurosurgery. 1979; 4(1):12–17

[30] Harris JH, Jr, Carson GC, Wagner LK. Radiologic diagnosis of traumatic occipitovertebral dissociation: 1. Normal occipitovertebral relationships on lateral radiographs of supine subjects. AJR Am J Roentgenol. 1994; 162(4): 881–886

[31] Harris JH, Jr, Carson GC, Wagner LK, Kerr N. Radiologic diagnosis of traumatic occipitovertebral dissociation: 2. Comparison of three methods of detecting occipitovertebral relationships on lateral radiographs of supine subjects. AJR Am J Roentgenol. 1994; 162(4):887–892

[32] Traynelis VC, Marano GD, Dunker RO, Kaufman HH. Traumatic atlanto-occipital dislocation. Case report. J Neurosurg. 1986; 65(6):863–870

[33] Dvorak J, Schneider E, Saldinger P, Rahn B. Biomechanics of the craniocervical region: the alar and transverse ligaments. J Orthop Res. 1988; 6(3):452–461

[34] Song WS, Chiang YH, Chen CY, Lin SZ, Liu MY. A simple method for diagnosing traumatic occlusion of the vertebral artery at the craniovertebral junction. Spine. 1994; 19(7): 837–839

[35] Bellabarba C, Mirza SK, West GA, et al. Diagnosis and treatment of craniocervical dislocation in a series of 17 consecutive survivors during an 8-year period. J Neurosurg Spine. 2006; 4(6):429–440

[36] Eismont FJ, Bohlman HH. Posterior atlanto-occipital dislocation with fractures of the atlas and odontoid process. J Bone Joint Surg Am. 1978; 60(3):397–399

[37] Montane I, Eismont FJ, Green BA. Traumatic occipitoatlantal dislocation. Spine. 1991; 16(2):112–116

[38] Frush TJ, Fisher TJ, Ensminger SC, Truumees E, Demetropoulos CK. Biomechanical evaluation of parasagittal occipital plating: screw load sharing analysis. Spine. 2009; 34(9): 877–884

[39] Levine AM, Edwards CC. Fractures of the atlas. J Bone Joint Surg Am. 1991; 73(5):680–691

[40] Spence KF, Jr, Decker S, Sell KW. Bursting atlantal fracture associated with rupture of the transverse ligament. J Bone Joint Surg Am. 1970; 52(3):543–549

[41] Dickman CA, Greene KA, Sonntag VK. Injuries involving the transverse atlantal ligament: classification and treatment guidelines based upon experience with 39 injuries. Neurosurgery. 1996; 38(1):44–50

[42] Bellabarba C, Bransford RJ, Chapman, JR. Occipitocervical and upper cervical spine fractures: textbook of the cervical spine. Saunders, Elsevier Inc.; 2014:167–183

[43] Fielding JW, Hawkins RJ. Atlanto-axial rotatory fixation: fixed rotatory subluxation of the atlanto-axial joint. J Bone Joint Surg Am. 1977; 59(1):37–44

[44] Tay BKB, Eismont FJ. Injuries of the upper cervical spine. Rothman-Simeone and Herkowitz's the spine. Elsevier, Inc.; 2017:1285–1309

[45] Anderson LD, D'Alonzo RT. Fractures of the odontoid process of the axis. J Bone Joint Surg Am. 1974; 56(8):1663–1674

[46] Clark CR, White AA, III. Fractures of the dens: a multicenter study. J Bone Joint Surg Am. 1985; 67(9):1340–1348

[47] Bednar DA, Parikh J, Hummel J. Management of type II odontoid process fractures in geriatric patients: a prospective study of sequential cohorts with attention to survivorship. J Spinal Disord. 1995; 8(2):166–169

[48] Levine AM, Edwards CC. Traumatic lesions of the occipitoatlantoaxial complex. Clin Orthop Relat Res. 1989(239): 53–68

[49] Starr JK, Eismont FJ. Atypical Hangman's fractures. Spine. 1993; 18(14):1954–1957

[50] Effendi B, Roy D, Cornish B, Dussault RG, Laurin CA. Fractures of the ring of the axis: a classification based on the analysis of 131 cases. J Bone Joint Surg Br. 1981; 63-B(3): 319–327

[51] Vaccaro AR, Hulbert RJ, Patel AA, et al. Spine Trauma Study Group. The subaxial cervical spine injury classification system: a novel approach to recognize the importance of morphology, neurology, and integrity of the disco-ligamentous complex. Spine. 2007; 32(21):2365–2374

[52] Vaccaro AR, Koerner JD, Radcliff KE, et al. AOSpine subaxial cervical spine injury classification system. Eur Spine J. 2016; 25(7):2173–2184

[53] Dvorak MF, Fisher CG, Fehlings MG, et al. The surgical approach to subaxial cervical spine injuries: an evidence-based algorithm based on the SLIC classification system. Spine. 2007; 32(23):2620–2629

[54] Eismont FJ, Arena MJ, Green BA. Extrusion of an intervertebral disc associated with traumatic subluxation or dislocation of cervical facets. Case report. J Bone Joint Surg Am. 1991; 73(10):1555–1560

[55] Vadera S, Ratliff J, Brown Z, et al. Management of cervical facet dislocations. Semin Spine Surg. 2007; 19:250–255

[56] Grant GA, Mirza SK, Chapman JR, et al. Risk of early closed reduction in cervical spine subluxation injuries. J Neurosurg. 1999; 90(1) Suppl:13–18

[57] Wiseman DB, Bellabarba C, Mirza SK, Chapman J. Anterior versus posterior surgical treatment for traumatic cervical spine dislocation. Curr Opin Orthop. 2003; 14:174–181

[58] Razack N, Green BA, Levi AD. The management of traumatic cervical bilateral facet fracture-dislocations with unicortical anterior plates. J Spinal Disord. 2000; 13(5): 374–381

[59] Banagan K, Gelb D. Surgical management of cervical spine fractures. In: Bridwell KH, eds. The Textbook of Spinal Surgery. Philadelphia: Lippincott Williams & Wilkins; 2011

[60] Seal C, Zarro C, Gelb D, Ludwig S. C1 lateral mass anatomy: proper placement of lateral mass screws. J Spinal Disord Tech. 2009; 22(7):516–523

[61] Puttlitz CM, Goel VK, Traynelis VC, Clark CR. A finite element investigation of upper cervical instrumentation. Spine. 2001; 26(22):2449–2455

[62] Harms J, Melcher RP. Posterior C1-C2 fusion with polyaxial screw and rod fixation. Spine. 2001; 26(22):2467–2471

[63] Schulz R, Macchiavello N, Fernández E, et al. Harms C1-C2 instrumentation technique: anatomo-surgical guide. Spine (Phila Pa 1976). 2011; 36(12):945–950

[64] Yeom JS, Buchowski JM, Park KW, Chang BS, Lee CK, Riew KD. Lateral fluoroscopic guide to prevent occipitocervical and atlantoaxial joint violation during C1 lateral mass screw placement. Spine J. 2009; 9(7):574–579

[65] Ebraheim NA, Misson JR, Xu R, Yeasting RA. The optimal transarticular c1–2 screw length and the location of the hypoglossal nerve. Surg Neurol. 2000; 53(3):208–210

[66] Punyarat P, Buchowski JM, Klawson BT, Peters C, Lertudomphonwanit T, Riew KD. Freehand technique for C2 pedicle and pars screw placement: is it safe? Spine J. 2018; 18(7):1197–1203

[67] Ma W, Feng L, Xu R, et al. Clinical application of C2 laminar screw technique. Eur Spine J. 2010; 19(8):1312–1317

[68] Merola AA, Castro BA, Alongi PR, et al. Anatomic consideration for standard and modified techniques of cervical lateral mass screw placement. Spine J. 2002; 2(6):430–435

[69] An HS. Internal fixation of the cervical spine: current indications and techniques. J Am Acad Orthop Surg. 1995; 3(4):194–206

11 Thoracolumbar Spine Injuries

Andrew Sinensky, William T. Li, Matthew Meade, Mayan Lendner, Barrett Boody, Dhruv K.C. Goyal, and Mark Kurd

Abstract

This chapter provides a broad overview of the epidemiology, pathomechanisms, clinical presentation, classification, and management of thoracolumbar injuries (TLIs). TLIs are the most common cause of spinal fracture in the United States. These injuries most often present subsequent to trauma, and commonly occur in a region of increased spinal mobility/instability known as the thoracolumbar (TL) junction (T11–L2). TLIs cause significant patient morbidity and disability. The most common subtypes of TLI are compression, burst, flexion-distraction, and fracture-dislocation fractures. Cauda equina syndrome (CES) and spinal/neurogenic shock are additional possible sequelae of TLI. The morphology of the TLI depends principally on the magnitude and types of force exerted on the spine. Radiographic imaging is the mainstay of diagnosis for TLIs, with X-ray, CT, and MRI being the most relevant modalities. Currently, there is no universal classification system for TLIs. The most commonly utilized systems are the TLICS, AO, and AOSpine systems. Generally accepted indications for surgical management of TLIs include spinal instability and neurological deficits. Patients with stable fractures and no neurological deficits can be managed nonoperatively, with braces and hyperextension casts for symptomatic relief. In these populations, there is questionable evidence that surgical intervention is superior to nonoperative management. There is a paucity of evidence regarding the optimal surgical approach for TLIs, and the choice is surgeon/institution specific. Finally, data regarding long-term outcomes of patients suffering from TLI is limited and highly dependent on the subtype of TLI.

Keywords: trauma, spine, thoracic, lumbar, thoracolumbar injury, TLICS, AO, AO spine, orthopaedic, injury

11.1 Introduction, Demographics, and Epidemiology/Prevalence

Thoracolumbar (TL) fractures are the most common type of spine fractures in the United States, with about 160,000 reported cases a year in North America.[1] These injuries often happen to otherwise young, healthy individuals and often have significant sequelae.[2,3,4] Thoracolumbar injuries (TLI) happen most often in individuals between 20 and 40 years old, affecting men twice as much as women.[5,6,7,8,9] Forty to 80% of these injuries are the result of high-energy traumas such as motor vehicle accidents, falls from heights, and direct blows to the spine.[10,11] Many of these injuries are unstable, with the possibility of resultant disability, deformity, and neurological deficit. In a multicenter study, the incidence of neurologic defect associated with spinal injury ranged from 22 to 51% depending on the specific fracture type.[7,12] Patients with TL fractures present with polytrauma up to 47% of the time, owing to the fact that a large portion of spinal trauma is associated with high-energy mechanism of injury.[13]

11.2 Functional Anatomy

The TL spine includes the thoracic spine, the TL junction (T11–L2), and the lumbar spine. The thoracic spine is unique, in that the ribs articulate here providing increased stability and subsequent restriction of flexion and extension. The rib cage also functions to increase the axial loading capacity of the thoracic region by three to fourfold.[14] In contrast to the superior thoracic spine, T11 and T12 have increased flexibility due to the fact that ribs 11 and 12 do not articulate with the sternum.[15] The TL junction is of significant interest as it is a unique transition zone between the more rigid thoracic spine and relatively mobile lumbar spine and is subject to significant biomechanical stress.[5] In contrast to the coronally oriented facets of the thoracic spine which limit anterior and posterior movement, those in the lumbar region are oriented more sagittally, considerably increasing anteroposterior mobility.[16] Upwards of 50% of all TL fractures occur within this three-segment area and are a major cause of disability.[17,18,19]

11.3 Mechanisms of Injury

The pathomechanisms of TL fractures can most easily be understood using Dennis's three-column classification for TLIs.[6] In this classification system, Dennis divides the individual vertebrae

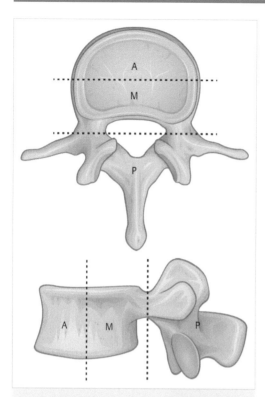

Fig. 11.1 Illustration of a lumbar vertebra divided into anterior (A), middle (M), and posterior (P) columns in accordance to the "three-column concept" introduced by Denis.[6]

anteroposteriorly into anterior, middle, and posterior "columns" (▶ Fig. 11.1).

The type of TLI suffered by the patient is largely dependent on the type/types and magnitude of forces they are subjected to. These forces are illustrated in ▶ Fig. 11.2 as well as summarized in (▶ Table 11.1).

11.3.1 Axial Compression

Axial compression occurs when compressive forces are exerted against the longitudinal axis of the vertebral column. Such forces may be seen with falls from a height, motor vehicle accidents, or following low-energy trauma in elderly osteoporotic populations.[20,21] **Compression fractures** are the most common type of spine fracture, representing over 50% of total spine fractures.[22] In a compression fracture, the compressive forces are generally located anterior to the axis of rotation of the vertebrae (back of middle column), resulting in mainly anterior column compression (▶ Fig. 11.2b).[6,23] When seen on

sagittal X-ray or CT imaging, there is loss of the anterior vertebral body height with preservation of the posterior vertebral body height, creating the appearance of a "wedge." There should be no retropulsion of bone into the spinal canal; thus, the risk of neurologic injury is minimal.[23] Axial compressive forces that occur in the TL junction are more evenly distributed across the vertebrae due to neutral alignment (lack of curvature).[24] This even distribution of force across the surface of the vertebral body predisposes the TL junction to **burst fractures** (▶ Fig. 11.2c). A burst fracture is a compression fracture of the anterior and middle vertebral columns.[6,23,25] This can cause retropulsion of posterior vertebral body fragments into the spinal canal and can be associated with cauda equina and/or spinal cord injury.[26,27] On sagittal X-ray and CT imaging, there is loss of the anterior vertebral body height, with bone fragmentation with radial distribution of fragments, and interpedicular widening can often be seen from the axial images.[23]

11.3.2 Extension/Flexion/ Distraction

The morphology of these injuries depends on the type of force applied to the spine. When a force is applied anterior to the vertebral body, they cause compression of primarily the anterior vertebral bodies as well as increasing tension on ligaments and structures of the posterior vertebral column (this tension is called a "distractive" force).[28] Flexion-distraction injuries are associated with sudden decelerations of a restrained passenger, often with motor vehicle accidents.[28,29] The resulting injury patterns from flexion forces on the anterior column can cause anterior wedge compression as well as lesions in intervertebral discs, while distraction forces on the middle and posterior columns cause rupture of posterior ligaments and facet joints.[30,31] This combination is referred to as a **flexion-distraction fracture** (▶ Fig. 11.2d).[32] Flexion-distraction fractures are frequently associated with intra-abdominal injuries.[11] Sagittal plane imaging may reveal decreased anterior vertebrae height in a similar pattern to a compression pressure. Additionally, the interspinous distance is widened in the coronal and sagittal planes. When a fraction-distraction fracture involves only the osseous structures, it is called a **Chance fracture**.[31] Chance fractures can be visualized as only involving the vertebral bone on sagittal imaging.[23] A **hyperextension injury** (▶ Fig. 11.2e) is a less

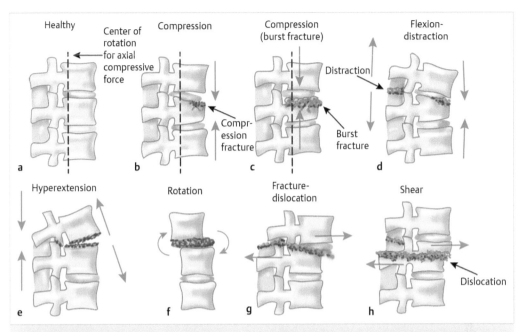

Fig. 11.2 Illustration of the different types of forces and injuries seen in thoracolumbar fractures, as described above. *Red arrows* indicate the direction and general location of forces being exerted on the thoracolumbar spine. (**a**) A healthy spinal column, with axial compression centered at the posterior aspect of the middle column. (**b**) A simple compression fracture resulting from an anterior compressive force. (**c**) A burst fracture, notice the compressive forces are centered around the middle column. (**d**) A flexion-distraction injury. Notice the anterior column is compressed, and the posterior ligamentous complex (PLC) has torn due to distractive forces. (**e**) A hyperextension injury, which results in compression of the posterior column and distraction of the anterior and middle columns, and can be associated with anterior longitudinal ligament disruption. (**f**) A rotation injury, which results from a rotational force along the long axis of the spinal column. (**g**) A fracture-dislocation injury, which results from primarily shear and rotative forces. (**h**) A shear injury, which results in translation perpendicular to the long axis of the spinal column.

Table 11.1 Summary of forces applied to different columns of the thoracolumbar spine and their associated injuries

Spine involvement of thoracolumbar injuries			
Injury type	Anterior column	Middle column	Posterior column
Compression fracture	Compression	Generally intact	Generally intact
Burst fracture	Compression	Compression	Generally intact
Flexion-distraction fracture	Compression	Distraction	Distraction
Fracture-dislocation fracture	Compression and/or rotation-shear	Distraction and/or rotation-shear	Distraction and/or rotation-shear

common TLI that results from forces posterior to the vertebral body axis of rotation that compress the posterior column and distract the anterior and middle column. The anterior longitudinal ligament is often disrupted.[11]

11.3.3 Rotational

Rotational injuries (▶ Fig. 11.2f) occur when rotational forces are applied along the long axis of the

spine, often concurrently with flexion-distraction and shear forces. Significant rotational forces commonly result in **fracture-dislocation fractures** (▶ Fig. 11.2g), an unstable injury with high risk of neurologic compromise.[33] These injuries often result in three-column complex failure of bony and ligamentous structures of the vertebrae.[34] In a fracture-dislocation fracture, the anterior spinal column is generally compressed and/or rotation-sheared, whereas the middle and posterior columns are generally distracted and/or rotation-sheared.[6,23] Anteroposterior listhesis can be seen on imaging in the sagittal plane, whereas lateral listhesis is observed in the coronal plane. Complete spinal cord transection at the level of fracture is common.

11.3.4 Shear

Shear forces cause vertebral displacement in the anterior, posterior, or lateral plane, and can cause severe disruption of the ligaments (▶ Fig. 11.2h).[25] Significant shear forces are associated with fracture-dislocation injuries.[35]

11.3.5 Conus Medullaris and Cauda Equina Syndromes

Conus medullaris syndrome (CMS) and CES are the result of compression of the caudal end of the spinal cord (L1–L2) and cauda equina (below L2), respectively. These are typically diagnosed clinically, and then confirmed with radiographic imaging.[36] Further information on differentiating these two syndromes can be found in the "Pearls" section at the end of this chapter. Imaging should be performed with MRI, as X-ray and CT cannot adequately visualize the spinal cord and cauda equina. There is general agreement that prompt surgical decompression is indicated.[37]

11.4 Clinical Presentation and Initial Evaluation

TLIs usually occur subsequent to high-energy trauma, are more common in men than women, and are more common in younger (15–29 years old) populations.[22,23,38,39,40] The majority of these injuries occur at the TL junction (>50%), and these patients often present with pain and point tenderness at the point of injury.[11,23,38,41] Polytraumas are extremely common in the setting of TLI, and common associated injuries include intra-abdominal bleeding, arterial/venous disruption, and pulmonary injuries.[11,39] For this reason, TLIs are often overlooked, especially in the context of more pressing, life-threatening injuries.[38] After life-threatening issues have been addressed, a full neurological work-up and imaging should be performed for patients with suspected TLI. In the setting of a suspected spinal injury, it is imperative to stabilize the spine, such as through the use of a cervical collar and backboard, to avoid further injury.[42]

Neurological function should be assessed using the ASIA classification system. If the level of neurological deficit is not in agreement with the suspected location of TLI (e.g., upper limb deficits in a suspected L1–L3 TLI), then MRI of the whole spinal column should be performed to identify the cause of the deficit.

All patients with suspected spinal trauma should receive a plain X-ray radiograph or CT scan of the entire vertebral column. Radiographs should include two views, anteroposterior and lateral.[41] CT is better than plain films at determining the bony morphology of TLIs, but neither can adequately visualize soft tissue structures.[11] MRI is superior for diagnosing soft tissue injuries such as disruption of the PLC, as well as assessing spinal cord integrity.[39,41]

Patients suffering from TLI may be in a state of spinal shock at presentation. Spinal shock refers to a temporary state of nonresponsiveness of spinal cord neurons below the level of the injury to CNS stimulation. In spinal shock, there is a temporary loss of all motor, sensory, and reflex function below the level of the TLI, likely due to effects of spinal cord contusion. Spinal shock typically lasts 1 to 3 days, after which, in the setting of an incomplete spinal injury, sensory, motor, and reflex function will begin to return. The bulbocavernous reflex (BCR), one of the first reflexes to return after spinal shock, can be used to identify whether spinal shock has subsided. The BCR is elicited by gently tugging on the glans penis or clitoris and testing for a reflexive increase in anal sphincter tone.[36] The absence of motor and sensory function below the level of TLI after a positive BCR test suggests a complete spinal cord injury, with no expectation of return of function.[41]

Special populations such as osteoporotic and pediatric patients often differ from the typical clinical and/or radiographic presentation in the context of trauma.[43,44] Osteoporotic patients with TLI are most commonly elderly, female patients, and present after low-energy, ground-level falls.[23,43] They often present with radiating leg pain and impaired mobility.[43] Pediatric TLIs, while rare, usually occurs in the context of trauma and can be difficult to diagnose on X-ray due in part to lack of calcification of their immature epiphyseal plates.[44]

11.5 Imaging Modalities and Findings

Radiographic imaging is the mainstay for confirmation of clinical suspicion of TLI. The choice of imaging modality utilized depends on institutional availability, time, clinical presentation, and cost.

11.5.1 Standard Radiographs (X-ray)

Generally, full spine anteroposterior and lateral X-rays are obtained first in setting of a suspected TLI. They are cheaper and faster than other modalities such as CT and MRI. Although time and cost effective, they are less sensitive than CT at identifying and classifying TL fractures.[45,46]

11.5.2 Computed Tomography (CT)

CT is superior to standard radiographs at identifying bone injuries subsequent to TLI.[45] Certain CT techniques, such as multislice spiral CT scans, have the added benefit of being able to screen for visceral and TLIs concurrently.[47]

11.5.3 Magnetic Resonance Imaging (MRI)

In the setting of neurological deficits, MRI is the imaging modality of choice. MRI is superior for identifying soft tissue structures, such as the spinal cord and PLC.

11.5.4 CT-Myelography (for those with Contraindications to MRI)

In patients with contraindications to MRI (e.g., Pacemaker), CT-myelography can be utilized to visualize soft tissue structures. It requires the injection of radiographic dye into the spinal canal, so it generally is not utilized unless there is contraindication to MRI.[11]

A summary of the most common TL fractures and their imaging findings can be summarized in ► Table 11.2.

11.6 Classification Systems

Currently, several systems are utilized to classify TLIs, often differing between institutions,[53] and few systems have been validated in a systematic manner.[54,55] In 1983, Dennis et al, published one

Table 11.2 Summary of image findings and management strategies of thoracolumbar injuries

Radiographic imaging and management of thoracolumbar injuries			
Injury type	Image findings	Management	Notes
Compression fracture	↓ anterior vertebral column height, preserved middle and posterior column height, creating "wedge" appearance on lateral imaging	Nonsurgical if no PLC or neurological involvement	Most common > 50% all thoracolumbar (TL) fractures,[22] minimal risk for neurological deficit
Burst fracture	↓ posterior vertebral column height, ↑ interpedicular distance	Nonsurgical if no PLC or neurological involvement. Otherwise posterior or combined approach[48]	Significant risk of neurological deficit
Flexion-distraction fracture	↓ anterior vertebral column height, ↑ interspinous distance	Surgery. Posterior or combined approach	
Flexion-dislocation	Anteroposterior listhesis and lateral listhesis of the spine	Surgery. Posterior or combined approach	Highly associated with spinal cord injury and cauda equina syndrome
Osteoporotic compression fracture	↓ anterior vertebral column height, often greater than 50%	Usually nonsurgical. If surgery undergone, generally vertebroplasty or kyphoplasty[49,50,51,52]	Common in elderly females
Cauda equina and conus medullaris syndrome	Visible compression of cauda equina on computed tomography (CT) or magnetic resonance imaging (MRI). Generally suspected clinically and confirmed radiographically[36]	Decompressive surgery as soon as patient is stable	Clinical suspicion should be raised if patient is presenting with saddle anesthesia and/ or urinary dysfunction

of the earliest classification systems, the three-column system, for classifying TLIs[6] (▶ Fig. 11.1). For clinical decision making, currently, surgeons most often use one of the following three classification systems: AO, TLCIS, and AOSpine.

11.6.1 AO Classification System

In 1994, Magerl et al proposed a classification system based on the AO Classification System.[9] Injuries were divided according to the mechanism of injury and split into three groups: type A (compression), type B (distraction), and type C (rotational). Although the AO Classification System was a major improvement from previous systems, its complexity and lack of reliability when applied in clinical situations has limited its utility.[56,57,58,59,60]

11.6.2 Thoracolumbar Injury Classification System (TLICS)

The Thoracolumbar Injury Classification System (TLICS) was a modification of the Thoracolumbar Injury Severity Score developed by Vaccaro et al.[54,58] It is a treatment algorithm that aimed to assist in directing patient management and treatment using three major categories: mechanism of injury, integrity of the posterior ligamentous complex (PLC), and neurologic status of the patient. Each of these major categories has subdivisions where a point value (1–4) is assigned to a certain variable reflective of injury severity (▶ Table 11.3).[58] Scores from the three major categories are summed in a final value that helps dictate treatment modalities (▶ Table 11.4).[58] Studies have shown that implementation of the TLICS better allows surgeons to identify unstable injuries requiring operative management with good interrater reliability.[61,62,63] Despite the external validity of the TLICS system, one commonly identified shortcoming is its inconsistency when used for grading and recommending treatment for burst fractures.[62]

11.6.3 AOSpine Injury Score

The Thoracolumbar AOSpine Injury Score was developed through a survey given out to surgeons worldwide and aimed to combine the AO classification and TLICS while eliminating their weaknesses (specifically the reliance on MRI for diagnosis).[64] It utilizes a hierarchical approach to the classification of fractures with types A, B, and C that are further divided into subgroups, while

Table 11.3 The thoracolumbar injury classification system (TLICS)

Variable	Qualifier	Score
Morphology		
Compression		1
	Burst	1
Translation/rotation		3
Distraction		4
PLC integrity		
Intact		0
Suspected/indeterminate		2
Injured		3
Neurological status		
Intact		0
Nerve root		2
Cord/conus	Complete	2
	Incomplete	3
Cauda equina		3

Table 11.4 Treatment recommendations based on the thoracolumbar injury classification system (TLICS) cumulative score

Score	Recommendation
≤3	Initial trial of nonoperative treatment recommended
4	Decision for operative vs. nonoperative treatment at the discretion of the surgeon
≥5	Surgical stabilization recommended

also taking patient's neurological status into account with a separate hierarchy (▶ Table 11.5).[64] Like the TLICS, the AOSpine Injury Score assigns numerical value to the fracture type and neurological status, summing them in a final number that helps dictate the treatment approach for a patient (▶ Table 11.6).[65,66] The AOSpine Injury Score demonstrates substantial interobserver reliability in classification of fracture morphology (A–C) and, moderate reliability in subgrouping the fractures (A0–A4, B1–B3, and C).[63]

11.6.4 Classification of Spinal Cord Injury: The ASIA Impairment Scale

While there are a number of classifications for vertebral injury, neurological assessment of traumatic spinal cord injuries is classified by the American Spinal Injury Association (ASIA) Impairment Scale

Table 11.5 The Thoracolumbar AOSpine Injury Score classification system

Classification	Score
Type A: compression injuries	
A0	0
A1	1
A2	2
A3	3
A4	5
Type B: tension band injuries	
B1	5
B2	6
B3	7
Type C: translational injuries	
C	8
Neurological status	
N0	0
N1	1
N2	2
N3	4
N4	4
NX (unknown neurological status)	3
Patient: specific modifiers	
M1	1
M2	0

grade.[67] The ASIA grade characterizes relative neural involvement and functional impairment at and below the level of injury and defines injury severity. That ASIA Impairment Scale is graded A–E based on the degree of injury (▶ Table 11.7).[67] The ASIA Impairment Scale is critical in assessing for severity of neurological damage following TL injury.

11.7 Treatment

11.7.1 Conservative Treatment

Compression and stable burst fractures can usually be managed nonsurgically.[11,23] Both molded braces and hyperextension casts have been shown to be suitable options for these types of

Table 11.6 Treatment recommendations based on AOSpine cumulative score

Score	Recommendation
< 4	Initial trial of nonoperative treatment recommended
4–5	Decision for operative vs. nonoperative treatment should be individualized based on patient variables and surgeon preference
> 5	Early operative treatment recommended

Table 11.7 The ASIA impairment scale (AIS)

Grade	Meaning	Definition
A	Complete	No sensory or motor function preserved in the sacral segments S4–S5
B	Sensory incomplete	Sensory but not motor function preserved below the neurological level and includes the sacral segments S4–S5 (light touch or pin prick at S4–S5 or deep anal pressure) AND no motor function is preserved more than three levels below the motor level on either side of the body
C	Motor incomplete	Motor function preserved at the most caudal sacral segments for voluntary anal contraction (VAC) OR the patient meets the criteria for sensory incomplete status (sensory function preserved at the most caudal sacral segments (S4–S5) by light touch, pin prick, or deep anal pressure), and has some sparing of motor function more than three levels below the ipsilateral motor level on either side of the body. (This includes key or nonkey muscle functions to determine motor incomplete status.) For AIS C—less than half of key muscle functions below the single neurological level of injury have a muscle grade ≥ 3
D	Motor incomplete	Motor incomplete status as defined above, with at least half (half or more) of key muscle functions below the single neurological level of injury (NLI) having a muscle grade ≥ 3
E	Normal	If sensation and motor function as tested with the International Standards for Neurological Classification of Spinal Cord Injury (ISNCSCI) are graded as normal in all segments, and the patient had prior deficits, then the AIS grade is E. Someone without an initial spinal cord injury does not receive an AIS grade

TLIs for symptomatic relief, but no brace is necessary for stability.[68,69,70] Nonoperative approaches also avoid the cost and morbidities associated with operative management.[11,71] The management of neurologically intact burst fractures is controversial, with conflicting views in the literature. In a prospective randomized study, Wood et al found no differences in functional outcomes between operative and nonoperative management for stable burst fractures without neurological deficit.[71] Conversely, in another prospective study of stable TL compression fractures without neurological deficits, Siebenga et al found improved outcomes and return to work in patients treated operatively vs. nonoperative management.[72]

11.7.2 Indication for Surgery

There are two main clinical indications for surgical management of TLI: neurologic impairment and instability.[11,23,60] The consensus among surgeons is that patients with TLICS scores greater than 4 would benefit from surgical management, as these patients commonly have significant PLC injury or neurologic compromise. Patients with neurologic injury and evidence of neurologic compression on imaging should undergo decompression. Additionally, mechanically unstable TLI should undergo surgical stabilization, commonly involving posterior pedicle screw and rod instrumentation with fusion.[11,23,60] However, significant controversy exists regarding the approaches for decompression and length of stabilization for these injuries. Long-segment instrumentation (> 1 level above and below the fracture) can be considered to improve the biomechanical stability with osteoporotic patients, three-column injuries, and TL junction injuries. Long-segment instrumentation is also recommended in patients with ankylosing spondylitis; however, further discussion of this condition is outside the scope of this chapter.

11.7.3 Surgical Options with Advantages/Disadvantages of Each Option

The absence of high-quality prospective studies makes clear clinical indications for different surgical approaches difficult.[11] Despite this major shortcoming, there are certain guidelines that are generally followed.[23,53,58]

TLIs that involve the PLC and/or neurologic compromise can be addressed via a posterior surgical approach.[23,53,58] Commonly, less than 50% canal stenosis from retropulsed fracture fragments can be addressed from posterior approaches. Indirect decompression through restoration of vertebral height through traction can be a useful adjunct in reducing anterior canal stenosis, but is only effective if done within 48 hours of injury.[73] For direct decompression, a laminectomy can remove any posterior canal compression and the addition of a facetectomy with or without pedicle removal (transpedicular approaches) can allow for a lateral trajectory for direct removal of retropulsed anterior fragments. Although some surgeons may prefer an anterior approach for significant (> 50%) anterior canal compromise, posterior transpedicular approaches can be used when polytrauma or medical contraindications preclude anterior approaches. Additionally, the posterior approach is also a useful approach for reducing displaced rotational and shear injuries through direct manipulation of proximal and distal vertebral segments.

Injuries with significant anterior compression of the spinal cord or cauda equina in addition to PLC injuries can be considered for circumferential (anterior and posterior based) approaches.[23,53,58] In general, when significant decompression of the anterior column is required, a posterior approach alone may be insufficient due to the difficulty in visualizing and accessing the anterior column. Another major drawback in a posterior-only approach is that it generally requires a longer surgical fixation construct, which limits mobility about the vertebral column.

While anterior approaches may be appropriate in certain contexts, it also generally requires a longer operative time, and is associated with larger intraoperative blood loss.[74,75] Anterior approaches allow for direct decompression of retropulsed bone and soft tissue from the canal as well as anterior column reconstruction. However, the anterior approach frequently requires a posterior approach as well for pedicle screw instrumentation, adding time and morbidity to the procedure. Multiple studies of patients with TL fractures undergoing combined anteroposterior surgeries have failed to find meaningful improvements in functional outcomes over posterior-only approaches.[7,76,77,78]

Percutaneous approaches are becoming increasingly popular due to their soft tissue sparing nature and decreased surgical morbidity.[79] Compared to conventional open techniques for pedicle screws, percutaneous techniques result in less postoperative pain, shorter duration of hospitalization, and lower intraoperative blood loss.[80,81,82] A recent meta-analysis assessing percutaneous vs. open approach in patients with intact neurological status and stable TL fracture found no difference between the groups in terms of long-term outcome.[83]

11.7.4 Surgical Techniques and Postoperative Care

The surgical techniques available can most simply be divided into four categories: anterior, posterior, paraspinal, and percutaneous. Anterior surgeries can be done in conjunction with a general, vascular, or thoracic surgeon. The anterior approach can be used to access the anterior aspects of the thoracic and lumbar spine from approximately the mid-thoracic spine to the lumbosacral junction. Anterior thoracic approaches can be performed from the left or right sides, but commonly a left-sided approach is utilized as the aorta is a more robust vascular structure to retract than the more delicate vena cava. Thoracic approaches use a lateral, oblique incision at the level of the TLI and often requires entering the thoracic cavity when accessing thoracic levels. For lumbar anterior approaches, an open retroperitoneal approach can access from the TL junction to the lumbosacral junction. When accessing the TL junction, the positioning and approach are similar to thoracic approaches, using lateral positioning and extensile oblique incisions. Conversely, for low lumbar spine access that requires access to the lumbosacral junction, supine positioning with an extensile midline incision for the open anterior retroperitoneal approach allows improved access to the L5–S1 disc space when compared to lateral positioning and approaches. Although extensile, open approaches to the thoracic and lumbar spine are the "workhorse" approach for anterior treatment of TLI, the development of minimally invasive approaches to the TL spine such as direct lateral/trans-psoas or oblique/anterior-to-psoas approaches with specialized retraction systems can minimize approach-related morbidity for the anterior treatment of TLI. Posterior approaches

involve a midline incision on the prone patient cut deep to the level of involved spinous process. The Wiltse paraspinal approach is a common subtype of posterior approach involving a more lateral pathway to the involved vertebral level.[75] Percutaneous approaches are variable, but are characterized by their less-invasive approach to access the TLI.[79] The posterior approach begins with a midline longitudinal incision. Intraoperative radiography is used to confirm operative levels prior to extensive exposure. The spine is exposed subperiosteally with electrocautery, beginning with the spinous process and proceeding deep and lateral to the lamina, pars articularis, and then transverse process. The facet capsules of joints not included in the fusion should be avoided. Muscle relaxant facilitates exposure but is contraindicated for cord-level decompressions with neuromonitoring. Care should be taken at levels with fractured lamina or ruptured PLC, as the standard anatomy may not be present to prevent inadvertent dural or neurologic injury during exposure.

Screw tracts are cannulated, tapped, and occluded with bone wax prior to decompression. Cord-level laminectomy decompressions are performed with a motorized burr using longitudinal troughs. The troughs are deepened to the level of the ligamentum flavum and/or dura and the lamina are removed en-bloc. The spinous processes are grasped with a sharp towel clamp and gently lifted to allow final soft tissue resection with a nerve hook and 2-mm kerrison rongeur. If fusion is concurrently performed, the lamina bone is separated from the soft tissues, morselized, and used as autologous local bone graft. After screw and rod placement, the transverse processes are decorticated, and bone graft is placed in the lateral gutters. Indirect decompression can be achieved by using monoaxial screws, bilaterally placing rods and endcaps loosely at the cephalad level and tightly at the caudad level. A distractor is used to distract between the screws spanning the injured segment, and the loose endcaps at the cephalad level are tightened.

To perform an anterior decompression through the posterior approach, first a facetectomy is performed on the side required to access anteriorly. After laminectomy decompression, osteotomes and kerrison rongeurs are used to remove the inferior and superior articular processes. Following this, Penfield 1 dissectors are used to protect the adjacent dura and exiting nerve root.

The pedicle is then decancellated with a burr down to the posterior vertebral body until the pedicle walls are paper-thin. The walls can then be removed either with a pituitary or impacted into the pedicle cavity. At this point the ventral aspect of the cauda equina or spinal cord can be accessed for fracture fragment removal. For removal of fragments causing significant anterior compression, the vertebral body can be decancellated through the resected pedicle and the compressive fracture fragments can be impacted into the vertebral body cavity.

Postoperatively, patients should have chemical (heparin) and mechanical (SCDs) DVT prophylaxis. Mobilization with physical therapy should begin day of surgery when possible. Antibiotics are continued postoperatively for 24 hours after surgery and the wounds are closely followed in the hospital to monitor for excessive postoperative drainage or signs of infection. Infections are relatively common in the setting of TLI surgeries, with incidence as high at 10% in some studies.[11] Overall, given the broad range of surgical options and diversity of TLIs, there is no universally adopted postoperative approach, and care should be tailored to the individual patient.

11.7.5 Expected Outcomes (Based on Recent Literature)

There is still a deficiency in high-quality literature regarding long-term patient outcomes due to the difficulty in conducting well-controlled studies in trauma populations.[11] Additionally, the heterogeneity of TLI radiographic and clinical presentations further complicated the generation of comprehensive outcome measures. Despite the difficulty of categorizing these injuries, it is clear that severe TLIs have substantial effects on functional and return to work status.[84] One study on patients with unstable TL fractures found that 70% of patients were able to return to work, with only approximately 50% able to return to their preinjury level of activity.[22,84]

11.8 Pearls

11.8.1 Cauda Equina (CES) and Conus Medullaris Syndrome (CMS)

CES is significantly more common than CMS, and is most commonly caused by central lumbar herniation.[36,85] However, CES and CMS can also present in the context of a TLI. There is significant overlap in clinical presentation, because compression of only the conus medullaris is highly unlikely. Classically, CES results from spinal canal compression between the L2 and L4 vertebrae. Patients present with asymmetric significant lower limb sensory/motor loss, saddle anesthesia, and lower motor neuron signs. Bladder dysfunction is a common later stage finding of CES. CMS, being due to compression of the caudal end of the spinal cord, presents with symmetric, mild lower limb sensory/motor loss, and mixed upper and lower motor neuron signs.[36,85] In contrast to CES, loss of bladder function is a consistent and early finding. The anatomical basis of this presentation of CMS lies in the fact that the cell bodies of the neurons in the L5–S3 nerve roots reside in the conus medullaris, and compression results in loss of voluntary control of micturition through the pudendal nerve.[79] In pure CMS, the cauda equina nerve roots are mostly spared.[36]

11.8.2 Osteoporotic Populations

In patients with normal bone density, anterior vertebrae compression of more than 40% is highly suggestive of a burst or flexion-distraction fracture. However, in patients with osteoporosis/osteopenia, anterior compression of greater than 50% is not at all uncommon.[23] These TLI populations are unique, in that they generally present without a preceding traumatic event, and are often managed with nonoperative or percutaneous approaches such as cement augmentation.[43,49,50,51]

11.8.3 Multiple Vertebral Fractures

Multiple noncontiguous vertebral fractures are common, presenting in as many as 15 to 20% of TLI patients with an identified vertebral fracture. For this reason, any patient with an identified fracture should undergo radiographic imaging of the entire spine, especially in the context of a polytrauma.[40,86]

11.8.4 Lack of High-Quality Scientific Evidence in Management

Despite advances in the surgical techniques and patient outcomes, there is still a lack of concrete evidence regarding proper patient management in the context of TLI. For this reason, management of these injuries remains highly surgeon specific, with physicians being guided by their familiarity and experience with certain treatment modalities.

11.8.5 Consider the Patient Preference

While surgical approaches are associated with considerably higher morbidity than conservative management, there are certain indications for surgical management of stable TLIs. Surgical approaches allow for faster return to activity, and this may be appropriate in patients for whom prolonged bed rest is unacceptable.

11.8.6 Methylprednisone in the Setting of SCI

High-dose steroids such as methylprednisone in the setting of SCI is highly controversial.[11] Theoretically, these steroids prevent and reduce inflammation, reducing the risk of further injury and facilitating recovery. However, treating patients with methylprednisone has not been shown to improve clinical outcomes, and is associated with significant complications, such as respiratory and urinary infections.[11,87,88] In light of this, the use of steroids in the setting of SCI has been decreasing.[89]

11.8.7 Neurogenic Shock

Neurogenic shock refers to the loss of sympathetic (SNS) innervation below the level of injury, resulting in unopposed parasympathetic (PNS) activity. It is a clinical diagnosis, and is usually seen in TLIs that occur above the T6 vertebral level.[42] Unopposed PNS activity results in systemic vasodilation and decreased cardiac sinoatrial node rate, resulting in hypotension and bradycardia. It is critical to maintain normal systemic blood pressure and sinus rhythm to avoid spinal and visceral hypoperfusion. This can be accomplished with a vasopressor such as norepinephrine.[42]

11.8.8 If All Else Fails, Consider the Clinical Manifestations

Injuries to the thoracic vertebrae will cause lower extremity weakness and segmental denervation of the abdominal muscles. Lumbar injuries will generally spare all but the lower motor extremities, and are likely to present with CES or CMS. Similarly, suspect CMS in the presence of saddle anesthesia and/or urinary dysfunction.

11.9 Board-style Questions

1. A radiology attending is discussing a sagittal CT revealing 50% compression of the anterior vertebral column of L4. Which of the following descriptions best characterizes a patient that is likely to present with a similar finding in the absence of a more severe TLI?
   a) 47-year-old woman presenting after fall from third-story building
   b) 74-year-old woman presenting in a nontraumatic context (osteoporotic fractures compress more easily)
   c) 30-year-old male presenting after a motor vehicle accident
   d) 6-year-old male presenting after a motor vehicle accident

2. A 43-year-old male presents to the emergency room after being involved in a motor vehicle collision. He has suffered significant blood loss, and a visible bulge is palpable in his lower back, highly suggestive of TLI. His breathing is labored, and he is oriented only to person. Which of the following is the next best step in management?
   a) Assess airway and vitals (vitals trump all)
   b) Plain X-ray film of entire spine to identify spinal injury
   c) Plain X-ray film of thoracolumbar spine to identify TLI
   d) MRI to access spinal cord integrity

3. Which of the following thoracolumbar vertebral fractures is most likely to present with complete neurologic impairment below the level of injury?
   a) Compression fracture
   b) Burst fracture
   c) Osteoporotic compression fracture
   d) Flexion-dislocation fracture

4. A 35-year-old male presents to the emergency room with a stable compression fracture of the L1 vertebrae after motor collision. There is no evidence of neurological involvement, and his vitals are otherwise unremarkable. Which of the following is the best course of management of this patient's TLI?
   a) Posterior vertebroplasty
   b) Anterior vertebroplasty

    c) Nonoperative management (stable fracture, no neurological impairment)

    d) L1–L2 fixation and fusion

5. Which of the following best characterizes the mechanism of a compression fracture?

    a) High-energy shear

    b) High-energy axial loading (pretty much what defines the compression fracture)

    c) Low-energy shear

    d) Low-energy axial loading

6. Which of the following is best representative of an indication for surgical management of a TLI?

    a) Damage to the PLC (need surgery if PLC is damaged, it is avascular and doesn't heal well)

    b) Involvement of the lumbar spine

    c) Involvement of T1–T6

    d) Compression of > 20% of any single vertebral level

7. Damage to the spinal cord can be most accurately assessed with which of the following imaging modalities?

    a) Plain X-ray film

    b) Spiral CT

    c) Ultrasound

    d) MRI

8. A 42-year-old woman presents to emergency room obtunded. While originally unstable, trauma care manages to stabilize her. Purely epidemiologically speaking, in the absence of additional information, which of the following TLIs is most likely?

    a) Burst fracture of L2 (by far most likely of choices)

    b) Chance fracture of T6

    c) Flexion-distraction of L1

    d) Chance fracture of T8

9. Which of the following TLIs is most likely to present with significant PLC failure?

    a) Compression fracture

    b) Flexion-distraction fracture

    c) Burst fracture

    d) Osteoporotic compression fracture

10. A 34-year-old woman presents with a burst fracture that has led to cauda equina syndrome. Which of the following vertebral levels were most likely involved in the burst fracture?

    a) L3 (spinal cord ends at L1–L2)

    b) T7

    c) T9

    d) L1

Answers

1. b
2. a
3. d
4. c
5. b
6. a
7. d
8. a
9. b
10. a

References

[1] Holbrook TL, Grazier KL. The frequency of occurrence, impact, and cost of selected musculoskeletal conditions in the United States. American Academy of Orthopaedic Surgeons; 1984. https://books.google.com/books?id=u0xsAAAAMAAJ

[2] Kato S, Murray J-C, Kwon BK, Schroeder GD, Vaccaro AR, Fehlings MG. Does surgical intervention or timing of surgery have an effect on neurological recovery in the setting of a thoracolumbar burst fracture? J Orthop Trauma. 2017; 31 Suppl 4:S38–S43

[3] Zhang C, Ouyang B, Li P, et al. A retrospective study of thoracolumbar fractures treated with fixation and nonfusion surgery of intravertebral bone graft assisted with balloon kyphoplasty. World Neurosurg. 2017; 108:798–806

[4] Ender SA, Eschler A, Ender M, Merk HR, Kayser R. Fracture care using percutaneously applied titanium mesh cages (OsseoFix®) for unstable osteoporotic thoracolumbar burst fractures is able to reduce cement-associated complications: results after 12 months. J Orthop Surg Res. 2015; 10: 175

[5] Gertzbein SD. Scoliosis Research Society. Multicenter spine fracture study. Spine. 1992; 17(5):528–540

[6] Denis F. The three column spine and its significance in the classification of acute thoracolumbar spinal injuries. Spine (Phila Pa 1976). 1983; 8(8):817–831

[7] Knop C, Blauth M, Bühren V, et al. Operative treatment of fractures and dislocations of the thoracolumbar spine—Part 1: epidemiology. Unfallchirurg. 1999; 102(12):924–935

[8] Reid DC, Hu R, Davis LA, Saboe LA. The nonoperative treatment of burst fractures of the thoracolumbar junction. J Trauma. 1988; 28(8):1188–1194

[9] Magerl F, Aebi M, Gertzbein SD, Harms J, Nazarian S. A comprehensive classification of thoracic and lumbar injuries. Eur Spine J. 1994; 3(4):184–201

[10] Dai LY, Yao WF, Cui YM, Zhou Q. Thoracolumbar fractures in patients with multiple injuries: diagnosis and treatment—a review of 147 cases. J Trauma. 2004; 56(2):348–355

[11] Wood KB, Li W, Lebl DR, Ploumis A. Management of thoracolumbar spine fractures. Spine J. 2014; 14(1):145–164

[12] Knop C, Fabian HF, Bastian L, et al. Fate of the transpedicular intervertebral bone graft after posterior stabilisation of thoracolumbar fractures. Eur Spine J. 2002; 11(3): 251–257

[13] Saboe LA, Reid DC, Davis LA, Warren SA, Grace MG. Spine trauma and associated injuries. J Trauma. 1991; 31(1):43–48

[14] Gray L, Vandemark R, Hays M. Thoracic and lumbar spine trauma. Semin Ultrasound CT MR. 2001; 22(2):125–134

[15] Wilke HJ, Herkommer A, Werner K, Liebsch C. In vitro analysis of the segmental flexibility of the thoracic spine. PLoS One. 2017; 12(5):e0177823

[16] Forseen SE, Gilbert BC, Patel S, Ramirez J, Borden NM. Use of the thoracolumbar facet transition as a method of identifying the T12 segment. Spine. 2015; 4(2):10–13

[17] Ghobrial GM, Maulucci CM, Maltenfort M, et al. Operative and nonoperative adverse events in the management of traumatic fractures of the thoracolumbar spine: a systematic review. Neurosurg Focus. 2014; 37(1):E8

[18] Dai LY, Jiang SD, Wang XY, Jiang LS. A review of the management of thoracolumbar burst fractures. Surg Neurol. 2007; 67(3):221–231, discussion 231

[19] Kraemer WJ, Schemitsch EH, Lever J, McBroom RJ, McKee MD, Waddell JP. Functional outcome of thoracolumbar burst fractures without neurological deficit. J Orthop Trauma. 1996; 10(8):541–544

[20] Ivancic PC. Hybrid cadaveric/surrogate model of thoracolumbar spine injury due to simulated fall from height. Accid Anal Prev. 2013; 59:185–191

[21] Nagaraja S, Awada HK, Dreher ML, Gupta S, Miller SW. Vertebroplasty increases compression of adjacent IVDs and vertebrae in osteoporotic spines. Spine J. 2013; 13(12):1872–1880

[22] Reinhold M, Knop C, Beisse R, et al. Operative treatment of 733 patients with acute thoracolumbar spinal injuries: comprehensive results from the second, prospective, Internet-based multicenter study of the Spine Study Group of the German Association of Trauma Surgery. Eur Spine J. 2010; 19(10):1657–1676

[23] Raniga SB, Skalski MR, Kirwadi A, Menon VK, Al-Azri FH, Butt S. Thoracolumbar spine injury at CT: trauma/emergency radiology. Radiographics. 2016; 36(7):2234–2235

[24] King AG. Burst compression fractures of the thoracolumbar spine: pathologic anatomy and surgical management. Orthopedics. 1987; 10(12):1711–1719

[25] Roaf R. A study of the mechanics of spinal injuries. J Bone Joint Surg Br. 1960; 42-B(4):810–823

[26] Zaryanov AV, Park DK, Khalil JG, Baker KC, Fischgrund JS. Cement augmentation in vertebral burst fractures. Neurosurg Focus. 2014; 37(1):E5

[27] Yüksel MO, Gürbüz MS, Gök Ş, Karaarslan N, İş M, Berkman MZ. The association between sagittal index, canal compromise, loss of vertebral body height, and severity of spinal cord injury in thoracolumbar burst fractures. J Neurosci Rural Pract. 2016; 7(5) Suppl 1:S57–S61

[28] Defino HLA, De Pádua MA, Shimano AC. Estudo experimental da aplicação das forças de compressão ou distração sobre o sistema de fixação pedicular. Acta Ortop Bras. 2006; 14(3):148–151

[29] Domenicucci M, Ramieri A, Lenzi J, Fontana E, Martini S. Pseudo-aneurysm of a lumbar artery after flexion-distraction injury of the thoraco-lumbar spine and surgical realignment: rupture treated by endovascular embolization. Spine. 2008; 33(3):E81–E84

[30] Grossbach AJ, Dahdaleh NS, Abel TJ, Woods GD, Dlouhy BJ, Hitchon PW. Flexion-distraction injuries of the thoracolumbar spine: open fusion versus percutaneous pedicle screw fixation. Neurosurg Focus. 2013; 35(2):E2

[31] Weitzman G. Treatment of stable thoracolumbar spine compression fractures by early ambulation. Clin Orthop Relat Res. 1971; 76(76):116–122

[32] Chance GQ. Note on a type of flexion fracture of the spine. Br J Radiol. 1948; 21(249):452

[33] Tian NF, Mao FM, Xu HZ. Traumatic fracture-dislocation of the lumbar spine. Surgery. 2013; 153(5):739–740

[34] Holdsworth FW. Fractures, dislocations, and fracture-dislocations of the spine. J Bone Joint Surg Br. 1963; 45-B (1):6–20

[35] Freeman BJC, Bisbinas I, Nelson IW. Shear fracture-dislocation of the lumbar spine without paraplegia. Injury. 1997; 28(8):563–564

[36] Orendácová J, Cízková D, Kafka J, et al. Cauda equina syndrome. Prog Neurobiol. 2001; 64(6):613–637

[37] Spector LR, Madigan L, Rhyne A, Darden B, II, Kim D. Cauda equina syndrome. J Am Acad Orthop Surg. 2008; 16(8):471–479

[38] Sherman SC. Simon's Emergency Orthopedics. McGraw-Hill; 2015

[39] An HS, Singh K. Synopsis of spine surgery. In: An HS, Singh K, eds. Synopsis of Spine Surgery. Georg Thieme Verlag; 2016

[40] Ghobrial GM, Jallo J. Thoracolumbar spine trauma: review of the evidence. J Neurosurg Sci. 2013; 57(2):115–122

[41] Rajasekaran S, Kanna RM, Shetty AP. Management of thoracolumbar spine trauma: an overview. Indian J Orthop. 2015; 49(1):72–82

[42] Dave S, Cho JJ. Neurogenic Shock. Treasure Island, FL: StatPearls Publishing; 2018

[43] Han S, Park H-S, Pee Y-H, Oh S-H, Jang I-T. The clinical characteristics of lower lumbar osteoporotic compression fractures treated by percutaneous vertebroplasty : a comparative analysis of 120 cases. Korean J Spine. 2013; 10(4):221–226

[44] Saul D, Dresing K. Epidemiology of vertebral fractures in pediatric and adolescent patients. Pediatr Rep. 2018; 10(1):7232

[45] Hauser CJ, Visvikis G, Hinrichs C, et al. Prospective validation of computed tomographic screening of the thoracolumbar spine in trauma. J Trauma. 2003; 55(2):228–234, discussion 234–235

[46] Krueger MA, Green DA, Hoyt D, Garfin SR. Overlooked spine injuries associated with lumbar transverse process fractures. Clin Orthop Relat Res. 1996; 327(327):191–195

[47] Leidner B, Adiels M, Aspelin P, Gullstrand P, Wallén S. Standardized CT examination of the multitraumatized patient. Eur Radiol. 1998; 8(9):1630–1638

[48] Atlas SW, Regenbogen V, Rogers LF, Kim KS. The radiographic characterization of burst fractures of the spine. AJR Am J Roentgenol. 1986; 147(3):575–582

[49] Klazen CA, Lohle PN, de Vries J, et al. LPNM. Vertebroplasty versus conservative treatment in acute osteoporotic vertebral compression fractures (Vertos II): An open-label randomised trial. Lancet. 2010; 376(9746):1085–1092

[50] Link TM, Guglielmi G, van Kuijk C, Adams JE. Radiologic assessment of osteoporotic vertebral fractures: diagnostic and prognostic implications. Eur Radiol. 2005; 15(8):1521–1532

[51] Liu JT, Liao WJ, Tan WC, et al. Balloon kyphoplasty versus vertebroplasty for treatment of osteoporotic vertebral compression fracture: a prospective, comparative, and randomized clinical study. Osteoporos Int. 2010; 21(2):359–364

[52] Patil S, Rawall S, Singh D, et al. Surgical patterns in osteoporotic vertebral compression fractures. Eur Spine J. 2013; 22 (4):883–891

[53] Vaccaro AR, Lehman RA, Jr, Hurlbert RJ, et al. A new classification of thoracolumbar injuries: the importance of injury morphology, the integrity of the posterior ligamentous complex, and neurologic status. Spine. 2005; 30 (20):2325–2333

[54] Vaccaro AR, Baron EM, Sanfilippo J, et al. Reliability of a novel classification system for thoracolumbar injuries: the Thoracolumbar Injury Severity Score. Spine. 2006; 31(11) Suppl:S62–S69, discussion S104

[55] Bono CM, Vaccaro AR, Hurlbert RJ, et al. Validating a newly proposed classification system for thoracolumbar spine trauma: looking to the future of the thoracolumbar injury classification and severity score. J Orthop Trauma. 2006; 20 (8):567–572

[56] Oner FC, Ramos LM, Simmermacher RK, et al. Classification of thoracic and lumbar spine fractures: problems of reproducibility. A study of 53 patients using CT and MRI. Eur Spine J. 2002; 11(3):235–245

[57] Patel AA, Vaccaro AR, Albert TJ, et al. The adoption of a new classification system: time-dependent variation in interobserver reliability of the thoracolumbar injury severity score classification system. Spine. 2007; 32(3):E105–E110

[58] Vaccaro AR, Zeiller SC, Hulbert RJ, et al. The thoracolumbar injury severity score: a proposed treatment algorithm. J Spinal Disord Tech. 2005; 18(3):209–215

[59] Joaquim AF, Lawrence B, Daubs M, et al. Measuring the impact of the Thoracolumbar Injury Classification and Severity Score among 458 consecutively treated patients. J Spinal Cord Med. 2014; 37(1):101–106

[60] Wood KB, Khanna G, Vaccaro AR, Arnold PM, Harris MB, Mehbod AA. Assessment of two thoracolumbar fracture classification systems as used by multiple surgeons. J Bone Joint Surg Am. 2005; 87(7):1423–1429

[61] Raja Rampersaud Y, Fisher C, Wilsey J, et al. Agreement between orthopedic surgeons and neurosurgeons regarding a new algorithm for the treatment of thoracolumbar injuries: a multicenter reliability study. J Spinal Disord Tech. 2006; 19(7):477–482

[62] Rihn JA, Yang N, Fisher C, et al. Using magnetic resonance imaging to accurately assess injury to the posterior ligamentous complex of the spine: a prospective comparison of the surgeon and radiologist. J Neurosurg Spine. 2010; 12(4): 391–396

[63] Kepler CK, Vaccaro AR, Koerner JD, et al. Reliability analysis of the AOSpine thoracolumbar spine injury classification system by a worldwide group of naïve spinal surgeons. Eur Spine J. 2016; 25(4):1082–1086

[64] Kepler CK, Vaccaro AR, Schroeder GD, et al. The thoracolumbar aospine injury score. Global Spine J. 2016; 6(4): 329–334

[65] Schroeder GD, Harrop JS, Vaccaro AR. Thoracolumbar trauma classification. Neurosurg Clin N Am. 2017; 28(1): 23–29

[66] Vaccaro AR, Schroeder GD, Kepler CK, et al. The surgical algorithm for the AOSpine thoracolumbar spine injury classification system. Eur Spine J. 2016; 25(4):1087–1094

[67] Dukes EM, Kirshblum S, Aimetti AA, Qin SS, Bornheimer RK, Oster G. Relationship of American Spinal Injury Association impairment scale grade to post-injury hospitalization and costs in thoracic spinal cord injury. Neurosurgery. 2018; 83 (3):445–451

[68] Weinstein JN, Collalto P, Lehmann TR. Thoracolumbar "burst" fractures treated conservatively: a long-term follow-up. Spine. 1988; 13(1):33–38

[69] Mumford J, Weinstein JN, Spratt KF, Goel VK. Thoracolumbar burst fractures: the clinical efficacy and outcome of nonoperative management. Spine. 1993; 18(8):955–970

[70] Shen WJ, Shen YS. Nonsurgical treatment of three-column thoracolumbar junction burst fractures without neurologic deficit. Spine. 1999; 24(4):412–415

[71] Wood K, Buttermann G, Mehbod A, Garvey T, Jhanjee R, Sechriest V. Operative compared with nonoperative treatment of a thoracolumbar burst fracture without neurological deficit: a prospective, randomized study. J Bone Joint Surg Am. 2003; 85(5):773–781

[72] Siebenga J, Leferink VJM, Segers MJM, et al. Treatment of traumatic thoracolumbar spine fractures: a multicenter prospective randomized study of operative versus nonsurgical treatment. Spine. 2006; 31(25):2881–2890

[73] Whang PG, Vaccaro AR. Thoracolumbar fracture: posterior instrumentation using distraction and ligamentotaxis reduction. J Am Acad Orthop Surg. 2007; 15(11):695–701

[74] Zhu Q, Shi F, Cai W, Bai J, Fan J, Yang H. Comparison of anterior versus posterior approach in the treatment of thoracolumbar fractures: a systematic review. Int Surg. 2015; 100 (6):1124–1133

[75] Wu H, Fu C, Yu W, Wang J. The options of the three different surgical approaches for the treatment of Denis type A and B thoracolumbar burst fracture. Eur J Orthop Surg Traumatol. 2014; 24(1):29–35

[76] Oprel P, Tuinebreijer WE, Patka P, den Hartog D. Combined anterior-posterior surgery versus posterior surgery for thoracolumbar burst fractures: a systematic review of the literature. Open Orthop J. 2010; 4(1):93–100

[77] Smits AJ, Polack M, Deunk J, Bloemers FW. Combined anteroposterior fixation using a titanium cage versus solely posterior fixation for traumatic thoracolumbar fractures: a systematic review and meta-analysis. J Craniovertebr Junction Spine. 2017; 8(3):168–178

[78] Mayer M, Ortmaier R, Koller H, et al. Impact of sagittal balance on clinical outcomes in surgically treated T12 and L1 burst fractures: analysis of long-term outcomes after posterior-only and combined posteroanterior treatment. BioMed Res Int. 2017; 2017:1568258

[79] Alander DH, Cui S. Percutaneous pedicle screw stabilization: surgical technique, fracture reduction, and review of current spine trauma applications. J Am Acad Orthop Surg. 2018; 26 (7):231–240

[80] Lau D, Khan A, Terman SW, Yee T, La Marca F, Park P. Comparison of perioperative outcomes following open versus minimally invasive transforaminal lumbar interbody fusion in obese patients. Neurosurg Focus. 2013; 35(2):E10

[81] Terman SW, Yee TJ, Lau D, Khan AA, La Marca F, Park P. Minimally invasive versus open transforaminal lumbar interbody fusion: comparison of clinical outcomes among obese patients. J Neurosurg Spine. 2014; 20(6):644–652

[82] Wang J, Zhou Y, Feng Zhang Z, Qing Li C, Jie Zheng W, Liu J. Comparison of the clinical outcome in overweight or obese patients after minimally invasive versus open transforaminal lumbar interbody fusion. J Spinal Disord Tech. 2014; 27(4):202–206

[83] McAnany SJ, Overley SC, Kim JS, Baird EO, Qureshi SA, Anderson PA. Open versus minimally invasive fixation techniques for thoracolumbar trauma: a meta-analysis. Global Spine J. 2016; 6(2):186–194

[84] McLain RF. Functional outcomes after surgery for spinal fractures: return to work and activity. Spine. 2004; 29(4): 470–477, discussion Z6

[85] Radcliff KE, Kepler CK, Delasotta LA, et al. Current management review of thoracolumbar cord syndromes. Spine J. 2011; 11(9):884–892

[86] Ruiz Santiago F, Tomás Muñoz P, Moya Sánchez E, Revelles Paniza M, Martínez Martínez A, Pérez Abela AL. Classifying thoracolumbar fractures: role of quantitative imaging. Quant Imaging Med Surg. 2016; 6(6):772–784

[87] Ito Y, Sugimoto Y, Tomioka M, Kai N, Tanaka M. Does high dose methylprednisolone sodium succinate really improve neurological status in patient with acute cervical cord injury?: a prospective study about neurological recovery and early complications. Spine. 2009; 34(20): 2121–2124

[88] Evaniew N, Noonan VK, Fallah N, et al. RHSCIR Network. Methylprednisolone for the treatment of patients with acute spinal cord injuries: a propensity score-matched cohort study from a Canadian Multi-Center Spinal Cord Injury Registry. J Neurotrauma. 2015; 32(21): 1674–1683

[89] Hurlbert RJ, Hamilton MG. Methylprednisolone for acute spinal cord injury: 5-year practice reversal. Can J Neurol Sci. 2008; 35(1):41–45

Suggested Readings

Raniga SB, Skalski MR, Kirwadi A, Menon VK, Al-Azri FH, Butt S. Thoracolumbar spine injury at CT: trauma/emergency radiology. Radiographics. 2016; 36(7):2234–2235

Reinhold M, Knop C, Beisse R, et al. Operative treatment of 733 patients with acute thoracolumbar spinal injuries: comprehensive results from the second, prospective, Internet-based multicenter study of the Spine Study Group of the German Association of Trauma Surgery. Eur Spine J. 2010; 19(10):1657–1676

Sherman SC, Sharieff GQ. Simons Emergency Orthopedics. New York: McGraw-Hill Medical; 2014

Vaccaro AR, Oner C, Kepler CK, et al. AOSpine Spinal Cord Injury & Trauma Knowledge Forum. AOSpine thoracolumbar spine injury classification system: fracture description, neurological status, and key modifiers. Spine. 2013; 38(23):2028–2037

Wood KB, Li W, Lebl DR, Ploumis A. Management of thoracolumbar spine fractures. Spine J. 2014; 14(1):145–164

12 Adolescent Idiopathic Scoliosis

Junyoung Ahn, Jannat M. Khan, Mark Berkowitz, Garrett K. Harada, and Christopher J. DeWald

Abstract

Adolescent idiopathic scoliosis (AIS) is one of the most common conditions treated by modern spinal deformity surgeons, and affects roughly 0.47 to 5.2% of the overall population. As such, mastery of appropriate history and physical condition is necessary to guide further diagnostic imaging and clinical management. Inquiry covering the patient's developmental history and symptoms combined with observation of any gait abnormalities, asymmetry, or neurologic defects may point towards a diagnosis of AIS. Positive findings can be further supplemented with more specialized maneuvers such as Adam's Forward Bend Test, leg length discrepancy measures, and full-body length radiographic evaluation. Nonoperative management of AIS is largely dependent upon the patient's skeletal maturity and/or severity of scoliotic deformity. Such patients may respond positively to a period of bracing with a thoracic-lumbar-sacral orthosis. Many AIS cases may be sufficiently treated with this approach, whereas surgical intervention is particularly complex and relies heavily upon appropriate classification and identification of major and minor structural spinal curvatures. Techniques such as interbody and instrumented fusions, osteotomies, anterior and posterior approaches, and mastery of three-dimensional manipulation maneuvers are key components of the deformity surgeon's armamentarium, allowing correction of complex multiplanar deformities. Irrespective, of the technique the primary goal for surgical management of AIS patients is to safely minimize risk of curve progression and to deliver lasting therapeutic relief of the associated symptoms.

Keywords: adolescent, scoliosis, deformity, AIS, spine

12.1 Introduction

Adolescent Idiopathic Scoliosis (AIS) is the most common form of scoliosis, characterized by a coronal curvature of the spine that is greater than 10 degrees.[1] In most cases of scoliosis, the cause is unknown which leads to the "idiopathic" designation in AIS.[2,3] In literature, the overall prevalence of AIS ranges between 0.47 and 5.2%.[2,4,5,6] The wide difference in prevalence is due to the heterogeneity in the literature in regards to the genetic makeup, age groups, definitions of scoliosis, investigational protocols, and genetic disorders associated with scoliosis.[1,2]

AIS is more common in adolescents than young children and is predominantly observed in females.[6,7] Studies suggest that incidence of AIS in females-to-males ranges from 1.5:1 to as high as 7.2:1 depending upon the severity of the deformity.[7,8,9]

The purpose of this chapter is to provide the tools required for obtaining a complete history and physical examination to develop a differential diagnosis that can lead to appropriate imaging and treatment modalities for AIS.

12.2 History and Examination

In general, patients with AIS may not experience any pain at all or may experience only mild back pain that does not deter them from performing daily tasks.[10] As such, routine screening has been historically recommended, allowing (1) early detection and (2) early implementation of conservative treatment.[11,12]

Obtaining an accurate history regarding age, pain, dysfunction, menarcheal status, birth history (hospitalization, developmental delay), family history of spinal deformity, and height is critical. In addition, during the initial consultation visit, it is important to thoroughly examine the patient for (1) any gait abnormality or neurologic defects, (2) asymmetry at the shoulder, breast, waist, and pelvis levels, (3) prominence/curvature involving the scapula/ribs/loss of lordosis, (4) skin abnormalities (i.e., hairy patches or sacral dimples), and (5) adolescent idiopathic scoliosis, which can accentuate deformities, if present (▶ Table 12.1).

During the Adam's FBT, the patient is asked to keep his or her feet together, knees straight, and bend forward 90 degrees at the waist, while the examiner assesses for irregular rotation of the rib cage or uneven shoulder height.[13,14] This position makes the deformities more pronounced, allowing

Table 12.1 Evaluation for adolescent idiopathic scoliosis (AIS)

	Assessment	Method
Observational evaluation	Upper body asymmetry	Patient, while standing upright, is visually assessed for asymmetry of shoulder level, breasts, waist, or pelvis.
	Protrusions and curvature	Upright patient is assessed for protruding scapula or ribs and loss of lordosis.
	Adam's forward bend test (FBT)	Patient is asked to keep his or her feet together, knees straight, and bend forward 90 degrees at the waist, while the examining physician can either look for irregular shape of the ribs bilaterally or an uneven shoulder height.
Specialized evaluation	Clinical plumb-line	Assessed in both coronal and sagittal planes by using a plumb bob. The bob is dropped from the C7 spinous process down and beyond the gluteal crease. In the normal spine, it will fall within 1–2 cm of the midline. Deviation is recorded.
	Leg length discrepancy (LLD)	Measure the discrepancy when patient is standing barefoot. Put a series of wooden blocks under the short leg until the hips are level, then measure the blocks to determine the discrepancy. Tape measurement from ASIS to medial malleolus bilaterally.
	Global pelvic balance	Examined by palpating both iliac crests.
	Neurological incongruity	Assess the patient's deep tendon flexes, and abdominal reflexes.

effective detection of scoliosis. Karachalios et al reported that the sensitivity and specificity of the Adam's FBT for patients with curves ≥ 10 degrees are 84.37% and 93.44%, respectively.[14] A meta-analysis by Fong et al demonstrated that utilizing the FBT alone as a screening tool increased the referral rate for further spine evaluation while the positive predictive values were 28.0% and 5.6% for curves ≥ 10 and ≥ 20 degrees, respectively.[15]

As such, although routine screening could increase the detection rate and early diagnosis for scoliosis, utilizing the FBT alone may be insufficient, *per se.* Accordingly, the United States Preventative Take Force recommends against routine screening for asymptomatic patients (due to the risk of increased radiation exposure) with the caution that patients with large curves should be carefully assessed and appropriately managed.[16]

To determine the significance of rotation of a scoliotic curve, a scoliometer may be used to measure the rib prominence or rotational deformity in the FBT for angle of trunk rotation (ATR). The clinical plumb-line should be assessed in both coronal and sagittal planes by using a plumb bob. The bob is dropped from the C7 spinous process down and beyond the gluteal crease. In the normal spine, it will fall within 1–2 cm of the midline. Global pelvic balance should be examined by palpating both iliac crests and if

obliquity and/or leg length discrepancy (LLD) are suspected, repeating the examination with small wooden blocks underneath the short extremity will allow elimination of the LLD's contribution to the pelvic obliquity.

A careful neurological examination assesses the patient's upper motor neurons (e.g., Babinski reflex or presence of clonus), deep tendon reflexes, and superficial abdominal reflexes. This allows the physician to check for symmetrical umbilical movement through lateral to medial light strokes on the abdomen. Asymmetrical movement correlates with neural axis pathology and typically warrants further evaluation with MRI, to rule out neurological causes of scoliosis, such as syringomyelia.[17]

By definition, the cause of AIS is unknown. However, it is generally believed to be related to patient's genetics. For example, patients with a family history of scoliosis have (1) 30% increased likelihood of presenting with a coronal curve of the spine and (2) a monozygotic twin concordance rate of 73%.[18]

12.3 Differential Diagnosis

The accepted approach to diagnosing AIS is by ruling out any other possible causes of pain and spinal deformity. In the adolescent, the differential diagnosis for back pain is wide ranging.[19]

Interestingly, correlating back pain to narrow down the differential diagnosis has had mixed results as back pain may be absent in the AIS patient.[10] Ramirez et al examined 2,442 patients with AIS, and only 23% of the patients presented with back pain.[10] In this study, the authors demonstrated a wide range of pathologies in patients who presented with scoliotic curves and back pain. The diagnoses included: (1) spondylolisthesis or spondylosis, (2) syrinx, (3) tethered cord, (4) tumor, (5) disc herniation, and (6) Scheuermann's kyphosis.

The associated spinal deformity can also have several etiologies: neurogenic scoliosis, thoracogenic scoliosis, congenital scoliosis, paralytic scoliosis, traumatic scoliosis, osteoid osteoma, Chiari I malformation, neuromuscular tumors, and other forms of idiopathic scoliosis such as infantile and juvenile idiopathic scoliosis. The age of onset may guide in distinguishing between the etiologies of the deformity. For example, infantile idiopathic scoliosis affects < 3 years old patients while juvenile idiopathic scoliosis occurs in 3–10 years old patients.

In summary, a careful and focused history, comprehensive physical examination, and appropriately guided imaging modalities are critical in determining the etiology as well as management of the patient's spinal deformity and pain, if present.

12.4 Diagnostic Imaging

Following careful assessment utilizing the history and physical examination, radiographs may be performed as the first line of diagnostic imaging modality. Standing radiographs (posteroanterior [PA] and lateral views) should be obtained to assess for the physiologic alignment of the patient while standing.

First, the skeletal maturity of the patient should be determined by characterizing the iliac crest apophysis. The Risser sign describes the progression of the ossification of the iliac crest apophysis. Grade 0 is the absence of any ossification. Ossification of 25%, 50%, 75%, and 100% describe grades I, II, III, and IV, respectively. Grade V describes complete fusion of the apophysis to the iliac crest and denotes the completion of spinal growth.[20,21,22]

Cobb angles are measured in the coronal plane to quantify the severity of the patient's deformity.[23] To obtain the Cobb angle, lines are drawn parallel to (1) superior endplate of the superior vertebral body and (2) inferior endplate of the inferior vertebral body at the top and bottom of the scoliotic curve on a standing PA radiograph. The vertebrae that produce the largest angle are chosen as the reference point. If measuring on plain radiographs, perpendicular lines are drawn from the endplate lines described above, and the angle created between the perpendicular lines is the Cobb angle. If digitally measuring the angle, tools are available to automatically assess the angle created between the two endplate lines.

A number of limitations of the Cobb angle are recognized and caution should be exercised in assuming that sequential measurements are correct when little change is evident. Some recognized limitations include: (1) intraobserver and interobserver variation; (2) rotation: minor rotation of patients between examinations can significantly change measurements (may be as high as 20 degrees variation); consistent positioning must, therefore, be obtained[23] and (3) diurnal variation: in the same patient on the same day, curvature increases during the day (~5 degrees variation).[24]

12.5 Classification

Two major classification systems have been described. In 1983, King et al introduced the King classification system to guide levels of fusion for scoliosis.[25] The system allowed for determination of appropriate surgical treatment for the thoracic curve and when to include instrumentation into concomitant lumbar deformities. However, the authors did not describe pure lumbar scoliotic curves or assess sagittal alignment of scoliotic deformity.[26]

As such, Lenke et al introduced the Lenke classification system in 2001.[26] The authors' objectives for the new system was to create a comprehensive classification system with (1) acceptable interobserver and intraobserver reliability, (2) reproducibility and ease of use in the clinical setting, and (3) inclusion of the sagittal alignment.[27]

The Lenke system classifies curves based on curve type, coronal lumbar modifier, and thoracic sagittal profile (▶ Table 12.2). For this system, four plain film spine radiographs are obtained: (1) standing PA, (2) standing lateral, (3) supine right-bending, and (4) supine left-bending.[26]

Table 12.2 Lenke classification for adolescent idiopathic scoliosis (AIS)

Curve type				
Type	Description	Proximal thoracic	Main thoracic	Thoracolumbar/lumbar
1	Main thoracic	–	Structural (major)[a]	–
2	Double thoracic	Structural (minor)[b]	Structural (major)	–
3	Double major	–	Structural (major)	Structural (minor)
4[c]	Triple major	Structural (minor)	Structural (major/minor)	Structural (major/minor)
5	Thoracolumbar/lumbar	–	–	Structural (major)
6	Thoracolumbar/lumbar-main thoracic	–	Structural (minor)	Structural (major)

Notes: [a] The curve with the largest Cobb angle is considered major and is always structural.
[b] A minor curve is considered structural if: (1) the curve is > 25 degrees in the coronal plane without correction on bending radiographs or (2) the curve is > 20 degrees in the sagittal plane.
[c] Type 4 curves may have either main thoracic or thoracolumbar/lumbar major curves.

Table 12.2 (Continued) Lenke classification for adolescent idiopathic scoliosis (AIS)

Lumbar modifier	Center sacral vertebral line (CSVL) to lumbar apex relationship
A	CSVL falls between pedicles of apicle vertebrae
B	CSVL touches apical concave pedicle
C	CSVL lies lateral to (or outside of) apical vertebrae

Thoracic sagittal profile	
– (Hypo)	< 10 degrees
N (Normal)	10–40 degrees
+ (Hyper)	> 40 degrees

Classification = curve type (1–6) + lumbar modifier (A–C) + thoracic sagittal profile (–, N, +)

First, the standing coronal radiograph is assessed for any pelvic obliquity > 2 cm. If present, a block should be applied under the shorter extremity to negate the pelvic obliquity and limb length discrepancy in the pelvis.

Second, the curve type is determined. A major curve is the curvature with the greatest angle. A minor curve (angulation less than the major curve) can be structural *versus* non-structural. A structural thoracic curve can be defined in one of the two ways: (1) a rigid curvature of > 25 degrees on the side-bending radiographs or (2) kyphosis of > 20 degrees in the lateral radiographs. The clinical application of structural curves is that a fusion procedure should only include the major curve and the structural minor curves. Utilizing this algorithm, the curves are categorized into six different types: (1) main thoracic, (2) double thoracic, (3) double major, (4) triple major, (5) thoracolumbar/lumbar, and (6) thoracolumbar/lumbar + main thoracic.

Third, a lumbar coronal modifier is utilized for major thoracic scoliotic curves (types 1–4) with a lesser lumbar curvature. It is determined by drawing a central sacral vertical line (CSVL) vertically in the superior direction from the midpoint of the S1 vertebra. The lumbar modifiers are categorized into A, B, and C. The CSVL is referenced against the "stable vertebra," which is designated as the most superior vertebra (thoracic or lumbar) that is closest to being bisected by the CSVL in the coronal plane, as well as the "apical vertebra," which is the vertebral body farthest from the CSVL. The pedicles of the apical vertebra are described as being either the convex or concave pedicle of the curvature. In those cases where a disc space is most closely bisected by the CSVL, the vertebra just above the disc is designated as the stable vertebra. Similarly, if a disc space aligns most closely to the apex of the curvature, the vertebral bodies above and below the disc can be designated as the apical vertebrae.

Lumbar modifiers are utilized for main thoracic curvatures (Lenke 1-4) and not used with main lumbar curvatures (Lenke 5 and 6). The modifiers are used to determine the significance of the secondary lumbar curve and is based on where the CSVL falls within the secondary lumbar curve. Lumbar modifier A describes an instance in which the CSVL lies between the two pedicles of the apical vertebra of the lumbar curve (seen with minimal secondary lumbar curves).

Lumbar modifier B describes the CSVL contained within (or touching) the concave pedicle of the secondary lumbar curve.

Lastly, lumbar modifier C describes the position of the CSVL that is lateral to the lateral border (or completely outside) of the apical vertebral body of the secondary lumbar curve (seen with larger lumbar curvatures). Again, these lumbar modifiers apply to the secondary lumbar curves of major thoracic type deformities (i.e., thoracic, double thoracic, double major and triple curves - Lenke Types 1-4). Importantly, if the position of CSVL is not fully touching the lateral aspect of the apical vertebra or if the apical vertebra is not obviously lateral to the CSVL, the B modifier is applied.

Finally, the Lenke classification system describes the sagittal thoracic alignment and categorizes the curvature into three types: (−, N or normal, and +). The Cobb angle is measured from T5 to T12; if this Cobb angle is between + 10 and + 40, then a normal modifier is applied. A minus sign indicates a Cobb angle < 10 degrees (hypokyphotic curve), while a plus sign indicates a cobb angle > 40 degrees (hyperkyphotic).

Additional imaging, such as MRI, may be warranted for patients who present with atypical characteristics. These presentations include unusual or significant pain, left thoracic curves, or concerning findings such as an abnormal abdominal reflex.[28] However, neurologic abnormalities which present as AIS prior to MRI evaluation have been reported to be as high as 7.8%.[29] Therefore, the diagnosis of an underlying neurological abnormality does not necessarily explain the cause for scoliosis and may not affect the patient's treatment plan.

The routine utilization of MRI for all cases of idiopathic scoliosis remains controversial.[28,29,30] Winter et al demonstrated that in 140 patients with AIS, 4 diagnoses were reached according to a pre-operative MRI.[30] Of these 4 patients, 1 patient had a small thoracic syrinx and 3 patients had Chiari type I malformations which did not require neurosurgical procedure. Thus, the routine use of MRI as an evaluation tool is not typically employed in clinical practice.

12.6 Treatment

The primary goals for the treatment of AIS are multifold: (1) prevent progression, (2) maintain balance, (3) preserve respiratory function, (4) reduce pain, (5) preserve neurological status, and (6) improve cosmesis. An accurate evaluation is required to assess the patient's potential for growth and progression of the deformity utilizing the following information: age, skeletal maturity, gender, and pattern of curve.

When considering the potential for progression of deformity in AIS, the age of the patient plays a significant role. Younger patients with many more years of growth will more likely experience progression in their deformity as compared to patients nearing skeletal maturity. Such patients usually require frequent monitoring to assess progression of their deformity with age. Conversely, older adolescents with AIS are less likely to realize significant curve progression and may be managed with less rigorous follow-up.

Carefully evaluating the skeletal maturity of the patient on radiographs can guide clinical decision-making. The Risser scale aims to quantify skeletal maturity according to fusion of the iliac crest apophysis on a standing radiograph of the spine and pelvis. The Risser sign is noted to correlate with the greatest velocity of linear skeletal growth.[31,32]

Patients with a score ≤ 2 are considered skeletally immature, and are typically followed up every 3 to 6 months for curve progression if their curve is < 25 degrees.[33] More skeletally mature patients (Risser ≥ 3) with a similar curvature can be followed up at longer intervals, typically every 6 to 9 months, until skeletal maturity is achieved. Once mature, curvatures < 30 degrees often require no additional monitoring, while those > 50 degrees require additional surveillance.[34]

For skeletally immature patients with a curve between 25 and 40 degrees or those patients with curve progression > 5 degrees per visit, brace therapy can be utilized.[35] Evaluation for progression should be conducted every 4-6 months for patients undergoing brace therapy until skeletal maturity is reached. There are a wide variety of bracing options, each designed to apply an external force to the trunk during the adolescent growth phase to prevent progression. The pressure on the concave aspect of the curvature is relieved while simultaneously increasing pressure on the convexity of the curvature. However, each brace option differs in its material, indications based upon curvature characteristics, and duration of wear. Hence, prescribing a proper brace for each patient is an important step in the treatment process.

12.6.1 Bracing

The first cervico-thoracic-lumbar-sacral orthosis (CTLSO) called the Milwaukee brace was invented in the 1940s by Drs. Blount and Schmidt.[33,34] This brace is generally used for thoracic and double curves. The brace includes a neck ring and a throat mold from which metal bars extend down and attach to a uniquely molded pelvic girdle. Slings are attached to the bars to provide coronal correction pressure on the convex portion of the curve or curves. The neck ring helps in keeping the patients head centered over the pelvis. Occipital pads are used to help relieve pressure in the neck. Additionally, custom corrective pads are used to help the girdle apply pressure in the correct areas. However, due to the bulkiness, visibility of the neck component, and availability of more modern and comfortable bracing options, the frequency of use of the Milwaukee brace has decreased.[36,37]

Another full-time brace recommended by orthopedics is the Wilmington brace which is a thoracic-lumbar-sacral orthosis (TLSO).[37] The idea behind this brace was to improve on the structure of the brace, making it less bulky and more inconspicuous, thereby improving patient compliance. This brace consists of a custom plastic orthosis, designed to fit snugly under the patient's arms. The mold can be made from a variety of plastics and is designed to be worn as a jacket which is closed by Velcro straps in the front. This allows the patient to easily open and remove the brace at any time, improving the odds that the patient will comply with the prescribed wear schedule.

The most commonly prescribed full-time brace is the Boston brace.[38] Similar to the Wilmington brace, the Boston brace is also a TLSO brace. The Boston brace is made from prefabricated polypropylene pelvic module with a soft foam polyethylene lining. First, a mold is selected that best fits the patient's size and curve type. Then, corrective pads and trim lines are strategically placed within the brace to best accommodate each patient's unique curvature. Similar to the Wilmington brace, the Boston brace is slim and inconspicuous. However, unlike the Wilmington brace, this brace is opened from the back, generally requiring a second person to help the patient open and remove the brace.

The goal of brace therapy is not necessarily to correct the curve, but to prevent further progression during growth.[39] Typically, braces are required to be worn 16 to 23 hours per day until 2 years after menarche or 1 year after achievement of Risser stage 4. Compliant patients often show decrease or halt in progression while some patients may demonstrate improvement in their curvatures.[38,40]

12.6.2 Surgical Treatment

Patients may be operative candidates if: (1) the curve presents with an angle of > 45 degrees in a skeletally immature patient, (2) bracing has failed, and (3) curves progress beyond 50 degrees in skeletally mature teenagers.[41] Halting the progression and obtaining spinal and pelvic balance is often prioritized over curve correction, prevention of back pain, and cosmesis. Surgical correction of the spinal deformity carries a number of risks including continued pain, infection, neurologic injury, and implant-related complications. However, during the discussions leading up to surgery, it should be noted that surgical intervention for the sequelae of the non-surgically treated AIS in an adult is likely to be more complex than in a teenager.

Essential principles guiding surgical intervention for AIS include fusion to correct and limit progression of the curve, minimizing loss of motion resulting from fusion, and rebalancing of the trunk. Although there is a consensus regarding the necessity of correcting the major curve, there is debate regarding the management of the minor curve and the levels which should be included in the fusion construct. The Lenke classification provides guidance regarding the minor curves by assessing the need for surgical fusion based on flexibility and curve pattern.[26] Many surgeons support the omittance of flexible minor curves from the fusion as these curves may spontaneously correct following surgical correction of the major curve alone, and fusion of fewer vertebrae may help to preserve spinal motion.

In surgical correction, three-dimensional forces are applied utilizing cables, hooks, wires, screws, or synthetic bands as anchors to the bony anatomy of individual vertebra within the scoliotic curvature. These anchors can then be connected to longitudinal rods which provide stabilization along with curve correction. Anterior or posterior approaches can be utilized to gain surgical access to the spine depending on the type of curve, and instruments being utilized for correction.[42]

Historically, an anterior approach is preferred in the setting of select thoraco-lumbar and lumbar types of AIS as it provides adequate exposure to conduct discectomies, which can allow for additional halting of vertebral growth. However, a posterior approach for instrumented fusion is more commonly utilized for scoliosis surgery for both thoracic and lumbar curvatures.[43,44] For posterior approaches, patients should be placed prone on a Jackson frame. Proper padding should include the chest, anterior superior iliac spine of the pelvis, thighs, legs, and elbows. The upper extremities should be partially abducted and externally rotated at the shoulder, and bent at the elbow for support on padded arm boards. The abdomen should be left free so as to minimize contribution of abdominal pressure to intraoperative bleeding.

During the procedure, the surgeon can consider different measures to minimize complications. In addition to thoughtful patient positioning, proper surgical dissection, intermittent packing, Bovie cauterization, and tranexamic acid medication has been shown to minimize blood loss in surgery for AIS.

Most importantly, there remains a risk of paralysis in surgical correction of scoliosis, albeit low. It is the greatest concern of the scoliosis surgeon to maintain the adolescent's neurologic function during the correction of the spinal deformity. The risk of spinal cord injury during scoliosis correction is estimated to be < 0.25%.[9] The intraoperative use of neuromonitoring during the correction of AIS deformities is imperative to help prevent neurologic injury. The combined use of continuous somatosensory evoked potentials (SSEP) and intermittent motor evoked potentials (MEP) aids the surgeon in detecting potential spinal cord injuries early, allowing for possible surgical changes to prevent permanent nerve injury or paralysis.

When concerns arise over intraoperative neuromonitoring, the surgeon and the anesthesiologist should conduct a Stagnara wake-up test by effectively reversing sedation and neuromuscular blockade to enable the patient to move his or her feet upon verbal command to demonstrate the function of the spinal cord. If spinal cord injury is confirmed or strongly suspected, the procedure can be discontinued to allow for further spinal cord evaluation. If spinal cord injury is ruled out, the surgeon can consider re-anesthetizing the patient to complete the spinal procedure. The patient, the surgeon, and the anesthesiologist should be aware of the possible need of the Stagnara wake-up test and should carefully rehearse the maneuver prior to surgery, so as to best prevent accidental extubation or bodily injury during the wake-up test.

In the majority of cases, the Lenke classification guides surgical planning.[26] For a patient with Lenke type 1 (major structural thoracic curves),

fusion of only the thoracic curve down to the stable vertebrae is recommended. One exception is Lenke type 1A, where the distal fusion level is the merely touching vertebra, which is typically one above the stable vertebra. In order to prevent postoperative coronal decompensation in a thoracic scoliosis when not instrumenting the minor lumbar curvature, overcorrection of the thoracic curve should be avoided. Patients with double thoracic or Lenke type 2 curves require fusion of both curves from T2 to the stable vertebra, particularly if the left shoulder is higher than the right shoulder. For Lenke type 3, a major thoracic and a major lumbar double curve, a fusion of both thoracic and lumbar curve is recommended. A triple major curve (Lenke type 4) may require fusion from T2 to L3 or L4, while a Lenke type 5 may be treated with a fusion via either the anterior or posterior approach from the lumbar stable vertebrae and cephalad up to the bending cephalad stable vertebra. For structural lumbar curves, the caudal instrumented vertebrae can be stopped short of the stable vertebrae by one or two levels if the end vertebra becomes better aligned or becomes stable and neutral on the supine bending radiographs. For a Lenke type 6 curve, it is necessary to include both the thoracic and lumbar spine in the fusion construct. It should be noted that junctional kyphosis may result if the fusion is stopped at T12 in those curves with preoperative kyphosis at the thoracolumbar junction.[45] Furthermore, the risk of degeneration of adjacent segment remains prevalent with any fusion technique.

In larger and more rigid spinal deformities, various techniques can be employed to aid in increasing mobility. Facetectomy involves the removal of the inferior facets from each vertebral segment to be included in the instrumented fusion and is performed to obtain partial release of the scoliotic deformity, allowing for increased mobility of a structural curve. This is typically performed in the majority of posterior spinal fusions for scoliosis deformities. If additional mobility is desired in a more rigid deformity, Ponte osteotomies are performed by removal of the ligamentum flavum, spinous processes, interspinous ligaments, and both the superior and inferior facets bilaterally at the apical 3–7 levels to provide additional release, and greater coronal and sagittal correction during surgery.

For curves with rotational axial plane deformities that develop a rib prominence or "rib hump," mono-axial and uni-axial screws, in addition to vertebral derotation towers, allow for segmental rotation of the apex to decrease rib humps by downward and clockwise pressure on the convex and upward force on the concave portions of the curve, respectively, while placing the posterior rods. In situ benders and compression/distraction techniques may then be used to achieve additional three-dimensional correction.

Technical Pearls   i

- **Surgical goals for AIS:** The ultimate surgical goals in AIS are to: (1) obtain *partial* balanced correction of the spinal deformity, (2) prevent progression secondary to adolescent skeletal growth and/or degeneration in adulthood, and (3) accomplish both safely with minimal risk for paralysis.
- **Standing X-rays:** PA and lateral radiographs are needed to determine the need for surgical correction (severity of the curve), curve pattern, and pedicle size and to look for congenital anomalies. These radiographs are not only needed to determine the length of spinal construct required but also to be aware of any congenital abnormalities suggesting further workup and the possible need for fixation other than pedicle screws due to extremely small pedicles (i.e., sublaminar bands or wires, or hooks).
- **Side bending X-rays:** Right- and left-side bending radiographs and/or AP traction plain radiographs determine structural versus compensatory spinal curves, flexibility of curves, and end vertebrae to be instrumented.
- **Blood loss control:** The use of tranexamic acid infusion has been shown to help control perioperative blood loss and decrease the need for blood transfusions in AIS surgery.
- **Spinal cord safety:** The intraoperative use of neuromonitoring during the correction of AIS deformities is imperative for the safe correction of the spinal deformity curve to help prevent nerve injury/paralysis. The combined use of continuous somatosensory evoked potentials (SSEP) and intermittent motor evoked potentials (MEP) aids the surgeon in detecting potential spinal cord injuries early, allowing for possible surgical changes to prevent paralysis.
- **Stagnara wake-up test:** AIS spinal deformity surgeons and anesthesiologists should be familiar with the Stagnara wake-up test, to preoperatively practice the test with the patient, and to perform it during surgery, if needed. This test is utilized when there are concerns regarding the intraoperative neuromonitoring or if neuromonitoring malfunctions.
- **Deformity correction maneuvers:** In general, it is understood that *Compression* across a section of vertebral levels should be done on the CONVEX side of a scoliotic curve to straighten the deformity and this will lead to relative decrease in kyphosis (or lordosis). *Distraction* across a section of vertebral levels should be performed on the CONCAVE portion of a scoliotic curve to straighten the deformity and this will lead to relative increase in kyphosis.
- **Facetectomies:** Removal of the inferior facets from each vertebral segment to be included in the fused segments provides for partial release/increased mobility of a structural spinal deformity.
- **Ponte osteotomies:** In larger and more rigid scoliotic deformities, a complete posterior single column osteotomy can be performed across the apical 3–7 levels to provide additional release of a more rigid deformity to allow better coronal and sagittal correction during surgery. Ponte osteotomies involve removal of the ligamentum flavum and superior and inferior facets bilaterally at each of the selected vertebral segments.
- **Vertebral derotation:** Use of mono-axial and uni-axial screws, in addition to derotation towers, allow for segmental vertebral rotation of the apex to decrease the rib hump by downward clockwise pressure on the convex portion of the scoliosis and upward force on the concave portion.
- **X-ray confirmation of screw placement:** Whether fluoroscopy or computerized assistance is utilized, intraoperative confirmation of screw placement is necessary in order to allow for possible implant changes.
- **Fusion:** To obtain a stable solid bony arthrodesis, multi-level decortication of the exposed laminae, transverse processes, and facet joints is required, plus the use of cancellous allograft bone grafting.

12.7 Case Examples

12.7.1 Case 1

A 16-year-old female high school player diagnosed with adolescent idiopathic scoliosis (AIS) 2 years ago was conservatively treated with a brace. She presented with progressively worsening back pain and deformity, and admitted that she has largely been non-compliant with the bracing regimen. Physical examination (PE) revealed mild shoulder asymmetry, with the left shoulder sitting slightly lower than the right, along with a positive Adam's forward bend test (FBT) for left-sided rotational thoracolumbar prominence. Anteroposterior and lateral scoliosis radiographs showed a flexible thoracic curve in T4–T10 measuring 45.7 degrees and a left lumbar curve in T10–L3 measuring 54.8 degrees (▶ Fig. 12.1). The bending radiographs showed a flexible thoracic curve (corrected to 23.1 degrees) and lumbar curve (corrected to 3.3 degrees) (▶ Fig. 12.2). Based on PE and imaging, the

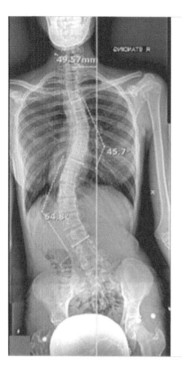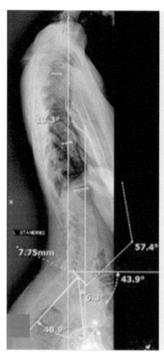

Fig. 12.1 Posteroanterior (PA) and lateral views of adolescent idiopathic scoliosis (AIS). Patient is a 16-year-old female with a 45.7 degrees right T4–T10 and 54.8 degrees left T10–L3 curve. A leftward truncal shift of 49.6 mm was observed. No sagittal plane deformity was observed.

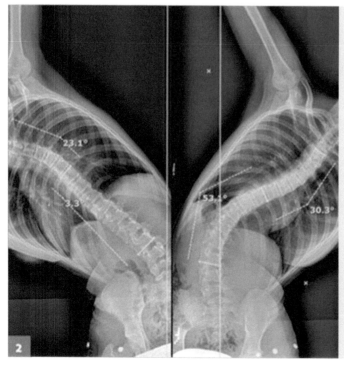

Fig. 12.2 Lateral bending films demonstrating flexibility of thoracic and lumbar curves. Thoracic and lumbar curves corrected to 23.1 and 3.3 degrees, respectively, upon bending to the left.

recommendation was made to perform posterior spinal fusion from T4 to L3 due to the progression risk of the thoracic and thoracolumbar (TL) curves in the setting of worsening back pain and recent brace wear.

12.7.2 Case 2

A 15-year-old girl presented with a Lenke 1BN curvature (▶ Fig. 12.3). Chest and abdominal asymmetry was demonstrated by soft-tissue silhouette on radiographs, in addition to the presence of a spondylolysis at L5 with a concomitant grade 1 spondylolisthesis. The patient's right-sided mid-thoracic (MT) curve was 43 degrees preoperatively. Pelvic incidence (PI) of 57 degrees, lumbar lordosis (LL) of 77 degrees (PI-LL mismatch of 20 degrees), thoracic kyphosis (TK) of 23 degrees, and sacral slope of 58 degrees were measured on additional examination. Posterior spinal instrumented fusion with pedicle screws from T2 to T12 was performed. Postoperatively, the patient appeared to be balanced coronally (0 mm) and soft-tissue silhouettes revealed chest and abdominal symmetry along with absence of preoperative rib hump in clinical examination. The MT was 3 degrees, a 91% correction. TK improved to 33 degrees; SVA, to 0.2 mm; LL, to 56 degrees; and PI, to 56 degrees (PI-LL mismatch of 0 degree). Soft-tissue silhouettes revealed chest and abdominal symmetry.

12.8 Board-style Questions

1. Which of the following patients most warrants a full spine MRI as a next step in his or her workup?
   a) 12-year-old female with no back pain and a 15-degree right-sided thoracic curve
   b) 8-year-old male with mild back pain and a 30-degree left-sided thoracic curve
   c) 15-year-old female with low back pain and a 35-degree right-sided thoracic curve and compensatory 30 degrees lumbar curve
   d) 13-year-old male with back pain and an 18-degree right-sided thoracic curve
   e) 18-year-old female with low back pain and a 30-degree main right-sided mid-thoracic curve, a 15-degree left-sided proximal thoracic curve, and a 20-degree left-sided lumbar curve

2. Your 14-year-old female patient, whom you have been following for AIS, returns to clinic. She has been wearing her brace compliantly for 15 months. Full-length standing spine radiographs reveal a 35-degree main right-sided thoracic curve. Evaluation of the iliac crests on those radiographs show that she is now at Risser stage 4. She is 2.5 years post-menarche. What will be your next steps in treatment?

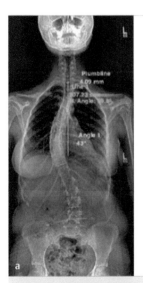
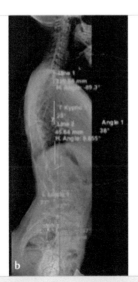
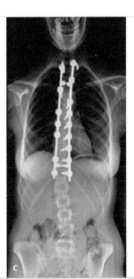
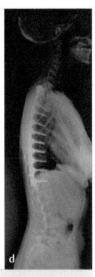

Fig. 12.3 Preoperative and postoperative anteroposterior (AP) and lateral views of adolescent idiopathic scoliosis (AIS) (Lenke 1BN). **(a)** The patient is a 15-year-old female with a 43 degrees right mid-thoracic curve. **(b)** Hyperlordosis of the lumbar spine is observed (77 degrees) with concomitant spondylolysis and spondylolisthesis at L5. PI-LL mismatch was 20 degrees. **(c)** Postoperative mid-thoracic curve measured 3 degrees, with **(d)** PI-LL mismatch of 0 degree.

a) Posterior instrumented spinal fusion
b) Obtain an MRI of the full spine to better evaluate the curve
c) Stop brace wear and continue activities as tolerated
d) Continue full-time brace wear for another 6 months
e) Wean the bracing down to just night-time brace wear for the next 12 months

3. At what stage is skeletal growth most rapid?
a) During Risser stage 2
b) After Risser stage 1 and menarche
c) Between Risser stage 1 and menarche
d) After menarche, but before Risser stage 1
e) Before Risser stage 1 and menarche

4. You are currently about to begin the de-rotation of portion of the posterior spinal instrumented fusion in a 13-year-old female with a Lenke 1 right-sided curve. What is the proper method to achieve improved rotational deformity?
a) Downward clockwise pressure on the convex portion of the scoliosis and upward force on the concave portion.
b) Upward clockwise pressure on the convex portion of the scoliosis and downward force on the concave portion.
c) Downward counter-clockwise pressure on the convex portion of the scoliosis and upward force on the concave portion.
d) Upward counter-clockwise pressure on the convex portion of the scoliosis and downward force on the concave portion.

Answers

1. b
2. c
3. e
4. a

References

[1] Konieczny MR, Senyurt H, Krauspe R. Epidemiology of adolescent idiopathic scoliosis. J Child Orthop. 2013; 7(1):3–9
[2] Asher MA, Burton DC. Adolescent idiopathic scoliosis: natural history and long term treatment effects. Scoliosis. 2006; 1(1):2
[3] Kleinberg S. The operative treatment of scoliosis. Arch Surg. 1922; 5(3):631–645
[4] Cilli K, Tezeren G, Taş T, et al. [School screening for scoliosis in Sivas, Turkey]. Acta Orthop Traumatol Turc. 2009; 43(5):426–430
[5] Kamtsiuris P, Atzpodien K, Ellert U, Schlack R, Schlaud M. [Prevalence of somatic diseases in German children and adolescents. Results of the German Health Interview and Examination Survey for Children and Adolescents (KiGGS)]. Bundesgesundheitsblatt Gesundheitsforschung Gesundheitsschutz. 2007; 50(5–6):686–700
[6] Soucacos PN, Soucacos PK, Zacharis KC, Beris AE, Xenakis TA. School-screening for scoliosis: a prospective epidemiological study in northwestern and central Greece. J Bone Joint Surg Am. 1997; 79(10):1498–1503
[7] Daruwalla JS, Balasubramaniam P, Chay SO, Rajan U, Lee HP. Idiopathic scoliosis: prevalence and ethnic distribution in Singapore schoolchildren. J Bone Joint Surg Br. 1985; 67(2):182–184
[8] Rogala EJ, Drummond DS, Gurr J. Scoliosis: incidence and natural history. A prospective epidemiological study. J Bone Joint Surg Am. 1978; 60(2):173–176
[9] Burton DC, Carlson BB, Place HM, et al. Results of the Scoliosis Research Society Morbidity and Mortality database 2009–2012: a report from the Morbidity and Mortality Committee. Spine Deform. 2016; 4(5):338–343
[10] Ramirez N, Johnston CE, Browne RH. The prevalence of back pain in children who have idiopathic scoliosis. J Bone Joint Surg Am. 1997; 79(3):364–368
[11] Wong H-K, Hui JHP, Rajan U, Chia HP. Idiopathic scoliosis in Singapore schoolchildren: a prevalence study 15 years into the screening program. Spine. 2005; 30(10):1188–1196
[12] Brooks HL, Azen SP, Gerberg E, Brooks R, Chan L. Scoliosis: a prospective epidemiological study. J Bone Joint Surg Am. 1975; 57(7):968–972
[13] Côté P, Kreitz BG, Cassidy JD, Dzus AK, Martel J. A study of the diagnostic accuracy and reliability of the Scoliometer and Adam's forward bend test. Spine. 1998; 23(7):796–802, discussion 803
[14] Karachalios T, Sofianos J, Roidis N, Sapkas G, Korres D, Nikolopoulos K. Ten-year follow-up evaluation of a school screening program for scoliosis: is the forward-bending test an accurate diagnostic criterion for the screening of scoliosis? Spine. 1999; 24(22):2318–2324
[15] Fong DYT, Lee CF, Cheung KMC, et al. A meta-analysis of the clinical effectiveness of school scoliosis screening. Spine. 2010; 35(10):1061–1071
[16] US Preventive Services Task Force. Screening for adolescent idiopathic scoliosis: policy statement. JAMA. 1993; 269(20):2664–2666
[17] Benli IT, Uzümcügil O, Aydin E, Ateş B, Gürses L, Hekimoğlu B. Magnetic resonance imaging abnormalities of neural axis in Lenke type 1 idiopathic scoliosis. Spine. 2006; 31(16):1828–1833
[18] An HS, Singh K. Synopsis of Spine Surgery. New York: Thieme; 2011
[19] Micheli LJ. Low back pain in the adolescent: differential diagnosis. Am J Sports Med. 1979; 7(6):362–364
[20] Nault M-L, Parent S, Phan P, Roy-Beaudry M, Labelle H, Rivard M. A modified Risser grading system predicts the curve acceleration phase of female adolescent idiopathic scoliosis. J Bone Joint Surg Am. 2010; 92(5):1073–1081
[21] Lonstein JE, Carlson JM. The prediction of curve progression in untreated idiopathic scoliosis during growth. J Bone Joint Surg Am. 1984; 66(7):1061–1071
[22] Sanders JO. Maturity indicators in spinal deformity. J Bone Joint Surg Am. 2007; 89 Suppl 1:14–20
[23] Carman DL, Browne RH, Birch JG. Measurement of scoliosis and kyphosis radiographs: intraobserver and interobserver variation. J Bone Joint Surg Am. 1990; 72(3):328–333

[24] Kim H, Kim HS, Moon ES, et al. Scoliosis imaging: what radiologists should know. Radiographics. 2010; 30(7): 1823–1842

[25] King HA, Moe JH, Bradford DS, Winter RB. The selection of fusion levels in thoracic idiopathic scoliosis. J Bone Joint Surg Am. 1983; 65(9):1302–1313

[26] Lenke LG, Betz RR, Harms J, et al. Adolescent idiopathic scoliosis: a new classification to determine extent of spinal arthrodesis. J Bone Joint Surg Am. 2001; 83(8): 1169–1181

[27] Ogon M, Giesinger K, Behensky H, et al. Interobserver and intraobserver reliability of Lenke's new scoliosis classification system. Spine. 2002; 27(8):858–862

[28] Zadeh HG, Sakka SA, Powell MP, Mehta MH. Absent superficial abdominal reflexes in children with scoliosis: an early indicator of syringomyelia. J Bone Joint Surg Br. 1995; 77(5): 762–767

[29] Qiao J, Zhu Z, Zhu F, et al. Indication for preoperative MRI of neural axis abnormalities in patients with presumed thoracolumbar/lumbar idiopathic scoliosis. Eur Spine J. 2013; 22 (2):360–366

[30] Winter RB, Lonstein JE, Heithoff KB, Kirkham JA. Magnetic resonance imaging evaluation of the adolescent patient with idiopathic scoliosis before spinal instrumentation and fusion: a prospective, double-blinded study of 140 patients. Spine. 1997; 22(8):855–858

[31] Biondi J, Weiner DS, Bethem D, Reed JF, III. Correlation of Risser sign and bone age determination in adolescent idiopathic scoliosis. J Pediatr Orthop. 1985; 5(6):697–701

[32] Sanders JO, Browne RH, McConnell SJ, Margraf SA, Cooney TE, Finegold DN. Maturity assessment and curve progression in girls with idiopathic scoliosis. J Bone Joint Surg Am. 2007; 89(1):64–73

[33] Blount WP, Schmidt AC, Keever ED, Leonard ET. The Milwaukee brace in the operative treatment of scoliosis. J Bone Joint Surg Am. 1958; 40-A(3):511–525

[34] Lonstein JE, Winter RB. The Milwaukee brace for the treatment of adolescent idiopathic scoliosis: a review of one thousand and twenty patients. J Bone Joint Surg Am. 1994; 76(8):1207–1221

[35] Richards BS, Bernstein RM, D'Amato CR, Thompson GH. Standardization of criteria for adolescent idiopathic scoliosis brace studies: SRS Committee on Bracing and Nonoperative Management. Spine. 2005; 30(18):2068–2075, discussion 2076–2077

[36] Schiller JR, Thakur NA, Eberson CP. Brace management in adolescent idiopathic scoliosis. Clin Orthop Relat Res. 2010; 468(3):670–678

[37] Howard A, Wright JG, Hedden D. A comparative study of TLSO, Charleston, and Milwaukee braces for idiopathic scoliosis. Spine. 1998; 23(22):2404–2411

[38] Wiley JW, Thomson JD, Mitchell TM, Smith BG, Banta JV. Effectiveness of the Boston brace in treatment of large curves in adolescent idiopathic scoliosis. Spine. 2000; 25 (18):2326–2332

[39] Danielsson AJ, Nachemson AL. Radiologic findings and curve progression 22 years after treatment for adolescent idiopathic scoliosis: comparison of brace and surgical treatment with matching control group of straight individuals. Spine. 2001; 26(5):516–525

[40] Weinstein SL, Dolan LA, Wright JG, Dobbs MB. Effects of bracing in adolescents with idiopathic scoliosis. N Engl J Med. 2013; 369(16):1512–1521

[41] Choudhry MN, Ahmad Z, Verma R. Adolescent idiopathic scoliosis. Open Orthop J. 2016; 10:143–154

[42] Lenke LG, Edwards CC, II, Bridwell KH. The Lenke classification of adolescent idiopathic scoliosis: how it organizes curve patterns as a template to perform selective fusions of the spine. Spine. 2003; 28(20):S199–S207

[43] Suk SI, Lee CK, Kim WJ, Chung YJ, Park YB. Segmental pedicle screw fixation in the treatment of thoracic idiopathic scoliosis. Spine. 1995; 20(12):1399–1405

[44] Luhmann SJ, Lenke LG, Erickson M, Bridwell KH, Richards BS. Correction of moderate (< 70 degrees) Lenke 1A and 2A curve patterns: comparison of hybrid and all-pedicle screw systems at 2-year follow-up. J Pediatr Orthop. 2012; 32(3):253–258

[45] Lonner BS, Ren Y, Newton PO, et al. Risk factors of proximal junctional kyphosis in adolescent idiopathic scoliosis—the pelvis and other considerations. Spine Deform. 2017; 5(3): 181–188

13 Adult Degenerative Scoliosis

Alexander Beschloss, Carol Wang, and Comron Saifi

Abstract

Adult degenerative scoliosis (ADS) is a deformity of the spine in the coronal plane that is defined as a Cobb angle > 10 degrees in a skeletally mature patient. Considering that the prevalence of ADS may be as high as 68% in the population, it is vital to understand how to approach this pathology both in the clinic and the operating room. Upon initial visit, patients who are suspected to have ADS will undergo a thorough history and physical exam, elucidating factors that would support the diagnosis. If suspected, this initial clinical visit will include a 36-inch posteroanterior and lateral radiograph. At this point, it is important to understand the factors that might influence decision-making to pursue a surgical, versus nonsurgical, approach with each individual patient. Nonoperative treatment is typically selected for patients who obtain sufficient pain relief with physical therapy, medications, or other nonoperative treatments and those with curves less than 30 degrees. Patients with severe pain that is not relieved by nonoperative treatments, with curves greater than 30 degrees, and with a T-score of greater than −2.5 are potential surgical candidates. The primary goals of surgery include correction of coronal and sagittal malalignment, decompression of neural elements, and typically achieving arthrodesis. The ADS classification by Lenke and Silva can assist in guiding treatment. The important factors in this classification system include neurogenic claudication, back pain, anterior osteophytes, olisthesis, > 30-degree coronal Cobb angle, lumbar kyphosis, and global imbalance. Providing patients with evidence-based data regarding surgical outcomes allows patients to make an informed decision regarding their treatment options.

Keywords: adult degenerative scoliosis, spine, fusion

13.1 Introduction

Adult scoliosis is a coronal plane deformity of the spine with a Cobb angle > 10 degrees in a skeletally mature patient.[1] The two most common forms of scoliosis in adults are (1) adult idiopathic scoliosis, which is the natural progression of adolescent idiopathic scoliosis, and (2) de novo adult degenerative scoliosis (ADS). ADS develops due to progressive age-related, asymmetric, degeneration of the intervertebral discs and facet joints.[2] The reported prevalence of ADS varies but has been reported to be as high as 68% in the adult population.[3,4,5] This high prevalence can be attributed to the fact that most cases of degenerative scoliosis are asymptomatic, with significantly lower degrees of curvature than are seen in adolescent or juvenile scoliosis. Per Silva et al, only 24% of degenerative scoliotic curves measure greater than 20 degrees.[1] Among symptomatic patients who present for evaluation, concomitant stenosis or abnormal vertebral rotation is frequently observed, at up to 97% and 39% incidence, respectively.[6,7]

13.2 History and Examination

The mean age at presentation of ADS is 70.5 years; however, the underlying pathologic processes often start developing around the age of 50.[1] Ninety percent of patients present with back pain as their chief complaint.[5,8,9]

Patients with ADS should be evaluated for sagittal malalignment, which often also affects this patient population. Adult spinal deformity (ASD) includes patients with coronal and/or sagittal malalignment. Coronal malalignment can lead to axial and/or central pain overlying the convexity of the scoliotic curve. This pain is hypothesized to be due to paraspinal musculature fatigue, often worsens upon maintaining an upright posture, and is relieved by lying down.[10] Patients who have both coronal and sagittal malalignment may have fatigue-related paraspinal pain secondary to either condition or both conditions, which can be challenging to differentiate. Sagittal malalignment is thought to be a stronger predictor of axial low back pain compared to coronal malalignment. Fatigued musculature can cause pain that is either pinpoint at muscle insertions along the iliac crest and the sacrum, or it can be diffuse in nature over the entire spine.[8]

Neurologic symptoms, including pain, occur in 47 to 78% of patients with ADS.[11] Foraminal stenosis in the concavity of the curve can compress nerve roots causing radiculopathy; much less commonly, nerve roots can be stretched through traction created by the curve along its convexity.[12] Both central and lateral recess stenosis can occur due to the degenerative nature of the condition with resulting facet hypertrophy, ligamentum flavum hypertrophy, and disc bulging, which, when paired with traction and/or compression, can result in radiculopathy or neurogenic claudication worsened with standing or walking.[8,13] Vertebral body rotation may worsen these symptoms. The onset of neurological symptoms tends to be more insidious in nature, due to the slow progression of the scoliotic curve. While fecal and urinary incontinence can occur, they are very infrequently reported.[10]

Although pain is by far the most common presenting symptom, other complaints include cosmesis and extraspinal complications. Patients may present with a visible deformity due to vertebral rotation, asymmetric back musculature, or the spinal curve. Although the cosmetic aspect of degenerative scoliosis has historically been well-tolerated by the elderly, increasing regard for quality of life in the aging US population has resulted in cosmetic correction playing a larger role in treatment decision-making.[10]

The primary goal of clinical evaluation is to determine the mechanism, onset, location, radiation, and aggravating/alleviating factors of the patient's pain.[11] The exam should include visual inspection of the spine, waist, pelvis, and shoulder for asymmetry.[7] Due to the potential for neurological deficits, it is necessary to perform a thorough neurologic exam to test for strength, balance, and reflexes in all muscle groups, as well as sensory examination of the lower extremities, back, and chest.[14] Strength and balance can be assessed by asking the patient to perform toe-walking, heel-walking, heel-to-toe walking, and one-foot balance tests. The sensory exam should evaluate light touch in each individual dermatome bilaterally. The motor exam should grade strength on a standard 0–5 scale. Further, the exam should include evaluation of potential pelvic obliquity as well as leg length discrepancy or hip/knee flexion contractures.[15]

13.3 Extraspinal Differential Diagnosis

As with all patients with low back pain, it is imperative that the clinician be alert for signs and symptoms associated with extraspinal pathology including abdominal aortic aneurysm, cholecystitis, pancreatitis, renal pathology, and malignancy.[10]

13.4 Diagnostic Imaging

To adequately assess the degree of deformity and establish a measure of baseline curvature that can be monitored over time, full-length standing 36-inch posteroanterior and lateral radiographs are mandatory upon clinical visit. It is vital that the hip joints and proximal femurs are included in the radiograph in order to assess pelvic tilt (PT), which is an important factor in guiding surgical planning.[16] If the decision is made to proceed with surgery, radiographs taken in the supine or prone position demonstrate a more accurate representation of the curve correction on the operating room (OR) table intraoperatively.[17] Bending films are typically only necessary if the surgeon needs additional data to assess curve flexibility for the purpose of upper instrumented level selection or need for posterior column osteotomy (PCO).

Although scoliosis is defined as a coronal malalignment of the spine, recent studies have shown the importance of both coronal and sagittal plane analysis in surgical planning and predicting disease progression.[18,19] Cobb angle, which is the most widely used measurement of coronal malalignment, can be assessed via AP radiographs. This is measured using a goniometer and marking parallel lines to the end plates of the two most angulated vertebrae included in the curve. The intersection angle between these lines is defined as the Cobb angle (► Fig. 13.1).

Sagittal malalignment is perhaps a greater predictor of health-related quality-of-life (HRQoL) scores and disease progression than coronal malalignment, with multiple studies citing sagittal abnormalities as close predictors of increased adjacent segment disease, increased risk of vertebral fracture, higher pain levels, and decreased function.[20,21,22] The sagittal Cobb angle is utilized to calculate both the thoracic kyphosis and lumbar lordosis on the lateral radiograph, whereas sagittal vertical axis (SVA) is utilized to calculate the overall sagittal malalignment in a single measurement. The SVA is measured by drawing a vertical plumb line starting at the middle of the C7 vertebral body going inferiorly to the level of the sacrum. Next, the sagittal offset in the horizontal direction between this line and the posterosuperior corner of the sacral end plate is measured. Reference values

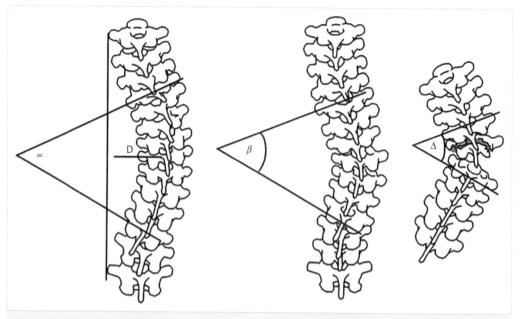

Fig. 13.1 Demonstration of Cobb angle measured from the superior end plate of T12 and inferior end plate of L3. (Reproduced with permission from Rotation deformations. In: Benzel E, ed. Biomechanics of Spine Stabilization. 3rd ed. Thieme; 2015.)

for SVA are primarily a function of age, with young healthy adults having an SVA of 0 to 1 cm.[23,24,25] However, a difference of up to 4 cm anterior of the sacral end plate is considered normal (▶ Fig. 13.2).[10,26]

Given that the pelvis is a key factor in spinal sagittal alignment, there are three related parameters that describe pelvic morphology as it pertains to spinal alignment; these are pelvic incidence (PI), pelvic tilt (PT), and sacral slope (SS). To measure PT, a line is drawn from the center of the S1 end plate to the center of the femoral head. A vertical line (parallel to the side margin of the radiograph) is then drawn that passes through the center of the femoral head. The angle between these two lines is defined as PT. To measure SS, a line is drawn parallel to the sacral end plate. Next, a horizontal line (perpendicular to the side margin of the radiograph) is drawn, and the angle between these two lines is defined as SS. Finally, PI is measured by drawing a line from the center of the S1 end plate to the center of the femoral head. The angle of intersection between this line and a perpendicular line to the S1 end plate is defined as PI (▶ Fig. 13.3). Additionally, the sum of the PT and SS equal the PI (PT + SS = PI).

The SVA, PI, PT, and lumbar lordosis are the cornerstone of the Scoliosis Research Society (SRS)-Schwab classification system, which is a widely accepted method of characterizing the nature of spinal curves in ASD and correlating radiographic parameters with quality of life. It has been repeatedly validated as a clinically relevant method of guiding treatment decisions, surgical planning, and patient counseling regarding outcome expectations.[27] The specific categories of spinal deformity under the SRS-Schwab classification system, along with their various modifiers, are shown in ▶ Fig. 13.4.

It is important to consider the increasingly large role of more modern radiographic techniques in diagnostic imaging. EOS, a form of X-ray technology introduced to clinical practice in 2007, is particularly suitable for visualizing spinal deformities. EOS allows simultaneous acquisition of full body AP and lateral films with the patient in the standing position, which can allow evaluation of hip and knee compensatory mechanisms. Notably, due to the significantly higher sensitivity of the detectors used in EOS imaging versus traditional X-ray imaging, the radiation exposure associated with EOS is six to nine times less than that of standard radiographs; this is an especially important consideration when serial imaging is required for monitoring disease course.[29,30,31,32]

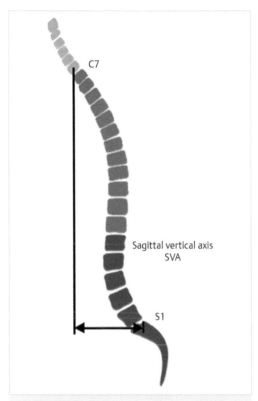

Fig. 13.2 Demonstration of measurement of sagittal vertebral alignment (SVA). (Reproduced with permission from Epidemiology. In: Brooks N, Strayer A, eds. Spine Surgery in an Aging Population. 1st ed. Thieme; 2019.)

Magnetic resonance imaging (MRI) is considered the gold standard in analyzing neural components, vasculature, soft tissue, and disc quality, and should be obtained for preoperative planning. The patient population that suffers from ASDs is often elderly, however, and may have comorbidities for which MRI is contraindicated, for example, cardiac pacemaker, prior instrumentation, aneurysm clip, etc. In these situations, a computed tomography (CT) myelogram is particularly useful in imaging bony anatomy and stenosis. Additionally, a preoperative CT scan aids in surgical planning.

Finally, a DEXA scan is important to assess bone density for surgical planning. Osteoporosis and osteopenia are risk factors strongly associated with postoperative complications including proximal junctional kyphosis and instrumentation failure.[33] Vitamin D, calcium, and pharmacologic therapy, such as bisphosphonates, danosumab, or teriparatide, should be initiated if needed to counter bone density loss in the preoperative period.[16]

13.5 Treatment

Both surgical and nonsurgical treatment options exist for increasing function and managing pain associated with degenerative scoliosis. The following section details several of these treatment types, followed by a discussion of the outcomes of surgical vs. nonsurgical management of ADS.

13.5.1 Nonsurgical Treatment Options

Due to the invasive nature of spinal fusion surgery for ADS and its associated complications, nonsurgical management is usually considered the first-line treatment for managing ASD. The exact nature of conservative treatment varies widely and includes physical therapy, bracing, chiropractic manipulation, epidural steroid injections, and pharmaceutical analgesics such as NSAIDs and opioids.

The most common goal for conservative management is symptomatic pain reduction. Bracing, which can prevent curve progression in infantile and juvenile idiopathic scoliosis, has not shown similar benefit in adults.[34,35] Rather, the role of bracing in adult scoliosis is limited to temporary relief of symptoms. Further, hard bracing is usually poorly tolerated by the ADS patient population, many of whom are elderly and may experience pain or cardiopulmonary restriction with rigid orthoses.[16,36]

Physical therapy is another nonoperative treatment method which has long been used for scoliosis care. Traditionally, the goal of physical therapy has been to strengthen the core muscles, hip abductors, and hamstrings to reduce load on paraspinal musculature, thereby decreasing pain and improving posture. Although this approach has enjoyed success among children and adolescents, a multicenter prospective study by Fritz et al showed no difference in levels of pain or opioid usage between symptomatic adult patients who received physical therapy for spinal deformity vs. those who did not.[37]

The Schroth method, a relatively less utilized style of physical therapy in the United States, is rooted in postural training which aims to elongate and de-rotate the scoliotic spine. It has shown promise for idiopathic scoliosis in adolescents and young adults; however, its role in ADS remains to be fully investigated. A retrospective 47-patient study by Jelačić et al revealed a 16% improvement

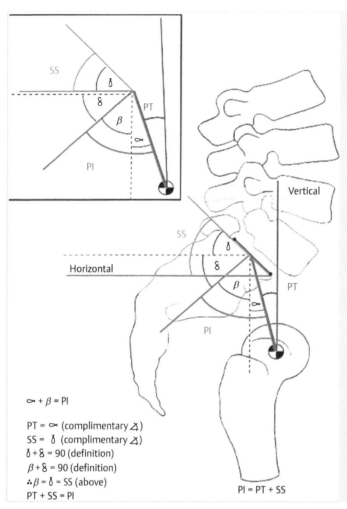

$\alpha + \beta = PI$

$PT = \alpha$ (complimentary $\angle$)
$SS = \delta$ (complimentary $\angle$)
$\delta + \gamma = 90$ (definition)
$\beta + \gamma = 90$ (definition)
$\therefore \beta = \delta = SS$ (above)
$PT + SS = PI$

$PI = PT + SS$

Fig. 13.3 Three measures of pelvic morphology and their relationship to each other are shown. (Reproduced with permission from Epidemiology. In: Brooks N, Strayer A, eds. Spine Surgery in an Aging Population. 1st ed. Thieme; 2019.)

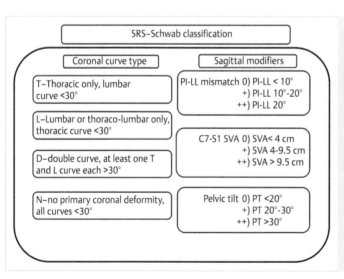

Fig. 13.4 SRS–Schwab classification system.[28] (Reproduced with permission from Modifiers. In: Ames C, Riew K, Abumi K, eds. Cervical Spine Deformity Surgery. 1st ed. Thieme; 2019.)

in trunk imbalance, 14% improvement in lateral deviation, and 5% improvement in surface rotation after 4 weeks of outpatient intensive rehabilitation.[38] Weiss et al retrospectively analyzed 113 patients with idiopathic scoliosis who received the therapy at the Schroth Institute in Germany and discovered an 18.94% increase in vital capacity.[39] A significant limitation of the studies listed here is that they are restricted to a young patient population with mean ages in the late teens to late twenties. To date, there are no studies to our knowledge with a high level of evidence evaluating the efficacy of the Schroth method in middle-aged or older adults. More work is required before it can be definitively recommended as an effective form of treatment for ADS.

Finally, narcotics have been demonstrated to not be effective in the treatment of low back pain. Opioid medications have a high risk for dependence and abuse, and as many as 36% of adults who carry a diagnosis of degenerative scoliosis are opioid-dependent prior to surgery.[40] Due to the complex and subjective nature of chronic pain, the role of cognitive behavioral therapy in relief of chronic pain may also warrant consideration, which was demonstrated in a study by Suska.[41]

13.5.2 Surgical Treatment Options

Symptomatic patients who have failed conservative management and do not have a medical contraindication should be considered for surgical treatment. Once the decision is made to pursue operative management, it is vital to understand the three primary goals of surgery. These goals include (1) correction of malalignment in the sagittal and coronal planes, (2) decompression of the neural elements, and (3) achieving arthrodesis.[42] The traditional surgical approach involves open posterior instrumented fusion to achieve stability, posterior column osteotomies to correct malalignment, and decompression to relieve pain from neurogenic claudication.[43,44] Three-column osteotomies are typically only necessary for fixed rigid deformities. The senior author (CS) typically utilizes three-column osteotomies as a procedure of last resort in patients with a rigid kyphotic deformity with a deformity angular ratio (DAR) greater than 20. The DAR is the magnitude of the curve divided by the number of levels involved in the curve. The surgical technique for vertebral column resection (VCR) is described in detail by Saifi et al.[45]

The classification for ADS by Lenke and Silva in 2010 stratifies patients into distinct treatment categories, ranging from Level I (decompression only) to Level VI (decompression with anterior and posterior instrumented fusion with osteotomies for correction of specific deformities). The clinical and radiographic criteria that characterize each treatment level, as well as the recommended surgical treatment corresponding to each, are shown in ▶ Table 13.1 and ▶ Table 13.2.

In general, decompression-only treatment is indicated for patients whose main complaints are consistent with neurogenic claudication without significant axial back pain and with a stable and balanced spine. Although decompression-only procedures are able to relieve symptoms of claudication, they may accelerate curve progression and/or spinal instability. Therefore, patients undergoing decompression-only should undergo

Table 13.1 Decision matrix for classifying the level of treatment warranted for degenerative scoliosis patients based on clinical symptoms and radiographic findings.

	Level I	Level II	Level III	Level IV	Level V	Level VI
Neurogenic claudication	+	+	+	+	+	+
Back pain	−	+/−	+	+	+	+
Anterior osteophytes	+	+	−	−	−	−
Olisthesis	−	−	+	+	+	+
Coronal Cobb angle > 30 degree	−	−	+	+	+	+
Lumbar kyphosis	−	−	−	+	+	+
Global imbalance	−	−	−	−	Flexible	Stiff/fused

Source: Modified from Silva FE, Lenke LG. Adult degenerative scoliosis: evaluation and management. Neurosurg Focus. 2010; 28(3):E1.

Table 13.2 Recommended operative treatment corresponding to each Lenke-Silva treatment level[1]

	Recommended operative treatment
Level I	Decompression only
Level II	Decompression + instrumented posterior spinal fusion limited to area of decompression
Level III	Decompression + instrumented posterior fusion of entire lumbar spine
Level IV	Decompression + instrumented anterior and posterior fusion of entire lumbar spine
Level V	Decompression + instrumented anterior and posterior fusion of lumbar spine + extension of fusion/instrumentation into thoracic region
Level VI	Decompression + instrumented anterior and posterior fusion of lumbar spine + extension of fusion/instrumentation into thoracic region + osteotomies for specific defects

routine postoperative monitoring to evaluate for signs of disease progression.[1,10,46]

When intolerable back pain is the chief complaint in ADS patients, fusion is generally indicated, which has the benefit of providing spinal stability and halting curve progression within the construct. Generally, patients with Cobb angles greater than 20 degree may benefit from an isolated posterior procedure. Patients with deformities greater than 40 degree may necessitate combined anterior–posterior instrumentation and fusion. The addition of the anterior procedure affords several advantages. First, it allows direct access to the intervertebral disc space and the anterior longitudinal ligament, which acts as an anterior tension band for the spine. The anterior approach allows improved visualization of disc space preparation and larger interbody cages compared to a posterior approach. Restoration in disc height may provide indirect decompression of nerve roots, obviating the need for a more extensive posterior decompression. Anterior interbody fusion with hyperlordotic cages is particularly helpful in restoring lordosis, which should represent approximately two-thirds of the patient's lumbar lordosis. Notably, anterior spinal fusion is associated with lower rates of pseudarthrosis and, when combined with posterior fusion, helps reduce rates of instrumentation failure. This is especially helpful for patients who are at the greatest risk of nonunion and instrumentation failure.

Despite the benefits of combined anterior–posterior fusion, an extended anterior approach has several disadvantages. First, access to the anterior spine may involve extensive vascular manipulation particularly at L4–L5 and above, which can lead to ischemia, thrombosis, or injury to the great vessels. Further, there is increased risk of damage to visceral organs and longer operative time than a posterior procedure alone. A retrospective cohort study by Pateder et al sought to determine whether the benefits of combined anterior–posterior approach outweighed the disadvantages of the additional procedure. Their results showed that for patients with Cobb angles between 40 and 70 degree who underwent posterior surgical correction vs. anterior–posterior combined surgical correction, there was no difference in sagittal or coronal correction or stability postoperatively. However, the complication rate for patients who underwent dual anterior–posterior approach was higher (45%) compared to patients who had a posterior-only approach (23%).[47] However, this is dependent on several factors such as the experience level of the exposure surgeon, the levels (L4–L5 vs. L5–S1) being fused, patient's body mass index (BMI) and vascular anatomy. The senior author (CS) performs anterior lumbar interbody fusion (ALIF) in ADS patients who have a PI minus lumbar lordosis mismatch greater than 40 degrees with disc collapse at L4–L5 and/or L5–S1. Patients with a mismatch of less than 45 degrees can typically be corrected with a deformity transforaminal lumbar interbody fusion (TLIF), which consists of a PCO and up to a 25-degree hyperlordotic TLIF cage at L5–S1 and to a lesser extent at L4–L5.

The overall complication rate for surgical correction of adult scoliosis varies based on patient age and number of fusion levels, but has been reported to be as high as 80%, with the rate of "major" complications (defined as excessive hospitalization time, need for reoperation, prolonged morbidity, or death) as high as 21%.[48,49] The two most common of these major complications are infection and high-volume blood loss, largely due to the nature of a long, midline incision.[50]

Any use of muscle sparing or minimally invasive techniques must be able to fully address the three goals of surgical management, which are restoration of sagittal and coronal alignment, decompression of the neural elements, and arthrodesis. A 2016 meta-analysis by Phan et al demonstrated that minimally invasive surgical techniques were successful in relieving back and leg pain and improving function, with an average decrease in visual analog scale (VAS) score of 54 points and an average decrease in Oswestry Disability Index (ODI) of 22.5 points. In this meta-analysis, all studies, but one, demonstrated that minimally invasive techniques were able to achieve equal decreases in Cobb angle when compared to open procedures. The pooled pseudarthrosis rate was 4.3%, while the incidence of pseudarthrosis in open procedures range between 5 and 35%.[51,52,53]

A retrospective study by Dakwar et al showed that one-third of their patients who underwent fusion via a minimally invasive lateral approach did not have adequate restoration of sagittal alignment.[54] The meta-analysis by Phan et al suggested that minimally invasive techniques are comparable to open techniques for decompressing neural elements, restoring coronal alignment, and achieving arthrodesis. More research is needed to evaluate the success of minimally invasive techniques in restoring sagittal alignment.

It is important to keep in mind that minimally invasive techniques come with their own unique set of complications. For example, lateral lumbar interbody fusion (LLIF) affords access to the anterior column through a lateral flank incision and allows interbody cage insertion and restoration of disc height. However, because this procedure requires dissection through the psoas muscle, it may be associated with dysesthesia, hyperesthesia, and motor palsy from the lumbar plexus nerves.[55] Minimally invasive procedures can be performed in conjunction with open procedures, which are described as hybrid procedures.

13.6 Outcomes

Despite the tendency to initiate treatment of degenerative scoliosis nonsurgically, evidence supporting the efficacy of conservative measures is sparse. The current literature includes level IV (very weak) evidence for bracing, physical therapy, or chiropractic manipulation as treatments for adult scoliosis and level III (weak) evidence for epidural steroid injections.[34] Patients who see the best results from nonoperative therapy are those who have small coronal deformities in the thoracolumbar region without any significant or progressive neurological deficits.[18] Further studies suggest that nonsurgical treatment of ASD is unlikely to *improve* the course of patients' disease, but may have some benefit to patients who are satisfied with and wish to maintain their current level of spine health.[56] It should be noted that approximately 30% of patients report an increase in pain levels after 2 years of nonoperative care, with 27% of patients reporting new-onset leg pain.[57]

Retrospective cohort studies comparing operative and nonoperative treatment of symptomatic ADS show significant improvement in operative groups vs. nonoperative groups in terms of pain, function, and long-term cost-effectiveness.[18,34,56,57] In 2019, Kelly et al published the first randomized control trial investigating surgical and nonsurgical outcomes in patients with adult symptomatic scoliosis. At 2-year follow-up, SRS-22 subscore increased by an average of 0.7 points and ODI score decreased by an average of 18 points in patients randomized to operative treatment, whereas there was no change in SRS-22 subscore and an average ODI decrease of only 2 points in patients randomized to nonoperative treatment. These data strongly suggest that symptomatic patients who desire improved HRQoL and decreased pain are more likely to benefit from surgical than from nonsurgical intervention.[58]

In terms of operative management, a successful outcome is defined as reduction in pain and gain in function as measured by various modalities (ODI, HRQoL, SRS-22, VAS, etc.). By these metrics, operative management is quite effective, with the literature unequivocally reporting average decreases in ODI and increases in HRQoL at 2-year follow-up.[59,60,61,62] A meta-analysis of the adult scoliosis literature shows that among surgical patients, 24% have complete resolution of back pain and 38% have complete resolution of leg pain at 2-year follow-up, with 73% and 57% reporting at least mild improvement in back pain and leg pain, respectively. Patients who have higher levels of pain and disability preoperatively, and patients whose deformities are mostly at lumbar levels, are more likely to report improvement in their pain postoperatively than patients with mild preoperative pain or thoracic malalignment.[57]

Finally, it should be noted that the range of surgical outcomes for ASDs is quite broad. Though most patients do report satisfaction after surgery, it is important to convey that not every patient may meet the average level of improvement postoperatively. No change in the patient's level of pain, or even a deterioration from preoperative pain, are not uncommon.[57] Therefore, it is important to temper expectations and convey to patients that surgery to correct spinal malalignment is likely to lead to a decrease in pain, but unlikely to lead to complete resolution of pain.

Clinical Pearls and Considerations

1. Postoperatively, patients who experience improvement in back pain but not in leg pain report significantly higher satisfaction with their outcomes than patients who experience improvement in leg pain but not back pain. This suggests that a focus on sagittal malalignment to reduce back pain may improve patient satisfaction.[61]
2. Once diagnosed, curves in ADS may progress at a faster rate (up to 3 degree/year) than those in idiopathic scoliosis. Risk factors for increased rates of progression include a curve greater than 30 degrees, greater than 30% apical vertebral rotation, greater than 6 mm of lateral listhesis, and presence of degenerative disease at the lumbosacral junction.[8]
3. It is important to identify and evaluate the *fractional curve* (▶ Fig. 13.5). Patients may develop isolated radiculopathy from neural compression at the concavity of the curve. Radiculopathy in isolation secondary to the fractional curve may be addressed with a limited indirect decompression and fusion. ▶ Fig. 13.5 demonstrates a patient with a right L4 radiculopathy due to superior–inferior foraminal stenosis from her fractional curve at L4–L5, which was completely relieved with an outpatient LLIF with percutaneous posterior instrumentation by the senior author (CS). At the 2-week follow-up, the patient reported full recovery and had ceased the use of opioid medication.
4. T1 pelvic angle (TPA) is a radiographic measure which incorporates global sagittal alignment and PT. Protopsaltis et al demonstrated that TPA has the strongest correlation to HRQoL outcomes compared to all other sagittal alignment values including LL-PI, PT, and SVA. A preoperative TPA greater than 20 degrees corresponds to severe disability and has the highest while a preoperative TPA of 14 degrees corresponds to an ODI of 20, which represents minimal disability. To calculate TPA, a line is drawn between the femoral head and the center of the T1 vertebral body and another line is drawn from the femoral head to the center of the center of the superior sacral end plate.[63] The angle between these two lines is defined as the TPA (▶ Fig. 13.6).
5. Global alignment and proportion score (GAP score) can be used to analyze spinopelvic alignment to determine the risk of mechanical complications after adult deformity surgery. The GAP score is calculated by adding the values of relative pelvic version (RPV), relative lumbar lordosis (RLL), relative spinopelvic alignment (RSA), lordosis distribution index (LDI), and an "age factor." Mechanical complications predicted by GAP score include proximal and distal junctional kyphosis and failure, rod breakage, and others. Scores of 0 to 2 reflect a proportioned spinopelvic state with a 6% complication rate. Scores of 3 to 6 reflect moderately disproportioned spinopelvic state with a 47% complication rate. Scores greater than or equal to 7 reflect severely disproportioned spinopelvic alignment with a 95% complication rate.[64]
   The radiographic parameters that comprise GAP score is:
   GAP = RPV + RLL + LDI + RSA + Age factor

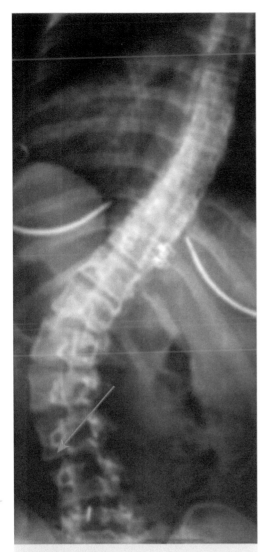

Fig. 13.5 X-ray of patient with scoliosis. *Red arrow* is indicating fractional curve.

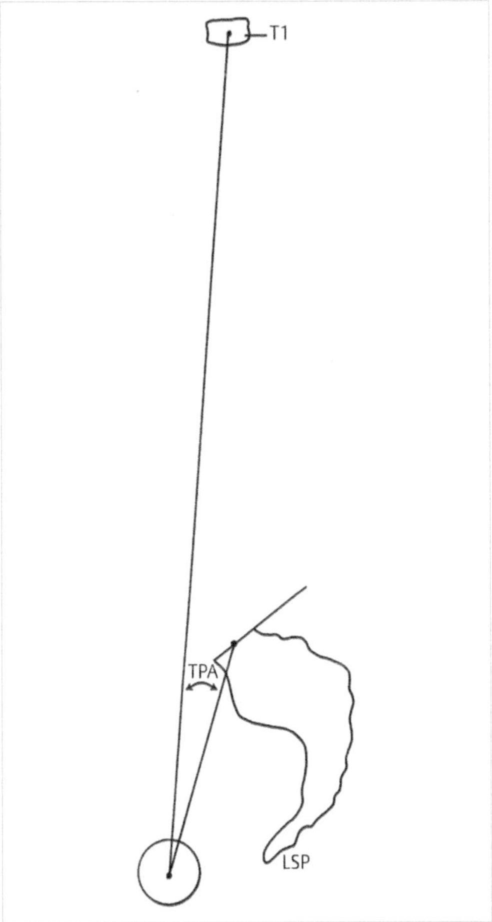

Fig. 13.6 A pictorial depiction of how to calculate T1 pelvic angle (TPA) is shown. One line is drawn between the femoral head and the center of the T1 vertebral body and another line is drawn from the femoral head to the center of the superior sacral end plate. (Reproduced with permission from Introduction. In: Weaver, Jr. E, ed. Surgical Care of the Painful Degenerative Lumbar Spine: Evaluation, Decision-Making, Techniques. 1st ed. Thieme; 2018.)

13.7 Case Example

This is a 69-year-old female with a history of L4–L5 posterior spinal fusion with instrumentation 10 years prior, status post intrathecal pain pump placement and spinal cord stimulator approximately 5 years prior and osteoporosis, who presented with intractable back pain secondary to ASD with coronal and sagittal malalignment (▶ Fig. 13.7).

She reports that her back pain worsens with activity and weightbearing and has been significantly interfering with activities of daily living. Her pain radiates from her low back down her left leg. She has had progressive difficulty with ambulation due to her posture. She also describes increasing difficulty breathing, which she feels is secondary to her spine deformity.

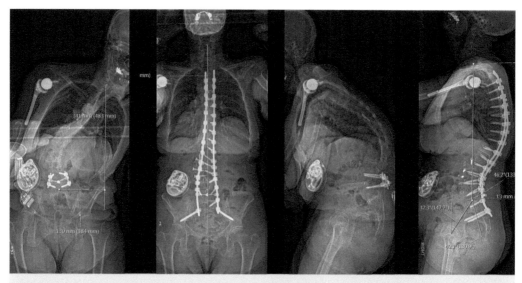

Fig. 13.7 Preoperative and postoperative thoracolumbar EOS anteroposterior (AP) and lateral imaging of the patient described.

Table 13.3 Preoperative and postoperative measurements of the patient described

	Coronal C7 PL (cm)	SVA (cm)	Lumbar lordosis (degree)	PI - LL mismatch (degree)	Pelvic tilt (degree)
Preop	13	30.0	0	48	40
Postop	0	1.3	46	2	32

Her physical exam yielded no deficits in strength or sensation. Her EOS imaging demonstrates both coronal and sagittal deformity. It demonstrates 65-degree (T10–L2) left-sided scoliosis and 52 degree (T11–L1) of thoracolumbar kyphosis with the apex at the T12–L1 disc space. Zero degree of lumbar lordosis. PI of 47 degree. PT of 40 degree. SVA of ~30 cm. She has significant coronal deformity to the right side. Her DEXA T-score is –2.2.

The patient underwent L1–L4 direct lateral interbody fusion followed by T2–pelvis posterior spinal fusion and instrumentation with removal of the spinal cord simulator. Preoperative and postoperative imaging is demonstrated in ▶ Fig. 13.7 with alignment parameters re-listed in ▶ Table 13.3. Postoperatively the patient is very pleased with her operation and states her quality of life has improved immensely.

References

[1] Silva FE, Lenke LG. Adult degenerative scoliosis: evaluation and management. Neurosurg Focus. 2010; 28(3):E1

[2] Phillips FM, Isaacs RE, Rodgers WB, et al. Adult degenerative scoliosis treated with XLIF: clinical and radiographical results of a prospective multicenter study with 24-month follow-up. Spine. 2013; 38(21):1853–1861

[3] Aebi M. The adult scoliosis. Eur Spine J. 2005; 14(10):925–948

[4] Anasetti F, Galbusera F, Aziz HN, et al. Spine stability after implantation of an interspinous device: an in vitro and finite element biomechanical study. J Neurosurg Spine. 2010; 13 (5):568–575

[5] Schwab F, Dubey A, Gamez L, et al. Adult scoliosis: prevalence, SF-36, and nutritional parameters in an elderly volunteer population. Spine. 2005; 30(9):1082–1085

[6] Fu K-MG, Rhagavan P, Shaffrey CI, Chernavvsky DR, Smith JS. Prevalence, severity, and impact of foraminal and canal stenosis among adults with degenerative scoliosis. Neurosurgery. 2011; 69(6):1181–1187

[7] Armstrong GW, Livermore NB, III, Suzuki N, Armstrong JG. Nonstandard vertebral rotation in scoliosis screening patients: its prevalence and relation to the clinical deformity. Spine. 1982; 7(1):50–54

[8] Ascani E, Bartolozzi R, Logroscino CA, et al. Natural history of untreated idiopathic scoliosis after skeletal maturity. Clin Biomech. 1987; 2(2):112

[9] Berven SH, Lowe T. The Scoliosis Research Society classification for adult spinal deformity. Neurosurg Clin N Am. 2007; 18(2):207–213

[10] Kotwal S, Pumberger M, Hughes A, Girardi F. Degenerative scoliosis: a review. HSS J. 2011; 7(3):257–264

[11] Graham RB, Sugrue PA, Koski TR. Adult degenerative scoliosis. Clin Spine Surg. 2016; 29(3):95–107

[12] Boachie-Adjei O, Gupta MC. Adult scoliosis + deformity. AAOS Instructional Course Lectures. 1999; 48(39): 377–391

[13] Ploumis A, Transfledt EE, Denis F. Degenerative lumbar scoliosis associated with spinal stenosis. Spine J. 2007; 7(4): 428–436

[14] Janicki JA, Alman B. Scoliosis: review of diagnosis and treatment. Paediatr Child Health. 2007; 12(9):771–776

[15] York PJ, Kim HJ. Degenerative scoliosis. Curr Rev Musculoskelet Med. 2017; 10(4):547–558

[16] Russo A, Bransford R, Wagner T, et al. Adult degenerative scoliosis insights, challenges, and treatment outlook. Curr Orthop Pract. 2008; 19(4):357–365

[17] Ferrero E. "Degenerative scoliosis: clinical presentation and diagnostic workup." Spine Surgery Education Programme, 2017, doi:10.28962/01.3.064

[18] Diebo BG, Varghese JJ, Lafage R, Schwab FJ, Lafage V. Sagittal alignment of the spine: what do you need to know? Clin Neurol Neurosurg. 2015; 139:295–301

[19] Glassman SD, Bridwell K, Dimar JR, Horton W, Berven S, Schwab F. The impact of positive sagittal balance in adult spinal deformity. Spine. 2005; 30(18):2024–2029

[20] Blondel B, Schwab F, Ungar B, et al. Impact of magnitude and percentage of global sagittal plane correction on health-related quality of life at 2-years follow-up. Neurosurgery. 2012; 71(2):341–348, discussion 348

[21] Baek S-W, Kim C, Chang H. The relationship between the spinopelvic balance and the incidence of adjacent vertebral fractures following percutaneous vertebroplasty. Osteoporos Int. 2015; 26(5):1507–1513

[22] Kumar MN, Baklanov A, Chopin D. Correlation between sagittal plane changes and adjacent segment degeneration following lumbar spine fusion. Eur Spine J. 2001; 10 (4):314–319

[23] Hasegawa K, Okamoto M, Hatsushikano S, Shimoda H, Ono M, Watanabe K. Normative values of spino-pelvic sagittal alignment, balance, age, and health-related quality of life in a cohort of healthy adult subjects. Eur Spine J. 2016; 25(11): 3675–3686

[24] Endo K, Numajiri K, Hasome T, et al. Measurement of whole spine sagittal alignment using the SLOT radiography of the SONIALVISION safire series clinical application. Medical Now, No. 78, 2018

[25] Bakouny Z, Assi A, Yared F, et al. Normative spino-pelvic sagittal alignment of Lebanese asymptomatic adults: comparisons with different ethnicities. Orthop Traumatol Surg Res. 2018; 104(5):557–564

[26] Oskouian RJ, Jr, Shaffrey CI. Degenerative lumbar scoliosis. Neurosurg Clin N Am. 2006; 17(3):299–315, vii

[27] Terran J, Schwab F, Shaffrey CI, et al. International Spine Study Group. The SRS-Schwab adult spinal deformity classification: assessment and clinical correlations based on a prospective operative and nonoperative cohort. Neurosurgery. 2013; 73(4):559–568

[28] Ames C, Riew K, Abumi K, ed. Cervical Spine Deformity Surgery. 1st ed. Thieme; 2019

[29] Maigne J-Y, Aivaliklis A, Pfefer F. Results of sacroiliac joint double block and value of sacroiliac pain provocation tests in 54 patients with low back pain. Spine. 1996; 21(16): 1889–1892

[30] Deschênes S, Charron G, Beaudoin G, et al. Diagnostic imaging of spinal deformities: reducing patients radiation dose with a new slot-scanning X-ray imager. Spine. 2010; 35(9): 989–994

[31] Somoskeöy S, Tunyogi-Csapó M, Bogyó C, Illés T. Accuracy and reliability of coronal and sagittal spinal curvature data based on patient-specific three-dimensional models created by the EOS 2D/3D imaging system. Spine. 2012; 12(11): 1052–1059

[32] Wybier M, Bossard P. Musculoskeletal imaging in progress: the EOS imaging system. Joint Bone Spine. 2013; 80 (3):238–243

[33] Bjerke BT, Zarrabian M, Aleem IS, et al. Incidence of osteoporosis-related complications following posterior lumbar fusion. Global Spine J. 2018; 8(6):563–569

[34] Everett CR, Patel RK. A systematic literature review of nonsurgical treatment in adult scoliosis. Spine. 2007; 32(19) Suppl:S130–S134

[35] Ailon T, Smith JS, Shaffrey CI, et al. Degenerative spinal deformity. Neurosurgery. 2015; 77 Suppl 4:S75–S91

[36] Frownfelter D, Stevens K, Massery M, Bernardoni G. Do abdominal cutouts in thoracolumbosacral orthoses increase pulmonary function? Clin Orthop Relat Res. 2014; 472(2): 720–726

[37] Fritz JM, Lurie JD, Zhao W, et al. Associations between physical therapy and long-term outcomes for individuals with lumbar spinal stenosis in the SPORT study. Spine J. 2014; 14 (8):1611–1621

[38] Jelačić M, Villagrasa M, Pou E, Quera-Salvá G, Rigo M. Barcelona Scoliosis Physical Therapy School (BSPTS)—based on classical Schroth principles: short term effects on back asymmetry in idiopathic scoliosis. Scoliosis. 2012; 7 Suppl 1:O57

[39] Weiss HR. The progression of idiopathic scoliosis under the influence of a physiotherapy rehabilitation programme. Physiotherapy. 1992; 78:815–821

[40] Sharma M, Ugiliweneza B, Sirdeshpande P, Wang D, Boakye M. Opioid dependence and health care utilization after decompression and fusion in patients with adult degenerative scoliosis. Spine. 2019; 44(4):280–290

[41] Suska J. Cognitive-behavioral-based physical therapy for patients with chronic pain undergoing lumbar spine surgery: a randomized controlled trial. Physioscience. 2017; 13(01):35–36

[42] Kretzer RM. Adult degenerative spinal deformity: overview and open approaches for treatment. Spine. 2017; 42 Suppl 7:S16

[43] Ali RM, Boachie-Adjei O, Rawlins BA. Functional and radiographic outcomes after surgery for adult scoliosis using third-generation instrumentation techniques. Spine. 2003; 28(11):1163–1169, discussion 1169–1170

[44] Bess RS, Lenke LG, Bridwell KH, Cheh G, Mandel S, Sides B. Comparison of thoracic pedicle screw to hook instrumentation for the treatment of adult spinal deformity. Spine. 2007; 32(5):555–561

[45] Saifi C, Laratta JL, Petridis P, Shillingford JN, Lehman RA, Lenke LG. Vertebral column resection for rigid spinal deformity. Global Spine J. 2017; 7(3):280–290

[46] Berven SH, Deviren V, Mitchell B, Wahba G, Hu SS, Bradford DS. Operative management of degenerative scoliosis: an evidence-based approach to surgical strategies based on clinical and radiographic outcomes. Neurosurg Clin N Am. 2007; 18(2):261–272

[47] Pateder DB, Kebaish KM, Cascio BM, Neubauer P, Matusz DM, Kostuik JP. Posterior only versus combined anterior and posterior approaches to lumbar scoliosis in adults: a radiographic analysis. Spine. 2007; 32(14):1551–1554

[48] Daubs MD, Lenke LG, Cheh G, Stobbs G, Bridwell KH. Adult spinal deformity surgery: complications and outcomes in patients over age 60. Spine. 2007; 32(20): 2238–2244

[49] Carreon LY, Puno RM, Dimar JR, II, Glassman SD, Johnson JR. Perioperative complications of posterior lumbar decompression and arthrodesis in older adults. J Bone Joint Surg Am. 2003; 85(11):2089–2092

[50] Smith JS, Shaffrey CI, Lafage V, et al. Prospective, multicenter assessment of nonoperative treatment outcomes and conversion to operative treatment for adult spinal deformity: minimum two-year follow-up. Spine J. 2014; 14(11): S98–S99

[51] Phan K, Huo YR, Hogan JA, et al. Minimally invasive surgery in adult degenerative scoliosis: a systematic review and meta-analysis of decompression, anterior/lateral and posterior lumbar approaches. J Spine Surg. 2016; 2(2):89–104

[52] Kim YJ, Bridwell KH, Lenke LG, Rhim S, Cheh G. Pseudarthrosis in long adult spinal deformity instrumentation and fusion to the sacrum: prevalence and risk factor analysis of 144 cases. Spine. 2006; 31(20):2329–2336

[53] Chun DS, Baker KC, Hsu WK. Lumbar pseudarthrosis: a review of current diagnosis and treatment. Neurosurg Focus. 2015; 39(4):E10

[54] Dakwar E, Cardona RF, Smith DA, Uribe JS. Early outcomes and safety of the minimally invasive, lateral retroperitoneal transpsoas approach for adult degenerative scoliosis. Neurosurg Focus. 2010; 28(3):E8

[55] Isaacs RE, Hyde J, Goodrich JA, Rodgers WB, Phillips FM. A prospective, nonrandomized, multicenter evaluation of extreme lateral interbody fusion for the treatment of adult degenerative scoliosis: perioperative outcomes and complications. Spine. 2010; 35(26) Suppl:S322–S330

[56] Kelly MP, Lurie JD, Yanik EL, et al. Operative versus nonoperative treatment for adult symptomatic lumbar scoliosis. J Bone Joint Surg Am. 2019; 101(4):338–352

[57] Teles AR, Mattei TA, Righesso O, Falavigna A. Effectiveness of operative and nonoperative care for adult spinal deformity: systematic review of the literature. Global Spine J. 2017; 7 (2):170–178

[58] Kelly MP, et al. Adult symptomatic lumbar scoliosis: randomized results from a dual-arm study. Scoliosis Research Society: 52nd Annual Meeting of SRS Conference in Philadelphia, 6 September 2017, Philadelphia, Philadelphia Marriott Downtown

[59] Yadla S, Maltenfort MG, Ratliff JK, Harrop JS. Adult scoliosis surgery outcomes: a systematic review. Neurosurg Focus. 2010; 28(3):E3

[60] Bridwell KH, Glassman S, Horton W, et al. Does treatment (nonoperative and operative) improve the two-year quality of life in patients with adult symptomatic lumbar scoliosis: a prospective multicenter evidence-based medicine study. Spine. 2009; 34(20):2171–2178

[61] Scheer JK, Smith JS, Clark AJ, et al. International Spine Study Group. Comprehensive study of back and leg pain improvements after adult spinal deformity surgery: analysis of 421 patients with 2-year follow-up and of the impact of the surgery on treatment satisfaction. J Neurosurg Spine. 2015; 22 (5):540–553

[62] Choi SH, Son SM, Goh TS, Park W, Lee JS. Outcomes of operative and nonoperative treatment in patients with adult spinal deformity with a minimum 2-year follow-up: a meta-analysis. World Neurosurg. 2018; 120:e870–e876

[63] Protopsaltis T, Schwab F, Bronsard N, et al. International Spine Study Group. The T1 pelvic angle, a novel radiographic measure of global sagittal deformity, accounts for both spinal inclination and pelvic tilt and correlates with health-related quality of life. J Bone Joint Surg Am. 2014; 96(19):1631–1640

[64] Yilgor C, Sogunmez N, Boissiere L, et al. European Spine Study Group (ESSG). Global Alignment and Proportion (GAP) Score: development and validation of a new method of analyzing spinopelvic alignment to predict mechanical complications after adult spinal deformity surgery. J Bone Joint Surg Am. 2017; 99(19):1661–1672

14 Kyphosis and Sagittal Plane Deformities of the Thoracolumbar Spine

Lawal A. Labaran, Khaled Kebaish, Francis Shen, and Hamid Hassanzadeh

Abstract

Sagittal imbalance (SI), the result of a defect in the natural kyphotic and lordotic curvatures of the spine, is most commonly seen in patients with multiple-level degenerative disc disease, severe osteoporosis, idiopathic scoliosis, and inflammatory arthropathies. Clinical symptoms of SI have been shown to be closely correlated to the degree of imbalance. All SI patients must undergo a standard musculoskeletal and neurologic exam in both the supine and standing positions. Patient's gait should be initially assessed for secondary compensatory mechanism in addition to hip range-of-motion exams for the presence of concomitant hip pathologies. The mainstay of sagittal plane deformity imaging is posteroanterior (PA) and lateral plain radiographs. Cobb angle measurements should be made on a PA film for assessment of coronal plane deformity and lateral films for sagittal plane deformity. Further evaluation of the severity of SI can be made using radiographic parameters such as sagittal vertical axis, T1 pelvic angle, pelvic incidence, pelvic tilt, and sacral slope. Thoracolumbar osteotomies remain the mainstay of treatment in correcting global SI. The posterior column Smith-Peterson/Ponte osteotomy, three-column pedicle subtraction osteotomy, and vertebral column resection are the most common types of osteotomies used till date. Complication rates in thoracolumbar osteotomies range from 25 to 40% in recent literature, with adults having higher complications compared to adolescents.

Keywords: sagittal plane deformity, sagittal imbalance, kyphosis, osteotomy, thoracolumbar spine deformity, sagittal vertical axis, posterior column osteotomy, pedicle subtraction osteotomy, vertebral column resection

14.1 Introduction

Sagittal plane deformity is an area of critical importance in spine surgery, with most cases resulting from kyphosis or hyperlordosis of the thoracolumbar spine. The natural kyphotic and lordotic curvatures of the spine permit the equal distribution of forces along the spinal column. Hence, the loss of curvature due to age and other spine pathologies can lead to significant sagittal plane deformity. Sagittal imbalance (SI) is most commonly seen in patients with multiple-level degenerative disc disease, severe osteoporosis, idiopathic scoliosis, and inflammatory arthropathies.[1,2,3,4,5] Clinical symptoms of SI have been shown to be closely correlated to the degree of imbalance.[5,6,7,8] SI patients have difficulty maintaining an upright posture, expend more energy during ambulation, and may have difficulty with respiration in some severe cases, which leads to a decrease in patient's perceived quality of life.[9,10,11] Due to the high degree of variation in reported normal sagittal balance parameters in both normal and spine deformity patients, SI may be difficult to detect among certain patients.[12,13,14]

14.2 History and Examination

Clinical evaluation includes a thorough history and physical examination. Patients may present differently based on the degree of SI and thoracolumbar kyphosis. These patients often present with symptoms that lead to poor quality of life (pain in the back, legs, and buttocks), decline in overall functional status, and/or loss of horizontal gaze.[14] SI patients develop a stooping posture and may become fatigued from efforts to maintain an upright posture.[14] Additionally, these patients develop a compensatory retroversion of their pelvis, hip extension, and knee flexion to maintain an upright posture and forward gaze.[13,14] The dysfunction caused by sagittal plane deformity have been described in terms of the primary deformity caused by imbalance and the compensatory changes to maintain posture in the pelvis.[14]

All SI patients must undergo a standard musculoskeletal and neurologic exam in both the supine and standing positions. The patient's gait should be initially assessed for secondary compensatory mechanism in addition to hip range-of-motion exams for the presence of concomitant hip pathologies. Nonetheless, further radiological imaging in addition to clinical examination is essential in the evaluation of SI.

Table 14.1 Summary of common causes and etiologies of sagittal imbalance

Deformity	Etiology of sagittal imbalance
Scheuermann kyphosis	Rigid spinal kyphosis with anterior wedging of the vertebra
Flatback syndrome	Iatrogenic loss of lumbar lordosis secondary to thoracolumbar instrumentation
Degenerative disc disease	Disc herniation, facet joint arthritis, hip and pelvic arthropathies, and loss of lumbar lordosis
Ankylosing spondylitis	Loss of lumbar lordosis due to destruction of intervertebral disc and vertebral body with progressive fusion of the spine
Posttraumatic kyphosis	Kyphotic deformity from spinal column injury
Iatrogenic causes	Proximal and distal junctional kyphosis from posterior instrumentation of the spine
Congenital causes	Klippel-feil syndrome, infantile scoliosis, osteogenesis imperfecta

14.3 Differential Diagnosis

In both young and elderly patients, the cause of SI is most likely multifactorial. Diagnoses that should be considered when evaluating patients with suspected SI include: Scheurmann kyphosis, iatrogenic flatback, post-traumatic deformity, neuromuscular disorders, congenital disorders such as infantile scoliosis and Down syndrome, degenerative disc disease, and inflammatory arthropathies.[9,15,16,17,18] Common causes and etiologies of SI are summarized in ► Table 14.1.

14.4 Diagnostic Imaging

The mainstay of sagittal plane deformity imaging is posteroanterior (PA) and lateral (standard full length and standing) plain radiographs (► Fig. 14.1). Cobb angle measurements should be made on a PA film for assessment of coronal plane deformity and lateral films for sagittal plane deformity, especially in patients with scoliosis. Dynamic flexion and extension radiographs should be obtained for evaluation of spine instability and flexibility. Additionally, a supine radiograph with a bolster can be used to evaluate the positional change in the degree of lumbar lordosis for optimal preoperative planning. Further evaluation of the severity of SI can be made using the following radiographic parameters: sagittal vertical axis (SVA), chin-brow vertical angle, C7 plumb line, T1 pelvic angle (TPA), pelvic incidence (PI), pelvic tilt

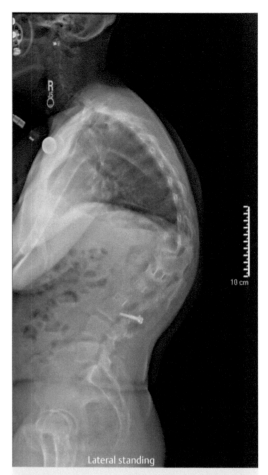

Lateral standing

Fig. 14.1 Standing lateral radiograph of a patient with thoracolumbar degenerative kyphosis causing sagittal malalignment.

(PT), and sacral slope (SS) (► Fig. 14.2). SI evaluation may also include advanced diagnostic imaging such as computed tomography (CT) and magnetic resonance imaging (MRI) for the assessment of associated spine pathology.

The C7 plumb line, a vertical line from C7 vertebral body from which SVA is derived, is critical in the radiographic evaluation of SI. The length of horizontal line connecting the C7 plumb line to the posterior superior sacral end plate is the SVA, one of the most widely used measurements of global sagittal alignment. Schwab et al described an SVA threshold of 47 mm or greater to be associated with severe disability.[19] The effect of age on sagittal balance is also important; for instance, SVA has been shown to increase with increasing age partly due to a loss of lumbar lordosis.[20] TPA is another

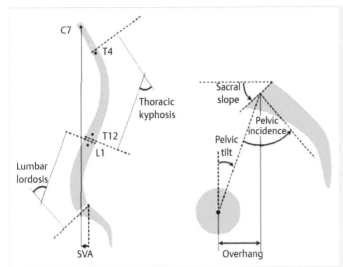

Fig. 14.2 Illustration showing pelvic parameters for measurements of global sagittal alignment. (Reproduced with permission from Newton P, O'Brien M, Shufflebarger H, et al. Idiopathic Scoliosis: The Harms Study Group Treatment Guide. 1st ed. 2010, Thieme Publishers, New York.)

spinopelvic parameter that describes the degree of SI by accounting for spine alignment and compensatory pelvic retroversion. It is defined as the angle formed by the line connecting the femoral head to the T1 vertebral body and the line from femoral head to the midpoint of S1 end plate. This angle has shown association with clinical outcomes.[21] Although TPA is related to SVA and PT, this measurement is not influenced by the compensatory changes of pelvic orientation, nor by the patient's posture compared to SVA.[22] Proposed target TPA ranges from less than 10° to 20°.[21,22,23] The chin-brow vertical angle is a postural angle that assesses a patient's horizontal gaze. It is the angle between a line from the chin to eyebrow and the vertical axis. A chin-brow vertical angle of 0° signifies a normal horizontal gaze. The relationship of pelvic orientation to the spine can be described by PI, PT, and SS.[24] PI is a static parameter that is significant during corrective spine surgery in determining required lumbar lordosis. SS is defined as the angle between the superior sacral end plate and the horizontal axis, which determines the position of the lumbar spine.[25] The relation of the pelvis to the axial spine as defined by PT, PI, and SS is summarized in following equation: SS + PT=PI. SS remains inversely proportional to PT due to the static nature of PI; thus, as PT increases to main upright posture, SS decreases, resulting in a horizontal L5–S1 angle.[13,14,26,27]

14.5 Treatments

Thoracolumbar osteotomies remain the mainstay of treatment in correcting global SI, although nonoperative management such as physiotherapy and bracing[28] may benefit a subset of patients with mild-to-moderate deformity. Deformity correction in the thoracolumbar region can be achieved with different types of osteotomies based on indication, degree of rigidity or flexibility, and the amount of correction needed.[4,9,29,30,31] The posterior column Smith-Peterson/Ponte osteotomy (PCO), three-column pedicle subtraction osteotomy (PSO), and vertebral column resection (VCR) are the most common types of osteotomies used till date (▶ Fig. 14.3).

First described by Smith-Peterson in 1945, PCO involves a single or multilevel posterior column release. This technique entails a resection of the inferior aspect of the spinous process, ligamentum flavum and intervening posterior spinal ligament, inferior lamina and superior articular processes. This leads to a shortening of the posterior column with about 10° to 15° of correction at the osteotomy level.[9,29,32] Indications of PCOs include pseudoarthrosis in ankylosing spondylitis (AS) patients (Anderson lesion), long smooth gradual kyphosis seen in Scheuermann disease, and degenerative flatback syndrome among others. PCO can be performed at a single level when a relatively small degree of correction is needed or at multiple levels for a more gradual correction of a larger deformity.

PSO, first described by Thomasen,[33] is a posterior closing-wedge osteotomy with an anterior cortical hinge that can provide up to 30° to 40° correction of kyphosis.[34] This technique functions to correct sagittal alignment at a single level without a concurrent

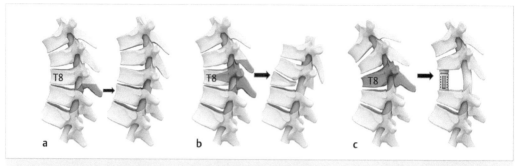

Fig. 14.3 Image showing three most commonly used osteotomies. **(a)** Posterior column osteotomy; **(b)** pedicle subtraction osteotomy; **(c)** vertebral column resection. (Reproduced with permission from Treatment. In: Vialle L, Berven S, de Kleuver M, eds. AOSpine Master Series, Vol. 9: Pediatric Spinal Deformities. 1st ed. Thieme; 2017.)

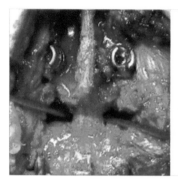

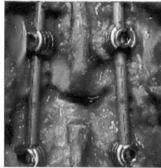

Fig. 14.4 Pedicle subtraction osteotomy with posterior spine instrumentation. (Reproduced with permission from Surgical techniques. In: Ames C, Riew K, Abumi K, eds. Cervical Spine Deformity Surgery. 1st ed. Thieme; 2019.)

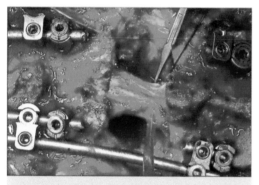

Fig. 14.5 Extensive single thoracic three-column osteotomy (VCR).

anterior approach. Indication of PSO as described by Gupta and Gupta include a desire for > 25° correction of lordosis, coronal malalignment, fixed SI, prior anterior column fusion, and > 10 cm SI among others.[34] PSO involves the removal of the posterior elements, bilateral pedicles, and a V-shaped

resection through the vertebral body that is closed anteriorly (▶ Fig. 14.4). Application of PSO is dependent on the nature of spine deformity; thus, PSO should be applied at the level of fixed-angled sagittal deformity if present.[34]

VCR, first described by Maclennan in 1922, is the most extensive approach of thoracolumbar osteotomies. While VCR can be performed via two approaches, anterior-posterior and posterior-only approach, the latter is more commonly utilized given its single-stage and shorter operative time advantage compared to the anterior-posterior approach.[35,36] Posterior-only VCR entails a resection of posterior elements including the spinous and transverse processes, facets and laminae, bilateral pedicles, and a gradual vertebral body resection in a "little-by-little" fashion (▶ Fig. 14.5). This technique results in about 50 to 70%[37] correction. A cage filled with bone chip, bone chip only, or titanium mesh may be used to fill in the resection gap depending on size.[35] Sharply angulated deformities may be corrected by a single vertebral

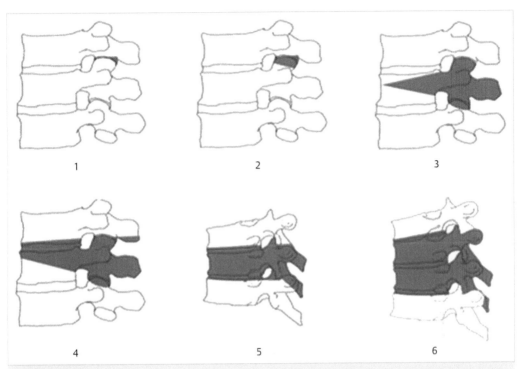

Fig. 14.6 Spinal osteotomy classification: Grade 1 showing partial facet joint resection to multiple vertebral and disc resection in Grade 6. (Reproduced with permission from Imaging of Spinal Deformity. In: Roussouly P, Pinheiro-Franco J, Labelle H, et al, eds. Sagittal Balance of the Spine: From Normal to Pathology: A Key for Treatment Strategy. 1st ed. Thieme; 2019.)

resection while multiple VCRs may be done at the apex of broad curvatures.[35] Indications of VCR include a fixed coronal plane deformity, sharply angulated deformities, a multiplanar spine deformity, spinal tumors, traumatic spondyloptosis, and others.[38] Obtaining a secure fixation, generally three vertebrae above and below the resection, extreme caution when handling exposed dura, and adequate surgeon comfort level among other technical considerations are advocated for a successful VCR.[9,10,29,39,40]

More recently, a six-grade standardized classification system by Schwab et al has been proposed to create a common language of osteotomy description among specialists. This classification also helps clarify the types of osteotomies based on the degree and location of bone resection (▶ Fig. 14.6). The Schwab classification covers the extent of osteotomy from a partial facet joint resection in Grade 1 classification to more than one vertebral and disc resection in Grade 6.[41]

14.6 Outcomes and Complications

Complication rates in thoracolumbar osteotomies range from 25 to 40% in recent literature, with adults having higher complications compared to adolescents.[9,10,29,40,42,43,44] In a retrospective series of 51 adult patients undergoing a three-column osteotomy for correction of spinal deformity by Hassanzadeh et al, 18% of patients developed major complications including motor deficits, deep wound infections, and epidural hematoma. Other reported complications of thoracolumbar osteotomies include instrumentation failure, commonly occurring at the site of osteotomy, and proximal junctional kyphosis, defined by a proximal sagittal Cobb > 10° as well as a 10 or more degree increase in the postoperative proximal sagittal Cobb angle compared to preoperative measurements. Proximal junctional kyphosis (PJK) can occur after adult and pediatric spinal deformity correction likely due to increased junctional stress concentrations, although the etiology may be multifactorial.[45,46,47] Despite the seemingly high reported complication rate, thoracolumbar osteotomies lead to a significant postoperative improvement in overall functional status.[48]

- Neural impingement due to a decrease in foraminal height can be mitigated by wide facetectomy in PCO.
- PCO can be performed at a single level when a relatively small degree of correction is needed or at multiple levels for a more gradual correction of a larger deformity.
- PSO should be applied at the level of fixed-angled sagittal deformity.
- To avoid buckling of the spinal cord in PSO, the extent of laminectomy should be limited to one level above and below the planned osteotomy site.[38]
- Obtaining a secure fixation, generally three vertebrae above and below the resection, extreme caution when handling exposed dura, and adequate surgeon comfort level among other technical considerations are advocated for a successful VCR.
- Sharply angulated deformities may be corrected by a single vertebral resection while multiple VCRs may be applied at the apex of broad curvatures.
- Extra attention should be given when assessing SI by correlating patients' standing radiographs with clinical examinations. SVA can be underdiagnosed in the patient with compensatory knee flexion to attain an upright posture or overdiagnosed SVA in patients with concomitant spinal stenosis. Many patients with spinal stenosis stoop forward to relieve the pressure of the nerve roots, and SI is partially functional in these patients.[49]
- In patients with Scheurmann kyphosis, the distal level of fusion should be the stable vertebra rather than the first lordotic vertebra.
- It should be noted that SI of one region affects adjacent regions, and surgical correction of the primary deformity also affects the adjacent vertebrae. For instance, thoracic hyperkyphosis due to conditions such as Scheurmann disease often causes hyperlordosis of the lumbar spine and cervical spine, and correction of thoracic hyperkyphosis decreases lumbar lordosis.

14.7 Case Examples

14.7.1 Case 1

This is a 58-year-old female with history of Scheuermann kyphosis and multiple prior spine surgeries at an outside hospital who presented with a long history of low-back pain. CT scan and MRI of the thoracolumbar spine reveals nonunion at T11–T12 and T12–L1 with significant collapse leading to severe kyphosis. She underwent PSO at T12 as well was posterolateral spine fusion at T8–L3 (▸ Fig. 14.7).

14.7.2 Case 2

This is a 62-year-old female with a history of low-back pain with neurogenic claudication, and spinal stenosis at L4–L5 and L5–S1. She underwent a three-column osteotomy/PSO at L5 and thoracic PCO at T8–T9 with segmental posterior spinal instrumentation from T4 to S1(▸ Fig. 14.8).

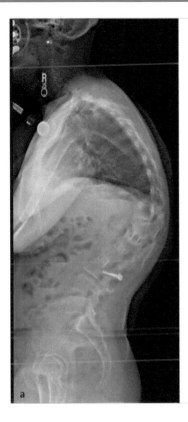

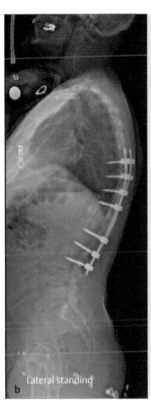

Lateral standing

Fig. 14.7 Patient with focal kyphosis at T12–L1 **(a)** undergoes a pedicle subtraction osteotomy at T12 with posterolateral spine fusion of T8–L3 **(b)**.

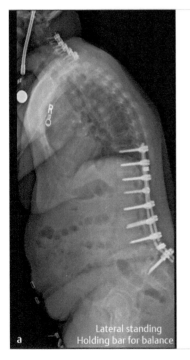

Lateral standing
Holding bar for balance

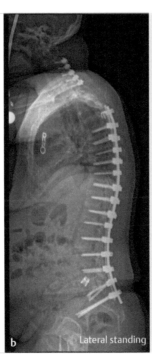

Lateral standing

Fig. 14.8 A 62-year-old with a history of T10–S1 instrumented fusion, kyphosis, and severe sagittal imbalance **(a)** undergoes a three-column osteotomy/pedicle subtraction osteotomy at L5 and thoracic posterior column osteotomy at T8–T9 with segmental posterior spinal instrumentation, T4–S1 **(b)**.

14.8 Board-style Questions

1. Which of the following radiographic parameters for assessing global sagittal imbalance describes the angle formed by the line connecting the femoral head to the T1 vertebral body and the line from femoral head to the midpoint of S1 end plate?
   a) Cobb angle
   b) Sagittal vertical angle
   c) T1 pelvic angle
   d) Pelvic tilt
   e) Sacral slope

2. A 67-year-old female patients with a history of multiple spine surgeries presents with poorly controlled low-back pain. Physical exams show a stooping posture and slightly flexed knees while standing. What threshold of pelvic incidence-lumbar lordosis mismatch is associated with increased disability in this patient?
   a) >11°
   b) >21°
   c) >5°
   d) >7°

3. Which of the following osteotomy approaches has been associated with the lowest neurological complications?
   a) Bone-disc-bone osteotomy
   b) Vertebral column resection
   c) Posterior column osteotomy
   d) Pedicle subtraction osteotomy

4. A complete vertebral resection including both adjacent intervertebral discs is indicative of which Schwab osteotomy classification?
   a) Grade 1
   b) Grade 2
   c) Grade 3
   d) Grade 4
   e) Grade 5

5. Which of the following is a compensatory mechanism commonly seen in SI patients to maintain an upright posture and a horizontal gaze?
   a) Hip extension
   b) Pelvic retroversion
   c) Knee extension
   d) Pelvic anteversion

Answers ✔

1. c
2. b
3. c
4. e
5. b

References

[1] Barrey C, Roussouly P, Perrin G, Le Huec J-C. Sagittal balance disorders in severe degenerative spine: can we identify the compensatory mechanisms? Eur Spine J. 2011; 20 Suppl 5: 626–633

[2] Barrey C, Jund J, Noseda O, Roussouly P. Sagittal balance of the pelvis-spine complex and lumbar degenerative diseases: a comparative study about 85 cases. Eur Spine J. 2007; 16 (9):1459–1467

[3] Acosta FL, Liu J, Slimack N, Moller D, Fessler R, Koski T. Changes in coronal and sagittal plane alignment following minimally invasive direct lateral interbody fusion for the treatment of degenerative lumbar disease in adults: a radiographic study. J Neurosurg Spine. 2011; 15(1):92–96

[4] Bridwell KH. Causes of sagittal spinal imbalance and assessment of the extent of needed correction. Instr Course Lect. 2006; 55:567–575

[5] Funao H, Tsuji T, Hosogane N, et al. Comparative study of spinopelvic sagittal alignment between patients with and without degenerative spondylolisthesis. Eur Spine J. 2012; 21(11):2181–2187

[6] Carreon LY, Smith CL, Dimar JR, II, Glassman SD. Correlation of cervical sagittal alignment parameters on full-length spine radiographs compared with dedicated cervical radiographs. Scoliosis Spinal Disord. 2016; 11:12

[7] Thoreson O, Beck J, Halldin K, Brisby H, Baranto A. A flat sagittal spinal alignment is common among young patients with lumbar disc herniation. Open J Orthop. 2015; 06(09)

[8] Chaléat-Valayer E, Mac-Thiong J-M, Paquet J, Berthonnaud E, Siani F, Roussouly P. Sagittal spino-pelvic alignment in chronic low back pain. Eur Spine J. 2011; 20 Suppl 5:634–640

[9] Kim K-T, Park K-J, Lee J-H. Osteotomy of the spine to correct the spinal deformity. Asian Spine J. 2009; 3(2):113–123

[10] Suk K-S, Kim K-T, Lee S-H, Kim J-M. Significance of chin-brow vertical angle in correction of kyphotic deformity of ankylosing spondylitis patients. Spine. 2003; 28(17):2001–2005

[11] Mummaneni PV, Dhall SS, Ondra SL, Mummaneni VP, Berven S. Pedicle subtraction osteotomy. Neurosurgery. 2008; 63(3) Suppl:171–176

[12] Berthonnaud E, Dimnet J, Roussouly P, Labelle H. Analysis of the sagittal balance of the spine and pelvis using shape and orientation parameters. J Spinal Disord Tech. 2005; 18(1):40–47

[13] Roussouly P, Gollogly S, Berthonnaud E, Dimnet J. Classification of the normal variation in the sagittal alignment of the human lumbar spine and pelvis in the standing position. Spine. 2005; 30(3):346–353

[14] Roussouly P, Nnadi C. Sagittal plane deformity: an overview of interpretation and management. Eur Spine J. 2010; 19 (11):1824–1836

[15] Vaz G, Roussouly P, Berthonnaud E, Dimnet J. Sagittal morphology and equilibrium of pelvis and spine. Eur Spine J. 2002; 11(1):80–87

[16] Van Royen BJ, De Gast A, Smit TH. Deformity planning for sagittal plane corrective osteotomies of the spine in ankylosing spondylitis. Eur Spine J. 2000; 9(6):492–498

[17] Van Royen BJ, De Gast A. Lumbar osteotomy for correction of thoracolumbar kyphotic deformity in ankylosing spondylitis: a structured review of three methods of treatment. Ann Rheum Dis. 1999; 58(7):399–406

[18] Farcy JP, Schwab FJ. Management of flatback and related kyphotic decompensation syndromes. Spine. 1997; 22(20): 2452–2457

[19] Schwab FJ, Blondel B, Bess S, et al. International Spine Study Group (ISSG). Radiographical spinopelvic parameters and disability in the setting of adult spinal deformity: a prospective multicenter analysis. Spine. 2013; 38(13): E803–E812

[20] Gelb DE, Lenke LG, Bridwell KH, Blanke K, McEnery KW. An analysis of sagittal spinal alignment in 100 asymptomatic middle and older aged volunteers. Spine. 1995; 20 (12):1351–1358

[21] Ryan DJ, Protopsaltis TS, Ames CP, et al. International Spine Study Group. T1 pelvic angle (TPA) effectively evaluates sagittal deformity and assesses radiographical surgical outcomes longitudinally. Spine. 2014; 39(15):1203–1210

[22] Protopsaltis T, Schwab F, Bronsard N, et al. International Spine Study Group. TheT1 pelvic angle, a novel radiographic measure of global sagittal deformity, accounts for both spinal inclination and pelvic tilt and correlates with health-related quality of life. J Bone Joint Surg Am. 2014; 96(19):1631–1640

[23] Banno T, Hasegawa T, Yamato Y, et al. T1 pelvic angle is a useful parameter for postoperative evaluation in adult spinal deformity patients. Spine. 2016; 41(21):1641–1648

[24] Legaye J, Duval-Beaupère G, Hecquet J, Marty C. Pelvic incidence: a fundamental pelvic parameter for three-dimensional regulation of spinal sagittal curves. Eur Spine J. 1998; 7(2):99–103

[25] Boulay C, Tardieu C, Hecquet J, et al. Anatomical reliability of two fundamental radiological and clinical pelvic parameters: incidence and thickness. Eur J Orthop Surg & Traumatol. 2005; 15:197–204

[26] Le Huec JC, Aunoble S, Philippe L, Nicolas P. Pelvic parameters: origin and significance. Eur Spine J : Off Publ Eur Spine Soc Eur Spinal Deform Soc Eur Sect Cerv Spine Res Soc. 2011;20 Suppl 5:564–571

[27] Schwab F, Patel A, Ungar B, Farcy J-P, Lafage V. Adult spinal deformity-postoperative standing imbalance: how much can you tolerate? An overview of key parameters in assessing alignment and planning corrective surgery. Spine. 2010; 35(25):2224–2231

[28] Weiss H-R, Werkmann M. Treatment of chronic low back pain in patients with spinal deformities using a sagittal re-alignment brace. Scoliosis. 2009; 4:7

[29] Bridwell KH. Decision making regarding Smith-Petersen vs. pedicle subtraction osteotomy vs. vertebral column resection for spinal deformity. Spine. 2006; 31(19) Suppl:S171–S178

[30] Voos K, Boachie-Adjei O, Rawlins BA. Multiple vertebral osteotomies in the treatment of rigid adult spine deformities. Spine. 2001; 26(5):526–533

[31] Cho K-J, Bridwell KH, Lenke LG, Berra A, Baldus C. Comparison of Smith-Petersen versus pedicle subtraction osteotomy for the correction of fixed sagittal imbalance. Spine. 2005; 30(18):2030–7

[32] McMaster MJ. A technique for lumbar spinal osteotomy in ankylosing spondylitis. J Bone Joint Surg Br. 1985; 67(2): 204–210

[33] Thomasen E. Vertebral osteotomy for correction of kyphosis in ankylosing spondylitis. Clin Orthop Relat Res. 1985; 0 (194):142–152

[34] Gupta S, Gupta MC. The nuances of pedicle subtraction osteotomies. Neurosurg Clin N Am. 2018; 29(3):355–363

[35] Smith JS, Wang VY, Ames CP. Vertebral column resection for rigid spinal deformity. Neurosurgery. 2008; 63(3) Suppl: 177–182

[36] Daubs MD. Commentary: is a two-staged anterior-posterior vertebral column resection (VCR) safer than a posterior-only VCR approach for severe pediatric deformities? Spine J. 2013; 13(5):487–488

[37] Saifi C, Laratta JL, Petridis P, Shillingford JN, Lehman RA, Lenke LG. Vertebral column resection for rigid spinal deformity. Global Spine J. 2017; 7(3):280–290

[38] Kose KC, Bozduman O, Yenigul AE, Igrek S. Spinal osteotomies: indications, limits and pitfalls. EFORT Open Rev. 2017; 2(3):73–82

[39] Bradford DS, Tribus CB. Vertebral column resection for the treatment of rigid coronal decompensation. Spine. 1997; 22 (14):1590–1599

[40] Hassanzadeh H, Jain A, El Dafrawy MH, et al. Three-column osteotomies in the treatment of spinal deformity in adult patients 60 years old and older: outcome and complications. Spine. 2013; 38(9):726–731

[41] Schwab F, Blondel B, Chay E, et al. The comprehensive anatomical spinal osteotomy classification. Neurosurgery. 2014; 74(1):112–20

[42] Kim H, Kim HS, Moon ES, et al. Scoliosis imaging: what radiologists should know—Erratum. Radiographics. 2015; 35(4): 1316

[43] Cho K-J, Bridwell KH, Lenke LG, Berra A, Baldus C. Comparison of Smith-Petersen versus pedicle subtraction osteotomy for the correction of fixed sagittal imbalance. Spine. 2005; 30(18):2030–2037, discussion 2038

[44] Thiranont N, Netrawichien P. Transpedicular decancellation closed wedge vertebral osteotomy for treatment of fixed flexion deformity of spine in ankylosing spondylitis. Spine. 1993; 18(16):2517–2522

[45] Kavadi N, Tallarico RA, Lavelle WF. Analysis of instrumentation failures after three column osteotomies of the spine. Scoliosis Spinal Disord. 2017; 12:19

[46] Kim HJ, Iyer S. Proximal junctional kyphosis. J Am Acad Orthop Surg. 2016; 24(5):318–326

[47] Yagi M, Akilah KB, Boachie-Adjei O. Incidence, risk factors and classification of proximal junctional kyphosis: surgical outcomes review of adult idiopathic scoliosis. Spine. 2011; 36(1): E60–E68

[48] Iyer S, Nemani VM, Kim HJ. A review of complications and outcomes following vertebral column resection in adults. Asian Spine J. 2016; 10(3):601–609

[49] Presciutti SM, Louie PK, Khan JM, et al. Sagittal spinopelvic malalignment in degenerative scoliosis patients: isolated correction of symptomatic levels and clinical decision-making. Scoliosis Spinal Disord. 2018; 13:28

15 Isthmic Spondylolisthesis

Jannat M. Khan, Steven T. Heidt, Howard S. An, and Matthew W. Colman

Abstract

The specific diagnosis of acute or chronic isthmic spondylolisthesis may be made when spondylolisthesis occurs in the setting of unilateral or bilateral fracture of the vertebral pars interarticularis. The generally chronic condition affects both children and adults and is thought to affect approximately 6% of the United States population. Acute presentations may be noted in young athletes who participate in sports requiring repetitive lumbar flexion, such as weight-lifting, gymnastics, or American football. This chapter focuses on the presentation, diagnosis, and management of this common spinal condition and offers an in-depth examination of surgical methods. Most operative approaches consist of neural decompression with posterior lumbar or circumferential fusion; risks and benefits of each method are discussed alongside outcomes from recent surgical research. Posterior lumbar fusion (PLF) is a common procedure performed for degenerative spinal etiology but can also be used for treatment of isthmic spondylolisthesis, given the findings that unilateral and bilateral PLFs decrease progression of slip more effectively than decompression alone. Circumferential fusion provides additional treatment options of isthmic spondylolisthesis by combining the use of interbody devices with posterior and anterior approaches for fusion, such as anterior lumbar interbody fusion (ALIF), transforaminal lumbar interbody fusion (TLIF), and posterolateral interbody fusion (PLIF). Some passive spondylolisthesis reduction can be obtained intraoperatively simply with anesthesia muscle relaxation, patient positioning, and/or decompression portions of the surgery. Active reduction of the spondylolisthesis can be attempted via pedicle screw instrumentation under neurologic monitoring and fluoroscopic guidance. However, additional attempts to improve the reduction need to be weighed against the potential risk of neurologic injury.

Keywords: isthmic spondylolisthesis, posterior spinal fusion, circumferential fusion, lumbar interbody fusion, lumbar back pain, lower extremity radiculopathy

15.1 Introduction

Spondylolisthesis is defined as a spinal condition in which a vertebra subluxates anteriorly (anterolisthesis) in relation to the caudal vertebra.[1,2] The cause of the malalignment is commonly related to chronic degenerative changes or trauma that results in variation of pars interarticularis defect; however, congenital, pathological, and/or iatrogenic etiologies can also be observed. Isthmic spondylolisthesis specifically occurs after fracture of unilateral or bilateral pars interarticularis in the lumbar spine (▶ Fig. 15.1). This condition can be appreciated in both children and adults, and is estimated to affect about 6% of the population.[3] Additionally, bilateral spondylolysis can progress to spondylolisthesis in 40 to 66% of patients.[1] While there is often no specific inciting event, the condition has been noted more commonly in those who participate in activities that require repetitive lumbar flexion, such as gymnastics or weightlifting. The condition most commonly affects the L5–S1 level, though may be found throughout the lumbar spine.[4] Symptoms are commonly

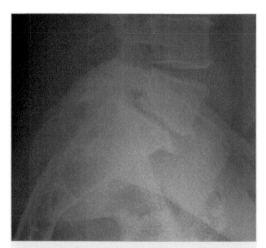

Fig. 15.1 Standing lateral plain radiograph of the lumbar spine demonstrating and isthmic spondylolisthesis of L5 on S1.

generalized back pain but can be accompanied by lower extremity pain and, at times, radicular symptoms. If isthmic spondylolisthesis is the result of acute trauma, neurological deficits such as incontinence may also be noted.

15.2 History and Physical Examination

Patients with isthmic spondylolisthesis will generally present with complaints of axial back pain. Radicular symptoms are also possible, though rarer, and, when these are present, are generally associated with pain or loss of sensation across the L5 dermatome due to compression of the nerve root at the L5–S1 spinal level. Patients with more severe disease may also complain of hamstring tightness. Finally, those who have both isthmic spondylolisthesis and spinal stenosis may present with neurogenic claudication, and those with cauda equina syndrome may present with bladder or bowel complaints.[4,5] Obtaining a proper history in patients with possible isthmic spondylolisthesis is critical, as the condition may present in a similar fashion to other spinal conditions.

The disease occurs in both men and women, as well as in both children and adults. Children with spondylolisthesis tend to present after the age of 10, and generally have a chief complaint of back pain radiating to the buttocks or upper thighs.[4] Symptoms have generally been present for some time, or may present as an acute exacerbation of a chronic condition. Children may have a history of activities that require repetitive extension of the lumbar spine, such as young football linemen or those participating in gymnastics. On examination, adolescents may assume a crouched appearance known as the Phalen-Dickson sign.[4] Children with the Phalen-Dickson sign present with knees bent, legs flexed, and a completely vertical spinal column. This presentation is thought to be related to a compensatory loss of lordosis of the lumbar spine following the onset of spondylolisthesis. Compensatory changes of the spine may also cause visible alterations to the spinous processes, creating a pronounced appearance of the L5 spinous process in those with spondylolisthesis at the L5–S1 level.[4] Additional findings indicative of isthmic spondylolisthesis in children are a positive straight leg test and impaired flexion or extension of the lumbar spine.[4]

Presentation of isthmic spondylolisthesis in adults is similar to that in children. Chronic back pain is the most common presenting symptom with about half of all patients also experiencing radiation of pain to the buttocks or lower extremities.[2,6] Neurologic findings such as radiculopathy, paresthesia, or sensory loss are less frequent symptoms, though sensory loss across the L5 dermatome is the most common of these symptoms.[7] Similar to the presentation in children, straight leg test is positive in about half of patients.[1] Neurogenic bladder or bowel symptoms are very rarely caused by isthmic spondylolisthesis.

15.3 Differential Diagnosis

The diagnosis of isthmic spondylolisthesis is made via clinical and radiographic evidence of disease. Differential diagnoses for isthmic spondylolisthesis include spondylolysis, disc herniation, osteomyelitis, and other types of spondylolisthesis, such as degenerative or dysplastic spondylolisthesis, among others. Spondylolysis is similar in presentation to spondylolisthesis, though without anterior movement of one vertebral body over another. Disc herniation can present with low-back pain and radicular symptoms, though these complaints are generally acute and following trauma or exertion, while the symptoms of isthmic spondylolisthesis are generally chronic. Osteomyelitis should be included in the differential diagnosis as well, though additional findings such as leukocytosis should also be present.

15.4 Diagnostic Imaging

A number of imaging techniques may be used in the diagnosis of isthmic spondylolisthesis. Patients with suspected disease should be imaged with standard standing radiographs in the lateral position.[1] Oblique views may enhance diagnostic capability. Pelvic tilt, pelvic incidence, sacral slope, and lumbar lordosis measurements are often used to quantify the severity of disease, given these parameters are found to be higher compared to patients without isthmic spondylolisthesis (▸ Fig. 15.2).[6] Patients in whom diagnosis is not

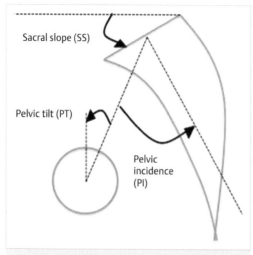

Fig. 15.2 Schematic diagram demonstrating pelvic tilt (PT), pelvic incidence (PI), and sacral slope (SS) measurements.

Labels within figure:
Sacral slope (SS)
Pelvic tilt (PT)
Pelvic incidence (PI)

Table 15.1 Wiltse-Newman classification of spondylolisthesis

Type I	Dysplastic	Congenital defect present in the pars articularis
Type II	Isthmic	Fracture of the pars articularis is present (subtypes are classified by type of fracture)
Type II-A		Fatigue fracture of the pars (Lytic)
Type II-B		Elongated by intact pars
Type II-C		Acute fracture of the pars
Type III	Degenerative	Instability without presence of acute fracture
Type IV	Traumatic	Vertebral fracture other than the pars articularis generating anterior movement
Type V	Neoplastic	Blastic or lytic destruction of the pars articularis

successfully made with standing radiographs should undergo computed tomography scanning for definitive diagnosis.[1] Patients who have neurologic complaints, such as sensory loss over the L5 dermatome or radiculopathy, should undergo further work-up with magnetic resonance imaging (MRI) in order to determine specific location of foraminal stenosis.[1]

Table 15.2 Meyerding classification

Grade I	<25% anterolisthesis
Grade II	25–50% anterolisthesis
Grade III	50–75% anterolisthesis
Grade IV	75–100% anterolisthesis
Grade V	Spondyloptosis

15.5 Classification

Classification of spondylolisthesis is important in terms of selection of treatment, and these classifications, originally devised by Wiltse and Newman, are generally based upon presence of fracture and method of injury (▶ Table 15.1; ▶ Fig. 15.3).[5] Meyerding classification is also commonly used, which allows for assessment of the severity of the spondylolisthesis as ratio of anterolisthesis to caudal vertebral body yielding a percentage representative of spondylolisthesis progression (▶ Table 15.2). Critical distinction is made between low- and high-grade spondylolisthesis using the Meyerding classification as high-grade (grade III–IV or > 50% slip) spondylolisthesis denotes higher risk of progression that helps navigate treatment. Additionally, Marchetti-Bartolozzi classification allows for distinguishing between developmental and acquired spondylolisthesis (▶ Table 15.3). Developmental etiology is further divided into low- and high-dysplastic while acquired slip is

sectioned into traumatic, postsurgical, pathologic, and degenerative forms of spondylolisthesis. This classification highlights the difference in the natural history of developmental versus acquired spondylolisthesis and helps to guide treatment strategies.[8] It is important to note that while these classifications aid in decisions regarding treatment, they do not account for global sagittal balance and are generally poor predictor of outcomes.

15.6 Treatment and Outcomes

Treatment for isthmic spondylolisthesis may either be operative or nonoperative. Nonoperative management is successful in many patients; however, cases that are refractory for at least six months may benefit from undergoing surgery. Nonoperative treatment generally consists of activity modification, typically 3 to 6 months, and use of nonsteroidal anti-inflammatory agents. Patients with greater pain may benefit from addition of muscle relaxants but narcotic analgesic

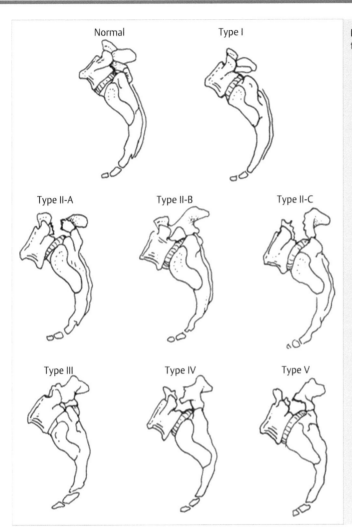

Fig. 15.3 Wiltse-Newman classification of spondylolisthesis.

Normal

Type I

Type II-A

Type II-B

Type II-C

Type III

Type IV

Type V

Table 15.3 Marchetti-Bartolozzi classification

Developmental	Acquired
Traumatic	Low-dysplastic
• Acute fracture	• With lysis
• Stress fracture	• With elongation
Postsurgical	High-dysplastic
• Direct	• With lysis
• Indirect	• With elongation
Pathologic	
• Local	
• Systemic	
Degenerative	
• Primary	
• Secondary	

should be limited in quantity and duration. Meanwhile, no clear evidence exists supporting the benefit of physical therapy, and other modalities of treatment, such as epidural injections. Studies comparing surgical treatment and conservative therapy have shown that while both therapies may improve levels of pain, surgical treatment alone may improve both pain and disability indices.[7] Specifically, Moller et al found that surgical intervention was more efficient in relieving pain and improving function after conducting a randomized control trial comparing 34 patients that participated in an exercise program and 77 patients that underwent posterolateral fusion (PLF). This study provided strong evidence in support of surgical intervention, which was in contrast to previous belief that surgery should be contraindicated for low-back pain that was not a result of nerve root compression. Although there is still a lack of agreement regarding the type of surgical intervention that should be used for treatment of isthmic spondylolisthesis, the benefit of surgery is recognized and intervention is supported in the literature.

Surgical treatment goals include stabilizing the affected spinal level and relieving any nerve compression, if present. A wide variety of surgical options exist, ranging from PLF to circumferential fusion techniques; however, there is a lack of consensus regarding the benefit of each procedure. Hence, the process of choosing a particular procedure incorporates the patient's presenting symptoms with radiographic findings. Typically, surgery is offered to patients who fail to improve clinically after 6 months of conservative treatment and report significant disability from neurogenic claudication or progression of neurologic deficit. Radiographic finding of grade III or greater slip in symptomatic adolescent is an additional indication for surgery, while the presence of cauda equina in a patient of any age requires immediate indication for surgical intervention.

Decompression of neural components is important for improvement of symptoms and is a consistent aspect of many techniques used for treatment of isthmic spondylolisthesis. The use of decompression alone is restricted because the procedure does not provide stability and, subsequently, can lead to rapid slip progression and disc degeneration. Specific populations such as elderly patients with stable anterior spinal column secondary to presence of anterior osteophytes may benefit from decompression alone. In particular, gill laminectomy can be performed before proceeding to fusion of symptomatic levels. The procedure begins with removal of interspinous ligament, zygapophyseal joint capsules, and loose posterior elements, specifically the lamina, along with any hypertrophic fibrocartilaginous masses at the pars defect. The ligamentum flavum and adhesions of the dura are also excised followed by careful dissection of the nerve root to confirm sufficient mobility through the intervertebral foramen. Partial removal of the pedicle can be incorporated to this technique if additional decompression of neural elements is necessary. Once decompression is successfully completed, fusion may be performed via the technique deemed suitable for the particular case. It is important to note that some cases may benefit from fusion alone without the need for decompression.[1]

Posterior lumbar fusion (PLF) is a common procedure performed for degenerative spinal etiology but can also be used for treatment of isthmic spondylolisthesis, given the findings that unilateral and bilateral PLFs decrease progression of slip more effectively than decompression alone. Specifically, PLF can be paired with trans-sacral L5 screw fixation for a high-grade L5–S1 spondylolisthesis. While trans-sacral screw fixation has been shown to be efficacious, evidence regarding the benefit of incorporating instrumentation, such as pedicle screws, or interbody in the fusion construct is less clear.[9,10] Endler et al compared 77 patients that underwent PLF to 86 patients that received posterolateral interbody fusion (PLIF) at an average of 11 years after initial treatment and found no difference in clinical or radiographic outcomes.[11] Despite the lack of difference in improvement, biomechanical studies suggest that the use of interbody allows for better anterior column support, reduction of the slip, and restoration of lordosis.[12]

Circumferential fusion provides additional treatment options of isthmic spondylolisthesis by combining the use of interbody devices with posterior and anterior approaches for fusion such as anterior lumbar interbody fusion (ALIF), transforaminal lumbar interbody fusion (TLIF), and PLIF. Techniques such as ALIF enable direct visualization of disc space that allows for complete removal of the disc while TLIF utilizes a lateralized portal to perform laminectomy and unilateral facetectomy allowing for less manipulation of the neural components and thecal sac. The placement of pedicle screws in combination with ALIF allows for successful treatment of isthmic spondylolisthesis without the need for posterior decompression, a procedure that requires wider muscle dissection and can therefore destabilize the spine. A study of patients who received ALIF with posterior pedicle screw placement revealed fusion in all patients at five-year follow-up, with an excellent or good clinical result in 88.9% of patients.[13] Several studies suggest that ALIF is comparable with PLIF and TLIF in terms of clinical improvement and fusion rate, despite allowing for greater improvements in disc height, lumbar lordosis, and whole spine lordosis than TLIF.[14,15,16] However, TLIF decreases the risk of injury to neural components when compared with PLIF and provides the advantage of decompressing the exiting and traversing nerve roots at once.

In 2016, North American Spine Society's (NASS) Evidence-Based Clinical Guideline for the Diagnosis and Treatment of Adult Isthmic Spondylolisthesis synthesized literature available as of 2013 into a beneficial decision-making tool for spine specialists.[1] The work group recommended the use of circumferential fusion, as these procedures result in higher fusion rates than PLF alone in low-grade spondylolisthesis. While improvement in clinical outcomes is seen with both circumferential fusions and PLF,

literature provides conflicting evidence regarding which procedure provides better clinical outcomes. Furthermore, the limited number of studies examining isthmic spondylolisthesis led the work group to neither refute nor support the benefit of surgical intervention versus conservative treatment; however, the group supported that surgical intervention is recommended to provide long-term improvement in clinical symptoms. There are many limitations to the guideline that highlight the paucity of literature examining isthmic spondylolisthesis.

Similarly, few studies have examined the benefit of reduction of the spondylolisthesis. In theory, reduction of high-grade spondylolisthesis allows for improvement of the sagittal alignment, number of segments to be fused, and mechanical environment for the fusion. However, it is vital to consider the risk of performing a reduction to the surrounding nerves. There is a component of passive reduction involved during all surgical intervention as the patient experiences intraoperative muscle relaxation via anesthesia, and physical manipulation during patient positioning but active reduction requires more preparation. Typically, active reduction is performed using pedicle screw instrumentation while somatosensory-evoked potentials, direct nerve stimulations, and electromyography data are collected for the patient to ensure proper neurologic monitoring. After reduction is performed, the patient typically undergoes an interbody fusion. Recent studies have found minimal complications as a result of reduction, commonly L5 root compression but rarely catastrophic injuries like cauda equina syndrome. Therefore, partial active posterior distractional reduction, under proper neurological monitoring, may be beneficial when paired with circumferential fusion.

General pearls for isthmic spondylolisthesis:
- Diagnostic imaging should begin with plain standing radiographs in the lateral position. CT imaging may be used to make a definitive diagnosis if radiographs are nonrevealing. MRI should be used in patients with neurologic symptoms to identify specific sites of damage.
- Nonoperative management with activity limitation and nonsteroidal anti-inflammatory drugs (NSAIDs) should be attempted prior to surgical management.
- The use of decompression alone is restricted because the procedure does not provide stability and, subsequently, can lead to rapid slip progression and disc degeneration.
- If indicated, surgical correction of isthmic spondylolisthesis should be attempted with ALIF or TLIF. ALIF is superior to TLIF in terms of restoring disc height and ensuring good clinical and radiographic outcomes.
- Techniques such as ALIF enable direct visualization of disc space which allows for complete removal of the disc while TLIF utilizes a lateralized portal to perform laminectomy and unilateral facetectomy allowing for less manipulation of the neural components and thecal sac.
- Some passive spondylolisthesis reduction can be obtained intraoperatively simply with anesthesia muscle relaxation, patient positioning, and/or decompression portions of the surgery. Active reduction of the spondylolistheis can be attempted via pedicle screw instrumentation under neurologic monitoring and fluoroscopic guidance. However, additional attempts to improve the reduction need to be weighed against the potential risk of neurologic injury.

Specific to a Gill laminectomy:
- The anteroposterior X-ray should be scrutinized for dysplastic posterior elements or spina bifida variants in order to avoid complications during exposure.
- Subperiosteal dissection is carried out down the cephalad and caudal laminae of the involved spinal level. Exposure of the lamina one segment higher than the isthmic segment (i.e., L4 for an L5/S1 isthmic spondylolisthesis) facilitates atraumatic exposure of the junctional facets. Special care is taken not to use monopolar cautery or penetrate near the pars of the cephalad (isthmic) segment, since this bone overlying the neural elements is not competent.
- Isthmic nature of the spondylolisthesis is confirmed by noting a relatively dorsally positioned, prominent, and mobile spinous process of the cephalad (isthmic) segment.
- Full exposure of the involved facets bilaterally is accomplished.
- Transection of the interspinous and supraspinous ligaments above and below the isthmic segment is accomplished.
- Typically, central and lateral recess stenosis is not high-grade. Tension on the ligamentum flavum is facilitated by using a lamina spreader above and below the isthmic segment.
- Ligamentum flavum and facet capsule is transected with a Kerrison rongeur above and below the isthmic segment.
- The isthmic lamina can be removed en bloc if the spinous process and lamina are confirmed to be mobile. This is facilitated by placing a Cobb elevator into the involved facet joints and using a gentle rotatory motion to further mobilize and release the dorsal segment. The segment is carefully removed while releasing any dural adhesions (commonly present due to inflammatory nature of isthmic motion at the zone of pars defect).
- Full exiting root exposure via extended atraumatic foraminotomy is accomplished bilaterally prior to performing spondylolisthesis manipulation.

15.7 Case Examples

15.7.1 Case 1

This is a 14-year-old female gymnast presenting with low-back pain. The insidious onset of low-back pain occurred one year ago in association with physical activities and worsened by impact activities. The low-back pain was accompanied by left lower extremity pain in the L5 distribution. She trialed physical therapy and other treatment modalities but did not notice any improvement in the low-back pain. Physical exam revealed limited range of motion in the lumbar spine with pain elicited at > 40 degrees of forward flexion and > 10 degrees of extension. Plain radiographs of the lumbar spine revealed grade III spondylolisthesis of L5 on S1 (▶ Fig. 15.4). MRI showed exaggerated lumbar lordosis with bilateral spondylolysis L5, mild posterior wedging of L5 and mild deformity of the superior S1 endplate, and severe stenosis at L5–S1 of the spinal canal and neural foramina, along with confirmation of grade III spondylolisthesis L5–S1 (▶ Fig. 15.5). She subsequently underwent L4–L5 posterior spinal decompression, laminectomy, L5–S1 bilateral lateral recess and foraminal decompression, sacral dome osteotomy to create a space to the L5 endplate, TLIF L5–S1, posterior segmental pedicle screw instrumentation with rod placement at L4–S1 and posterior spinal fusion using autograft and allograft at L4–S1 (▶ Fig. 15.6).

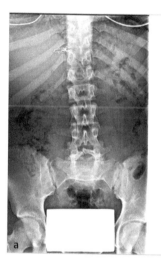
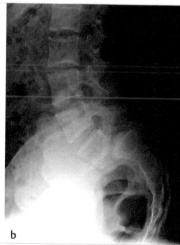

Fig. 15.4 A 14-year-old female gymnast presenting with low-back pain. Preoperative standing plain anteroposterior (a) and lateral (b) radiographs of the lumbar spine showing a Meyerding Grade III spondylolisthesis of L5 on S1.

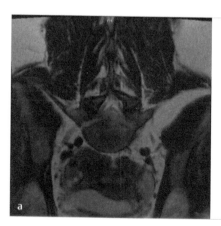
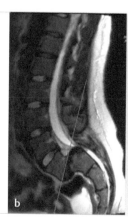

Fig. 15.5 T2-weighted coronal (a) and sagittal (b) magnetic resonance imaging demonstrating exaggerated lumbar lordosis with bilateral spondylolysis of L5, grade III spondylolisthesis L5–S1 mild posterior wedging of L5 and mild deformity of the superior S1 endplate, degenerative disc disease of L5–S1, and severe central and foraminal stenosis at L5–S1.

15.7.2 Case 2

This is a 49-year-old male presenting with low-back pain accompanied by plantar foot numbness and pain in bilateral buttocks and posterior thighs and calves. His past medical history is notable for a known diagnosis of spondylolisthesis at the age of 13-year-old. Physical exam was unremarkable.

Plain radiographs showed evidence of isthmic spondylolisthesis at L5–S1 (▶ Fig. 15.7). MRI also demonstrated evidence of isthmic spondylolisthesis at L5–S1 along with left worse that right lateral recess stenosis at L5–S1. He subsequently underwent L5–S1 ALIF with posterior segmental pedicle screw instrumentation (▶ Fig. 15.8).

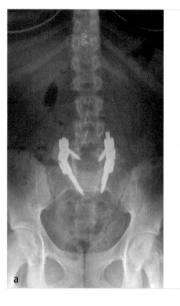
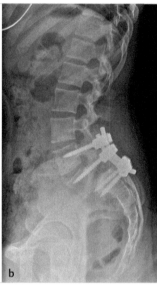

Fig. 15.6 Postoperative standing plain anteroposterior (**a**) and lateral (**b**) radiographs of the lumbar spine after L4–L5 posterior spinal decompression, laminectomy, L5–S1 bilateral lateral recess and foraminal decompression, sacral dome osteotomy (performed to create a space to the L5 end plate), transforaminal lumbar interbody fusion (TLIF) L5–S1, posterior segmental pedicle screw instrumentation with rod placement L4–S1, and posterior lumbar fusion (PLF) autograft and allograft L4–S1.

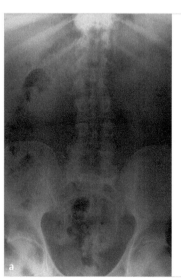
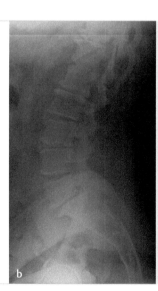

Fig. 15.7 A 49-year-old male presenting with low-back pain accompanied by plantar foot numbness and pain in bilateral buttocks and posterior thighs and calves. Preoperative standing plain anteroposterior (**a**) and lateral (**b**) radiographs of the lumbar spine showing spondylolisthesis of L5 on S1.

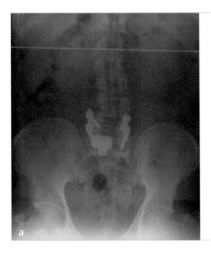
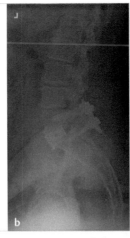

Fig. 15.8 Postoperative standing plain anteroposterior (**a**) and lateral (**b**) radiographs of the lumbar spine showing an L5–S1 anterior lumbar interbody fusion (ALIF) with posterior segmental pedicle screw instrumentation.

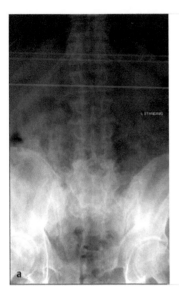
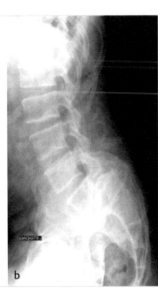

Fig. 15.9 A 56-year-old male presenting with chronic low-back and left leg pain. Preoperative standing plain anteroposterior (**a**) and lateral (**b**) radiographs of the lumbar spine showing a Meyerding Grade III/IV spondylolisthesis of L5 on S1.

15.7.3 Case 3

This is a 56-year-old male presenting with chronic low-back and left lower extremity pain which has progressively worsened over the past four years. He complains of difficulty ambulating and standing due to these symptoms. For the past several months, he has also experienced difficulty in controlling his bladder and bowel movements. Physical exam demonstrated mild weakness (4 out of 5)

in the extensor hallucis longus. Plain radiograph revealed L5–S1 grade III/IV spondylolisthesis that appeared to be chronic (▶ Fig. 15.9). Given the presenting symptoms, and subsequent findings, he underwent a laminectomy from L3 to S2 followed by L3–S1 PLF, trans-sacral screws, sacral dome osteotomy (dysplastic dome appeared to be tethering the dural sac), L5–S1 discectomy, right L5 pediculectomy, segmental instrumentation, and L3–S1 bilateral iliac screw fixation (▶ Fig. 15.10).

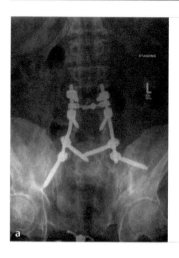
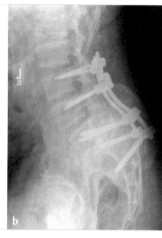

Fig. 15.10 Postoperative standing plain anteroposterior (**a**) and lateral (**b**) radiographs of the lumbar spine showing L3–S1 posterior lumbar fusion (PLF) with L5 trans-sacral screws, sacral dome osteotomy, segmental instrumentation, and L3–S1 bilateral iliac screw fixation.

15.8 Board-style Questions

1. A 24-year-old female presents with chronic back and bilateral leg pain that has not improved with extensive nonoperative management including physical therapy, oral medications, and corticosteroid injections. Radiographs reveal high-grade isthmic spondylolisthesis at L5–S1. What is the most appropriate next step in treatment?
   a) Minimally invasive direct lateral interbody fusion with percutaneous pedicle screw placement
   b) Lumbar decompression, L4 to S1 posterior lumbar fusion, and anterior column support
   c) Placement of epidural spinal stimulator
   d) Lumbar decompression alone
   e) Lumbar decompression with L5 to S1 posterior lumbar fusion

2. A 14-year-old female presents with severe back and radiating right leg pain after falling from the back of a pickup truck 4 days ago. She can walk only short distances with her hips in extension and her knees flexed. Straight-leg raise and crossed straight-leg raise findings are positive; motor and sensory examination findings are otherwise within normal limits. Radiographs taken in the emergency department are negative for fracture or dislocation. What is the best next step?
   a) Observation
   b) Direct L5 pars repair
   c) Rest, activity modification, and bracing
   d) L5–S1 decompression with instrumented posterior spinal fusion
   e) L5–S1 discectomy with foraminotomy

3. A 19-year-old female presents with chronic low-back pain. Physical exam reveals normal motor examination findings but diminished light touch sensation in an L5 distribution. Her back pain is reproduced with lumbar extension. Radiographs show isthmic spondylolisthesis at L5–S1. Which morphologic parameter has been correlated with the severity of her spinal condition?
   a) Slip angle
   b) Pelvic tilt
   c) Pelvic incidence
   d) Sacral slope
   e) Slip percentage

Answers ✓

1. b
2. c
3. c

References

[1] Kreiner DS, Baisden J, Mazanec DJ, et al. Guideline summary review: an evidence-based clinical guideline for the diagnosis and treatment of adult isthmic spondylolisthesis. Spine J. 2016; 16(12):1478–1485

[2] Lauerman WC, Cain JE. Isthmic spondylolisthesis in the adult. J Am Acad Orthop Surg. 1996; 4(4):201–208

[3] Kalichman L, Kim DH, Li L, Guermazi A, Berkin V, Hunter DJ. Spondylolysis and spondylolisthesis: prevalence and association with low back pain in the adult community-based population. Spine. 2009; 34(2):199–205

[4] Mataliotakis GI, Tsirikos AI. Spondylolysis and spondylolisthesis in children and adolescents: current concepts and treatment. Orthop Trauma. 2017; 31:395–401

[5] Wiltse LL, Newman PH, Macnab I. Classification of spondylolisis and spondylolisthesis. Clin Orthop Relat Res. 1976 (117):23–29

[6] Lee JH, Kim KT, Suk KS, et al. Analysis of spinopelvic parameters in lumbar degenerative kyphosis: correlation with spinal stenosis and spondylolisthesis. Spine. 2010; 35(24): E1386–E1391

[7] Möller H, Hedlund R. Surgery versus conservative management in adult isthmic spondylolisthesis: a prospective randomized study: part 1. Spine. 2000; 25(13):1711–1715

[8] Mac-Thiong JM, Labelle H, Parent S, Hresko MT, Deviren V, Weidenbaum M, members of the Spinal Deformity Study Group. Reliability and development of a new classification of lumbosacral spondylolisthesis. Scoliosis. 2008; 3:19

[9] Palejwala A, Fridley J, Jea A. Transsacral transdiscal L5-S1 screws for the management of high-grade spondylolisthesis in an adolescent. J Neurosurg Pediatr. 2016; 17(6): 645–650

[10] Endler P, Ekman P, Möller H, Gerdhem P. Outcomes of posterolateral fusion with and without instrumentation and of interbody fusion for isthmic spondylolisthesis: a prospective study. J Bone Joint Surg Am. 2017; 99(9):743–752

[11] Endler P, Ekman P, Ljungqvist H, Brismar TB, Gerdhem P, Möller H. Long-term outcome after spinal fusion for isthmic spondylolisthesis in adults. Spine J. 2019; 19(3):501–508

[12] Sudo H, Oda I, Abumi K, Ito M, Kotani Y, Minami A. Biomechanical study on the effect of five different lumbar reconstruction techniques on adjacent-level intradiscal pressure and lamina strain. J Neurosurg Spine. 2006; 5(2): 150–155

[13] Kim J-S, Choi WG, Lee S-H. Minimally invasive anterior lumbar interbody fusion followed by percutaneous pedicle screw fixation for isthmic spondylolisthesis: minimum 5-year follow-up. Spine J. 2010; 10(5):404–409

[14] Kim JS, Kang BU, Lee SH, et al. Mini-transforaminal lumbar interbody fusion versus anterior lumbar interbody fusion augmented by percutaneous pedicle screw fixation: a comparison of surgical outcomes in adult low-grade isthmic spondylolisthesis. J Spinal Disord Tech. 2009; 22(2):114–121

[15] Jones TR, Rao RD. Adult isthmic spondylolisthesis. J Am Acad Orthop Surg. 2009; 17(10):609–617

[16] Jacobs WC, Vreeling A, De Kleuver M. Fusion for low-grade adult isthmic spondylolisthesis: a systematic review of the literature. European Spine Journal. 2006; 15: 391–402

16 Spinal Infections

Harish Kempegowda and Chadi Tannoury

Abstract

Spinal infections represent an important clinical condition presenting with diagnostic challenge and variable prognosis. Unfortunately, the presentations have been commonly misdiagnosed on initial presentation. The conditions are caused by various pathogenic infections, including bacterial (pyogenic), tubercular, fungal (granulomatous) and parasitic infestations. The most common spinal infections encountered during routine practice are spinal epidural abscess, discitis, and/or vertebral osteomyelitis. Physicians should be aware of the various presentations of a spinal infection in order to make timely diagnosis using laboratory investigations and neuroimaging, thus preventing long-term sequel. Once a proper diagnosis has been made, spinal infections often require both medical and surgical modalities of treatment.

Keywords: spinal infections, spinal epidural abscess, discitis, vertebral osteomyelitis

16.1 Introduction

Spinal infections comprise a wide spectrum ranging from discitis, osteomyelitis, to abscess collection in the perivertebral and epidural spaces. The incidence of spinal infections has been trending upward due to increased recreational intravenous (IV) drug use and immunosuppression due to a growing population of patients with diabetes, HIV, cancer, and organ transplants.[1,2] Spinal infections are associated with significant morbidity and mortality in the affected patients and add significant financial burden to the healthcare system.[1,2,3,4] The treatment strategy of spinal infections can be complex and often multidisciplinary with a concerted effort from infectious disease, internal medicine, and spine surgery specialists.

16.2 Spinal Epidural Abscess (SEA)

This is a potentially devastating infection with abscess formation in the epidural space and within the non-expandable spinal canal. Hence, depending on the size of the SEA and its location, direct spinal cord and/or neural elements compression may occur with the potential for long-term neurologic sequelae.[1,2,3,4,5,6] The currently reported SEA incidence rate is 2–12.5 per 10,000 admissions.[3] The advancement in imaging technologies and heightened awareness have led to its earlier detection. The standard of care generally includes timely surgical decompression with debridement and systemic antibiotic therapy for long duration, especially in symptomatic patients with signs of systemic infections, sepsis, and/or neurologic deficits.[6]

16.2.1 Pathogenesis

In patients with SEA, risk factors include: IV drug use, spinal interventions (epidural steroid injections, spinal surgery, epidural catheters, etc.), spinal trauma, diabetes mellitus, chronic alcoholism, hepatic disease, immunosuppressive status, and local or systemic infections such as cellulitis, urinary tract infections, osteomyelitis, pneumonias, perinephric abscess etc.[4] Hematogenous spread following bacteremia remains the most common mode of infection (~50%), followed by direct spread (~33%), and in the remaining cases (~17%) the source could not be identified.[4,5]

The most common pathogen isolated from the blood or tissue culture is *Staphylococcus aureus* (63.6%) followed by negative cultures or no growth (13.9%), gram-negative bacteria (8.1%), coagulase-negative *Staphylococcus* (7.5%), and *Streptococcus* species (6.8%).[4,7] Among the *S. aureus* infection group, the data is not clear whether methicillin resistant (MRSA) or methicillin sensitive (MSSA) bacteria is predominant, with incidence reports ranging between 19–40% and 28–40% respectively.[8,9,10] Additionally, rare species such as actinomycosis, nocardiasis, mycobacteria, and fungi including candida and aspergillus and parasites such as echinococcus and dracunculus have been reported.[10]

With regards to the neurologic deterioration associated with SEA, direct mechanical compression caused by the space occupying abscess and/or indirect vascular damage with ischemic changes, are considered responsible (individually or in combination) for the neurologic insult.[5,9,10,11] SEAs are mostly found in either the lumbar (32–48%) or the thoracic regions (28–40%), followed by the cervical spine (18–24%).[1,3,12] Often times, SEAs are found in multiple segments and around transitional areas (mostly thoracolumbar junction); however, pan-spinal SEAs (involving cervical, thoracic, and lumbar spine) are relatively uncommon.[13,14]

16.2.2 Clinical Presentation

The most frequent presenting symptom in SEA is site-specific axial back pain (67%). The classical "triad" of pain, fever, and neurologic deficit are typical, but not the universal presentation.[4] Other presenting symptoms include motor weakness (52%), fever (44%), sensory abnormalities (40%), and bladder/bowel incontinence (27%).[1,4,5] The most common examination findings include spinal tenderness, focal weakness, radiculopathy, and myelopathy. Heusner's 1948 classic description of different stages of SEAs is based on symptomatology[15]:

- *Stage 1*: Axial back pain corresponding to the affected site.
- *Stage 2*: Neural elements irritation signs such as positive Lasègue, Kernig, and L'hermitte tests, positive Brudzinski reflex, neck stiffness, and radicular pain.
- *Stage 3*: True motor deficit, sensory deficit, and bladder or bowel incontinence.
- *Stage 4*: Advanced condition with complete paralysis.

The duration of, and time to transition between, the different stages may vary from hours to days. Hence, close clinical observation is strongly recommended.[1]

16.2.3 Diagnosis

The diagnosis of SEA is usually formulated based on the clinical presentation in a patient with associated risk factors, supplemented with abnormal laboratory parameters (elevated white blood cell (WBC) count, erythrocyte sedimentation rate [ESR], and C-reactive protein [CRP]), and confirmed through advanced imaging studies.[4] The gold standard is positive microbiological culture of the organism isolated from the abscess area or the blood. Blood culture is strongly recommended at the time of admission when SEA is suspected before administration of any antibiotics. Bacteremia is seen in nearly 60% of the *S. aureus* related SEAs. The inflammation parameters such as WBC, CRP, and ESR are elevated in 68–95% of cases. Following the trend of the lab parameters, specifically the CRP, after therapy is valuable in view of their

temporal patterns and restoration to normal values with effective treatment.[16,17]

Imaging studies have always remained the main modality of diagnosing SEA in any given circumstance. Magnetic resonance imaging (MRI) with and without contrast is considered as the standard imaging study in diagnosing and characterizing SEA and its extent.[18] The sensitivity and specificity of the MRI with gadolinium contrast is more than 90%. On T1-weighted (T1W) images, SEA and cerebrospinal fluid (CSF) yield similar intensity whereas in post-contrast T1W images, SEA appears bright and CSF remains the same which helps in clear delineation of the infection. T2-weighted (T2W) images also help to identify ischemic changes or myelomalacia within the spinal cord, and define the presence of bony edema denoting osteomyelitis and any perivertebral fluid collection (▶ Fig. 16.1).[18,19]

Computed tomography (CT) scan may not have a great role in the early detection of SEA but CT technologies are helpful in defining osteolytic changes associated with discitis-osetomyelitis. On the other hand, CT myelography can help define SEA with sensitivity nearly similar to MRI; nonetheless, it is an invasive technique and should be used with caution in patients with suspected lumbar SEA and in patients with contraindications for MRI.[20] Finally, plain radiographs are not helpful in early diagnosis of SEA but rather late finding of bone involvement.

16.2.4 Treatment

Despite advancements in diagnosis and treatment, SEA remains as a potentially devastating condition with permanent neurological deficit in the range of 12–27% and reported mortality in the range of 1.5–16%.[6,21] Therefore, early diagnosis is crucial for a timely management and to help prevent long-term sequelae. Given the low likelihood of a "classic triad" presentation (back pain, fever, and neurological involvement), when evaluating a patient with back pain, one should not overlook any risk factors (IV drug abuse, diabetes mellitus, immunocompromised status, recent spine surgeries, steroid injections, or other active infection) that may be associated with SEA.

Surgical decompression remains the mainstay of treatment for patients presenting with SEA and neurologic changes. While there is no clear guideline on timing of the surgery, any acute deficit of less than 72-hour onset is a clear indication for early surgical decompression.[6] Most available data

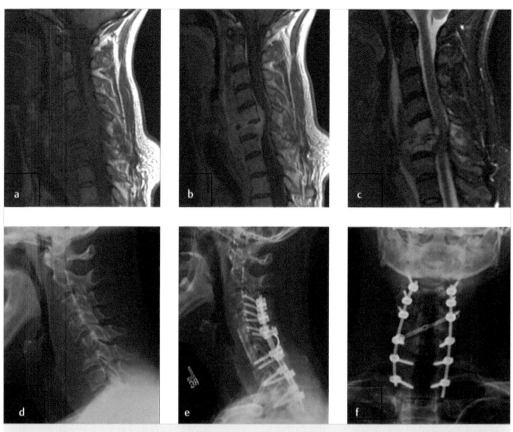

Fig. 16.1 A 35-year-old male with history of intravenous (IV) drug use with severe neck pain, and weakness in bilateral upper and lower extremity. (**a**) T1-weighted (T1W) sagittal image shows evidence of soft tissue/fluid collection in the epidural area but it is difficult to differentiate from cerebrospinal fluid (CSF). (**b**) Post-contrast T1 W image showing clear delineation of the epidural abscess. (**c**) T2-weighted (T2W) sagittal images showing osteomyelitis, prevertebral and epidural abscess. (**d**) Plain lateral radiograph showing C5 and C6 vertebral body destruction. The patient was treated with combined anterior and posterior decompression with fusion including corpectomy, fibular allograft, laminectomy, and posterior fusion. Postoperative images (**e, f**) showing anterior and posterior reconstruction with fibular allograft and posterior fixation.

on the indication and timing of surgical treatment are based on level III and level IV studies, hence the lack of strong evidence. However, most institutions do favor urgent decompression of SEA, supplemented with systemic IV antibiotics therapy for at least 6 weeks duration.[4] The surgical approach can be determined based on the involved spinal region (cervical, thoracic, or lumbar) and the location of the SEA within the spinal canal (anterior, posterior, or circumferential). Regardless of the selected approach (anterior vs. posterior), the ultimate goals should include: satisfactory neurologic decompression, adequate drainage of pus, debridement of granulation tissue, and safe placement of suction drainage if necessary.[22] Regarding

antibiotic therapy, it is preferable to start with a broad-spectrum antibiotics and then titrate according to the culture results. While Vancomycin is preferred as empirical therapy for suspected MRSA infections, Cefazolin or Nafcillin are preferred for MSSA, and gram-negative bacilli are treated with 3rd or 4th generation Cephalosporins.[4]

Few recent studies show increasing trends in the non-operative management of SEA.[6,12] This may be applicable to the early diagnosis of small and non-compressive SEA on advanced imaging in neurologically intact patients. Connor et al retrospectively compared patients with SEA treated with operative ($n = 57$) and non-operative ($n = 20$) management and found no significant difference in outcomes.[6] However, besides the significantly lower number of patients treated conservatively in this study, patients with motor deficits were more likely to have received surgery.[6] On the other hand, Kim et al reported risk factors for failure of non-operative management; these include diabetes, elevated CRP level (> 115 mg/L), leukocytosis (> 12,000 white blood cells/L), positive blood cultures, > 65 years of age, MRSA, and advanced neurological deficit.[23]

16.3 Vertebral Discitis and Osteomyelitis

Vertebral spondylodiscitis/osteomyelitis encompasses several types of spinal infections affecting the vertebral body, vertebral endplate, and intervertebral disc, and may be associated with adjacent compartment infections (paravertebral, prevertebral, psoas or secondary SEA). These infections can be the result of bacterial (pyogenic), tubercular, fungal (granulomatous), or parasitic spinal infestation. The incidence of vertebral osteomyelitis varies by geographic location and age group with reported incidence of 2.4/ 100,000, which represents 2–8% of all cases of musculoskeletal osteomyelitis.[24,25,26] Despite the low incidence of spondylodiscitis, the long-term outcomes can be devastating and may include chronic pain, spinal deformity, and permanent neurologic deficits.[27]

16.3.1 Pyogenic Vertebral Osteomyelitis

Pyogenic Vertebral Osteomyelitis (PVO) is the result of bacterial infection secondary to hematogenous seeding, direct inoculation from any spinal procedure, or contiguous spread from an infected adjacent tissue.[26] The incidence of PVO is rising due to improved longevity of the general population, widespread use of chemotherapy and immunotherapy, recreational IV drug use, increased awareness, and improved neuroimaging.[17]

Pathology

Staphylococcus aureus is the most common pathogen associated with PVO, followed by *E. coli*. However, in patients who have undergone a spinal procedure or an epidural catheter, coagulase-negative staphylococci and *Propionibacterium*

acnes have been implicated.[24] In hematogenous dissemination, the microbes reach small metaphyseal vessels either through arterial or venous channels to set up a nidus of infection and eventual avascular necrosis with further exponential growth and potential spread to the adjacent intervertebral disc. Additionally, the blood supply to the intervertebral disc becomes hampered, resulting in further metabolic disc deterioration and discitis progression. Hence, some authors believe that discitis and osteomyelitis represent various stages of the same disease.

The most common primary source of hematogenous spread include infections of the urinary tract, skin, and soft tissue, site of previous vascular access, endocarditis, bursitis, and septic arthritis.[24] Patients with underlying medical comorbidities such as diabetes, cancer patients on chemotherapy and immunotherapy, patients with renal failure on hemodialysis, and IV drug users are at a greater risk of developing hematogenous infections. The primary source of hematogenous infection is identified in 50% of PVO cases.[24]

On the other hand, infections by direct inoculation occur subsequent to spinal procedures with or without instrumentation, epidural catheters placement, steroid injections, and lumbar punctures. The least common mode of infection is contiguous in the site of adjacent infection such as retropharyngeal abscesses, esophageal ruptures, infections of aortic implants, or chest infections.[28]

Clinical Presentation

The clinical presentation of PVO is often non-specific axial pain in 86% of the cases.[24,28] The axial pain is of insidious onset, constant, and worsens during night time, and can be associated with radicular symptoms to the chest, abdomen, or extremity depending on the spinal segments involved. Hematogenous PVO commonly affect the lumbar region (58%), followed by the thoracic (30%) and the cervical spine (11%).[24,25] Fever is seen in nearly 48% of the cases. The lumbar PVO may present with weakness in hip flexion secondary to associated psoas abscess. Cervical osteomyelitis may be associated with dysphagia and torticollis, and sometimes may present as occipital headache when the occipitocervical junction is involved.[29] Nearly 33% of the PVO cases are associated with neurologic impairment including motor weakness, sensory loss, bowel/bladder symptoms, and radiculopathy.[28] Neurologic deficits are more often associated with the cervical spine due to small cross-sectional diameter of the spinal canal relative to the diameter of the cervical spinal cord.[29]

On physical examination, spinal tenderness to palpation is a common finding, while spinal deformity is a sign of advanced infection. Patients should also be auscultated for cardiac murmurs and peripheral signs of endocarditis.[26]

Laboratory Testing

An elevated WBC count is seen in > 80% of cases; however, CRP and ESR elevations are highly sensitive (98 and 100% respectively).[24] Serial CRP and ESR levels and trends are preferred for monitoring the success of any therapeutic intervention. Therefore, laboratory tests (including ESR, CRP, and WBC) are preferably repeated on a weekly basis for the inpatient and then on monthly basis during outpatient follow-up.[30] The blood culture is an essential part of workup with positive results seen in 30 to 78% of the cases.[30] The gold standard method of diagnosis is tissue culture of a biopsy specimen obtained either through image-guided method or open technique.[28]

Imaging

The provisional diagnosis of PVO is based on imaging studies including plain radiographs, CT scans, and MRI with and without contrast, with definite diagnosis based on histopathology and biopsy cultures. Unlike primary SEA, in PVO plain radiographs can be helpful in highlighting paravertebral soft tissue edema or abscess, disc height loss, vertebral destruction, and spinal deformity. Despite their low diagnostic specificity (57%), plain radiographs should be the considered first line in the imaging workup.[18,28] The main limitation with plain radiographs is the timeline to delineate the lesion, which takes approximately 2 to 4 weeks for any changes to be noticeable.[31] The initial signs of radiographic changes include discrete radiolucency in the anterior subchondral bone with loss of clear discretion of the bone endplate and narrowing of disc space. With further progression of infection, vertebral body destruction becomes more visible with opposition to the adjoining vertebrae.[18]

Compared to plain radiographs, CT scan provides much better delineation of bone and soft tissue changes because of its high soft tissue resolution. Epidural abscess extension with compression of

spinal cord, thecal sac, and nerve root, along with bone sequestration and calcification changes can be visible on CT scan.[18] In addition, CT scan can be utilized for the surgical plan during spinal reconstruction following bone destruction. Nowadays, CT scan is routinely utilized to guide bone biopsy for tissue-based diagnosis in neurologically intact patients. In patients who are not candidates for surgical debridement/stabilization, it is preferable to initially obtain tissue for culture through CT-guided biopsy. Also, CT-guided percutaneous drainage of perivertebral abscesses can be therapeutic as well.[18]

MRI with gadolinium contrast is the gold standard imaging technique in the assessment of the spondylodiscitis at any given stage of infection. The notable early finding can be seen in T2W images, and short time inversion recovery (STIR) sequence with inflammatory edema appears as bright signal at the infection sites.[18,32] Post-contrast T1W series provides clear view of the anatomy and differentiation between vascularized and nonvascular necrotic inflammatory components (abscess, phlegmon). Post-contrast T1W images also help to distinguish infections from degenerative Modic endplate changes and tumors (▶ Fig. 16.1 and ▶ Fig. 16.2).[32]

Treatment

The basic principles of PVO treatment comprises antibiotic therapy for eradication of infection, decompression of neural elements, and spinal stabilization with restoration of spinal alignment, if necessary.

Medical Treatment

The acute PVO can be managed with antibiotic therapy, provided the underlying pathogen is identified and the patient is neurologically intact without any spinal instability. Unless patient is in an uncontrolled sepsis or with an unknown infective pathogen, it is strongly recommended to initiate antimicrobial therapy; the therapy should only be undertaken after the underlying pathogen is identified.[24,28] The infection pattern varies geographically and also with age; hence, it is strongly recommended to involve the infectious disease specialists regarding the choice and duration of the antibiotic therapy. The preferred route of administration during initial phase is intravenous for 6 weeks period.[33] Further antibiotics administration, most commonly oral,

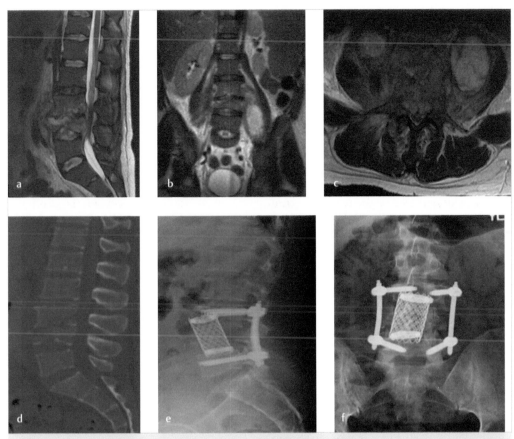

Fig. 16.2 A 28-year-old male with history of intravenous (IV) drug use with severe back pain, and weakness in bilateral hip flexion and left-side foot drop. **(a–c)** Pre-operative MRI images showing osteomyelitis of the L4 and L3 vertebrae with bilateral psoas abscess. Computed tomography (CT) scan sagittal image **(d)** showing osteolytic destruction of L4 vertebral body and L3 inferior vertebra endplate. The patient was treated with anterior decompression, drainage of bilateral psoas abscess, corpectomy, and percutaneous posterior fixation. One year post-operative anteroposterior and lateral view **(e, f)** of the lumbar spine showing cage and screw intact with well-maintained alignment.

depends on the individual response and lab results.[27] McHenry et al proposed that a 50% reduction in the CRP quantitative value/week is suggestive of appropriate therapy. Normalization of CRP and ESR values, along with clinical improvement, is indication for antibiotics discontinuation.[27]

Surgical management

Surgical treatment is indicated in the presence of symptomatic spinal cord compression, radicular neurologic deficit, spinal instability with kyphotic deformity, chronic pain related to deformity, septicemia despite antibiotic treatment, or to establish microbiological diagnosis. It is safe to perform decompression and instrumentation in the presence of acute infection if there is underlying stability.[24,34] Any standard surgical approach such as anterior, posterior, combined, or minimally invasive approaches can be utilized. The surgical strategy should be tailored according to the location of infection, the presence of neural elements compression with deficits, and the extent of bone destruction and/or associated spinal deformity.[24]

For cervical PVO requiring surgical management, the anterior approach is preferred for ventral cord compression and the posterior approach is reserved for lesions causing compressions on the dorsal part of the spinal cord and in conditions with multiple vertebrae involved requiring posterior supplemental fixation.[29] For isolated discitis with minimal endplate changes, anterior discectomy and fusion with bone graft are most commonly utilized. In case of multi-level involvement with bone destruction, anterior corpectomy and fusion supplemented with posterior instrumentation and posterior decompression are preferred.[24]

The treatment of thoracic PVO is slightly different from cervical spine PVO because of its inherent stability provided by the rib cage. If there is osteomyelitis without much destruction of the vertebral body then posterior decompression with or without instrumentation may be performed.[35] Mohamed et al reported on the technique of only posterior fixation without debridement or decompression which yielded good results in their patients; however, the study included only 15 patients.[36] The posterior only approach, including transpedicular or transfacetal approach, can also be used in the treatment of thoracic osteomyelitis involving both ventral and dorsal compression of the spinal cord. Alternatively, thoracotomy or transthoracic approach can be used for one- or two-level disease without the involvement of posterior elements.[24] In such scenarios, minimally invasive fixation plays a great role in providing stabilization through percutaneous pedicle screws and rods.[37]

In the lumbar spine, the treatment principles revolve around achieving neurologic decompression, structural stability, and proper spinal alignment. Si et al compared the anterior vs. posterior approach for the treatment of lumbar osteomyelitis with similar long-term fusion rates. Anterior surgery had better outcomes in pain control and overall well-being.[38] Minimally invasive surgical approach utilized in the treatment of degenerative spine such as ante-psoas approach or direct lateral approach supplemented with percutaneous pedicle screws may be used in the treatment of lumbar osteomyelitis with decreased surgical morbidity (▶ Fig. 16.2).[39]

16.3.2 Granulomatous Vertebral Osteomyelitis

Granulomatous Vertebral Osteomyelitis (GVO) is a slow subacute spinal infection characterized by the presence of granulomas. The most commonly responsible pathogens are *mycobacterium tuberculosis* and *Brucella* species followed by some fungal and parasitic infections. Tubercular (TB) is more common in developing countries; however, its incidence is globally increasing due to the growing number of patients with immunosuppressive conditions (e.g., AIDS immunotherapy, cancer chemotherapy, etc.).[40] Tubercular spondylitis constitutes 1% of all tuberculosis infections, but spine infections represent 25–60% of all osteoarticular TB.[41]

Pathology

TB osteomyelitis is the result of a hematogenous dissemination from a primary focus infection in the viscera. The primary focus may be active or quiescent, apparent or latent, often located either in the lungs or in the lymph glands of the mediastinum, mesentery, cervical region, or other viscera. Similar to PVO, the infection spreads to the spine through vascular channels including the systemic arteries (following bacteremia) and sometimes veins (e.g., Batson's plexus).[41,42] The most common type of TB spondylodiscitis is paradiscal (adjacent to endplate), and TB does not have direct effect on the disc itself. However, by indirect mechanism of hampering blood supply, eventual loss of disc space may occur. TB osteomyelitis is noted for marked exudative reaction associated with cold abscess formation. Regarding the location, the thoracic spine or thoracolumbar junction is the most common followed by lumbar and cervical spine.[42]

Clinical Features

The clinical presentation of tubercular vertebral osteomyelitis is related to both systemic illness and/or local infection with the most common symptom being pain (84%) corresponding to the affected area. A fever is observed in 40% of cases.[42] Other non-specific systemic symptoms such as weight loss, loss of appetite, night sweats, and malaise are seen in less than 30% of cases. Wide variation in the neurologic involvement ranges between 16 and 89% and is attributed to spinal kyphotic deformity, spinal abscess, and/or granulation tissue compressing the spinal cord or the cauda equina.[42,43]

Diagnosis

Delayed diagnosis of TB spine is most common because of the slow indolent course and variable nature of presentation.[42,44] The only specific diagnostic method is histopathological biopsy of the affected vertebrae. Laboratory studies including CBC, ESR, and CRP, although supportive to the diagnosis, have more important prognostic value. Mantoux skin test and interferon gamma-release

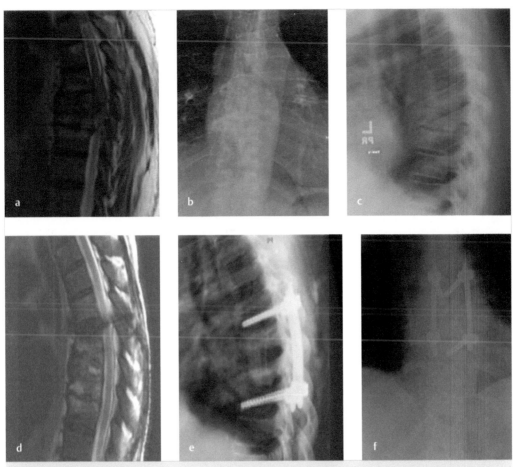

Fig. 16.3 A 64-year-old female with history of back pain with weakness in bilateral lower extremity diagnosed as tubercular spondylodiscitis based on tissue biopsy. T2-weighted (T2W) sagittal imaging (**a**) showing compression of the spinal cord with discitis, osteomyelitis, and epidural abscess. Anteroposterior and lateral plain radiographs (**b, c**) showing paravertebral soft tissue shadow secondary to abscess. The patient was treated with anterior decompression, corpectomy of T7 and T8 and rib graft. MRI 6 months post operation (**d**) showing complete resolution of abscess and decompression of the spinal cord. Anteroposterior and lateral views (**e, f**) of the thoracic spine obtained 6 months post-op showing bone graft in well-placed position with posterior instrumentation.

assays (IGRA) can be used for diagnosis but they do not differentiate active from latent infections. Imaging studies are paramount to establish the diagnosis and help guide the biopsy. Plain radiographic findings include loss of disc space, paravertebral abscess, soft tissue calcification, erosion of the vertebral body, and loss of vertebral height. CT scans help in specific evaluation of vertebral destruction and calcification of the surrounding soft tissue. MRI is the radiological investigation of choice which helps to evaluate spinal cord compression or myelopathic changes, osteolytic changes, disc involvement, and vertebral endplate erosions (▶ Fig. 16.3).

Treatment

The principle of tubercular vertebral osteomyelitis treatment is similar to that of PVO with goals to eradicate the infection, prevent or treat neurological deficit, and correct or prevent the occurrence of a focal kyphotic spinal deformity. Despite global presence of TB spine infections, there is no consensus on the duration of the treatment. According to the British Infection Society, TB spine infections should be treated by a combination of four drugs (isoniazid, rifampicin, pyrazinamide, and ethambutol) for the initial 2 months, followed by two drugs (isoniazid and rifampicin) as maintenance therapy for at least 10 months.[45] Jain suggested that chemotherapy duration may be tailored according to the patient's symptoms, lab parameters, and imaging.[46]

Surgical treatment is reserved for patients with neurologic deficits and underlying spinal cord compression, spinal deformity with instability, severe or progressive kyphosis, failure of anti-TB therapy, neurologic weakness despite medical treatment,

presence of large paraspinal abscesses, and non-diagnostic biopsies.[46] TB spine infections mostly affect the anterior/middle spinal columns; hence, conventional surgery included anterior transthoracic decompression. However, satisfactory anterior decompression can also be performed through a posterior transpedicular approach or extrapleural anterolateral approach.[47,48]

Pearls i

- *Staphylococcus aureus* is the most common organism causing spinal infections.
- Diagnosis of SEA is based on clinical presentation, lab parameters, and imaging studies.
- MRI with and without contrast is an imaging investigation of choice. Modic I changes in the endplates should not be confused with discitis in that the disc itself is not edematous (high signal intensity in T2-weighted image), usually associated with disc degeneration.
- Surgical decompression is the standard care for primary SEA with neurological involvement.
- Surgical strategy is based on location of spinal abscess, compression of neural elements, any associated spinal instability, destruction, and/or deformity.
- The key to outcome success for the surgical patients is adequate debridement of the infected and devitalized tissues and a stable biomechanical construct and biological fusion.
- Spinal instrumentation is safe in the presence of infection with instability.
- Surgical management of cervical spine infections should be tailored as per underlying conditions; for isolated discitis, anterior discectomy and fusion is recommended; if there is single level vertebral osteolysis, then corpectomy with anterior stabilization may suffice, whereas if multiple levels are involved warranting two level corpectomy, then supplementation with posterior instrumentation is preferred.
- Surgical management of lumbar spine infections include laminectomy along with thorough debridement if there are no signs of instability, whereas lumbar osteomyelitis with instability requires reconstruction which can be performed anteriorly, posteriorly, or both. Newer, minimally invasive anterior reconstruction approach along with percutaneous pedicle screw fixation seems to aid in faster recovery.
- CT-guided biopsy is the preferred approach to obtain tissue diagnosis in vertebral osteomyelitis without neurological deficits.
- Parenteral antibiotics administration for 6 weeks is preferred for medical treatment. Consultation with an infectious disease specialist is recommended for all cases of spinal infections.
- Serial monitoring of CRP and ESR is very helpful in evaluating treatment efficacy.

16.4 Case Examples

16.4.1 Case 1

A 31-year-old female presents to emergency department (ED) with complaints of progressive back pain for 2 months with fever of 103 °F and chills for 2 days. The patient denies any weakness, bowel/bladder retention or incontinence, or

ambulating pain. Her social history is significant for intravenous (IV) drug abuse. Her neurological examination is stable with grade 5 strength in bilateral lower extremity with tenderness corresponding to lower lumbar area. Lab values include white blood cell (WBC) count of 11,400, C-reactive protein (CRP) of 73, and erythrocyte sedimentation rate (ESR) of 89. Her plain radiographs are shown on the next page.

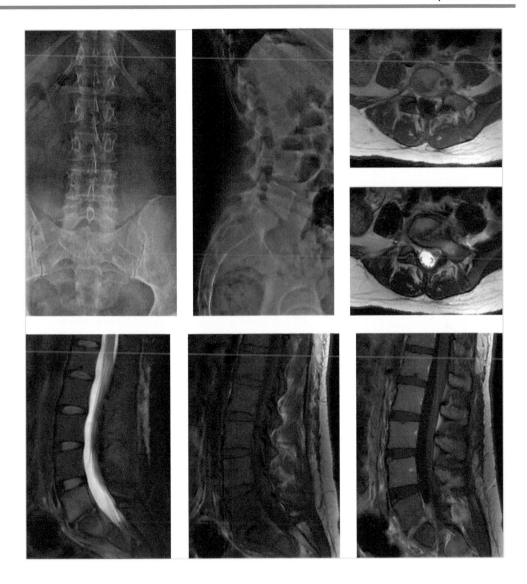

16.4.2 Case 2

A 34-year-old female presents to ED with complaints of progressive back pain for 1 week along with high grade fever and chills for 2 days. The patient describes new onset of right-side foot drop of 1 day. Her social history is significant for intravenous (IV) drug abuse. Her neurological examination is grade 2 ankle dorsiflexion, great toe extension, and plantar flexion in right lower extremity with grade 5 strength in left lower extremity. Lab values include white blood cell (WBC) count of 16,200, C-reactive protein (CRP) of 113, and erythrocyte sedimentation rate (ESR) of 92. Her imaging studies are shown on the next page.

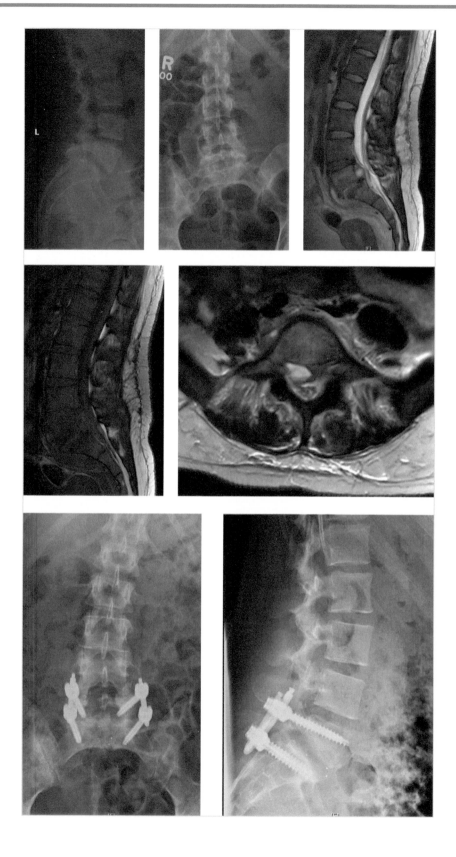

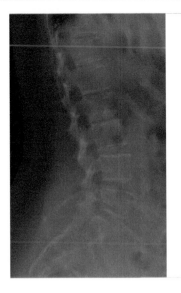
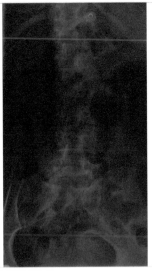
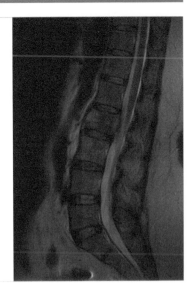

16.4.3 Case 3

A 64-year-old female admitted to the hospital with complaints of back pain for 3 months along with low grade evening fever. The patient denies any weakness or paresthesia or bowel/bladder involvement. The patient is a recent immigrant from India. Her neurologic examination is normal. Lab values include white blood cell (WBC) count of 9,200, C-reactive protein (CRP) of 53, and erythrocyte sedimentation rate (ESR) of 62. Her imaging studies are shown above.

16.5 Board-style Questions

1. In Case 1, what is the next most appropriate step in management?
   a) Reassurance and rest
   b) Physical therapy and nonsteroidal anti-inflammatory drugs (NSAIDS)
   c) Immediate surgical decompression
   d) MRI of lumbar spine with and without contrast
   e) Diskography

2. The images of MRI of lumbar spine are shown here. What is the best possible description of underlying diagnosis?
   a) Lumbar disc herniation
   b) Degenerative disc disease
   c) Primary epidural abscess
   d) Discitis/Osteomyelitis
   e) Secondary epidural abscess

3. What is the next most appropriate step in management?
   a) Surgical decompression
   b) Surgical fusion
   c) Physical therapy and NSAIDS
   d) CT-guided tissue biopsy and antibiotics as per sensitivity
   e) Not enough details available to comment on management

4. In Case 2, what is the next most appropriate step in management?
   a) Broad spectrum IV antibiotics only
   b) CT-guided tissue biopsy and antibiotics as per sensitivity
   c) Emergency surgical treatment
   d) Blood culture and appropriate antibiotics
   e) Immobilization and bed rest

5. What is the best surgical strategy for the scenario in Case 2?
   a) Percutaneous drainage under fluoroscopy
   b) Surgical decompression with irrigation and drainage
   c) Microdiscectomy of L5–S1 from either a midline approach or far lateral approach
   d) Surgical decompression with irrigation and drainage and fusion
   e) Percutaneous pedicle screw fixation

6. Post-operative images are shown here. What is the rationale behind the chosen treatment?

a) Lumbar infections invariably require instrumented fusion

b) Pathological fracture

c) Spinal instability along with abscess

d) Infection across lumbosacral junction

e) Surgeon's preference

7. After surgical decompression and fusion, the tissue sample was sent for culture. What is the most common underlying pathogen?

a) Staphylococcus aureus

b) Streptococcus viridans

c) Candida albicans

d) Klebsiella pneumoniae

e) Mixed culture

8. Culture samples were noted to grow methicillin-resistant *Staphylococcus aureus* (MRSA). What would be the next most appropriate step in management?

a) IV Vancomycin for 6 weeks

b) Surgical fixation is sufficient, no need for antibiotics

c) IV Ancef for 6 weeks

d) Oral Vancomycin for 6 weeks

e) IV Clindamycin for 6 weeks

9. In Case 3, what is the most likely diagnosis?

a) Degenerative disc disease

b) Pyogenic osteomyelitis

c) Tubercular osteomyelitis

d) Metastatic lesion

e) Both c & d

10. What is the most appropriate next step of management in Case 3?

a) Brace and bedrest with spinal precautions

b) Percutaneous pedicle screw fixation

c) CT-guided biopsy and antimicrobial therapy

d) Corpectomy

e) None of the above

Answers ✓

1. d
2. d
3. d
4. c
5. d
6. c
7. a
8. a
9. e
10. c

References

[1] Arko L, IV, Quach E, Nguyen V, Chang D, Sukul V, Kim BS. Medical and surgical management of spinal epidural abscess: a systematic review. Neurosurg Focus. 2014; 37(2):E4

[2] Eltorai AEM, Naqvi SS, Seetharam A, Brea BA, Simon C. Recent developments in the treatment of spinal epidural abscesses. Orthop Rev (Pavia). 2017; 9(2):7010

[3] Adogwa O, Karikari IO, Carr KR, et al. Spontaneous spinal epidural abscess in patients 50 years of age and older: a 15-year institutional perspective and review of the literature: clinical article. J Neurosurg Spine. 2014; 20(3):344–349

[4] Darouiche RO. Spinal epidural abscess. N Engl J Med. 2006; 355(19):2012–2020

[5] Reihsaus E, Waldbaur H, Seeling W. Spinal epidural abscess: a meta-analysis of 915 patients. Neurosurg Rev. 2000; 23 (4):175–204, discussion 205

[6] Connor DE, Jr, Chittiboina P, Caldito G, Nanda A. Comparison of operative and nonoperative management of spinal epidural abscess: a retrospective review of clinical and laboratory predictors of neurological outcome. J Neurosurg Spine. 2013; 19(1):119–127

[7] Zimmerer SM, Conen A, Müller AA, et al. Spinal epidural abscess: aetiology, predisponent factors and clinical outcomes in a 4-year prospective study. Eur Spine J. 2011; 20(12):2228–2234

[8] Huang PY, Chen SF, Chang WN, et al. Spinal epidural abscess in adults caused by Staphylococcus aureus: clinical characteristics and prognostic factors. Clin Neurol Neurosurg. 2012; 114(6):572–576

[9] Lechiche C, Le Moing V, Marchandin H, Chanques G, Atoui N, Reynes J. Spondylodiscitis due to Bacteroides fragilis: two cases and review. Scand J Infect Dis. 2006; 38(3):229–231

[10] Feldenzer JA, McKeever PE, Schaberg DR, Campbell JA, Hoff JT. Experimental spinal epidural abscess: a pathophysiological model in the rabbit. Neurosurgery. 1987; 20(6):859–867

[11] Hlavin ML, Kaminski HJ, Ross JS, Ganz E. Spinal epidural abscess: a ten-year perspective. Neurosurgery. 1990; 27(2):177–184

[12] Patel AR, Alton TB, Bransford RJ, Lee MJ, Bellabarba CB, Chapman JR. Spinal epidural abscesses: risk factors, medical versus surgical management, a retrospective review of 128 cases. Spine J. 2014; 14(2):326–330

[13] Kikuchi Y, Suzuki J, Onishi T, Morisawa Y. Pan-spinal epidural abscess in a diabetic patient. Intern Med. 2017; 56(15):2081

[14] Ju KL, Kim SD, Melikian R, Bono CM, Harris MB. Predicting patients with concurrent noncontiguous spinal epidural abscess lesions. Spine J. 2015; 15(1):95–101

[15] Heusner AP. Nontuberculous spinal epidural infections. N Engl J Med. 1948; 239(23):845–854

[16] Curry WT, Jr, Hoh BL, Amin-Hanjani S, Eskandar EN. Spinal epidural abscess: clinical presentation, management, and outcome. Surg Neurol. 2005; 63(4):364–371, discussion 371

[17] Hsieh PC, Wienecke RJ, O'Shaughnessy BA, Koski TR, Ondra SL. Surgical strategies for vertebral osteomyelitis and epidural abscess. Neurosurg Focus. 2004; 17(6):E4

[18] Jevtic V. Vertebral infection. Eur Radiol. 2004; 14(3) Suppl 3: E43–E52

[19] Shifrin A, Lu Q, Lev MH, Meehan TM, Hu R. Paraspinal edema is the most sensitive feature of lumbar spinal epidural abscess on unenhanced MRI. AJR Am J Roentgenol. 2017; 209(1):176–181

[20] Sendi P, Bregenzer T, Zimmerli W. Spinal epidural abscess in clinical practice. QJM. 2008; 101(1):1–12

[21] Davis DP, Wold RM, Patel RJ, et al. The clinical presentation and impact of diagnostic delays on emergency department patients with spinal epidural abscess. J Emerg Med. 2004; 26(3):285–291

[22] Hadjipavlou AG, Mader JT, Necessary JT, Muffoletto AJ. Hematogenous pyogenic spinal infections and their surgical management. Spine. 2000; 25(13):1668–1679

[23] Kim SD, Melikian R, Ju KL, et al. Independent predictors of failure of nonoperative management of spinal epidural abscesses. Spine J. 2014; 14(8):1673–1679

[24] Zimmerli W. Clinical practice: vertebral osteomyelitis. N Engl J Med. 2010; 362(11):1022–1029

[25] Grammatico L, Baron S, Rusch E, et al. Epidemiology of vertebral osteomyelitis (VO) in France: analysis of hospital-discharge data 2002–2003. Epidemiol Infect. 2008; 136(5):653–660

[26] Berbari EF, Kanj SS, Kowalski TJ, et al. Infectious Diseases Society of America. Infectious Diseases Society of America (IDSA) clinical practice guidelines for the diagnosis and treatment of native vertebral osteomyelitis in adults. Clin Infect Dis. 2015; 61(6):e26–e46

[27] McHenry MC, Easley KA, Locker GA. Vertebral osteomyelitis: long-term outcome for 253 patients from 7 Cleveland-area hospitals. Clin Infect Dis. 2002; 34(10):1342–1350

[28] Duarte RM, Vaccaro AR. Spinal infection: state of the art and management algorithm. Eur Spine J. 2013; 22(12):2787–2799

[29] Acosta FL, Jr, Chin CT, Quiñones-Hinojosa A, Ames CP, Weinstein PR, Chou D. Diagnosis and management of adult pyogenic osteomyelitis of the cervical spine. Neurosurg Focus. 2004; 17(6):E2

[30] Mylona E, Samarkos M, Kakalou E, Fanourgiakis P, Skoutelis A. Pyogenic vertebral osteomyelitis: a systematic review of clinical characteristics. Semin Arthritis Rheum. 2009; 39(1):10–17–. Elsevier

[31] Gupta A, Kowalski TJ, Osmon DR, et al. Long-term outcome of pyogenic vertebral osteomyelitis: a cohort study of 260 patients. Open Forum Infect Dis. 2014; 1(3):ofu107:. Oxford University Press

[32] Dunbar JAT, Sandoe JAT, Rao AS, Crimmins DW, Baig W, Rankine JJ. The MRI appearances of early vertebral osteomyelitis and discitis. Clin Radiol. 2010; 65(12):974–981

[33] Bernard L, Dinh A, Ghout I, et al. Duration of Treatment for Spondylodiscitis (DTS) study group. Antibiotic treatment for 6 weeks versus 12 weeks in patients with pyogenic vertebral osteomyelitis: an open-label, non-inferiority, randomised, controlled trial. Lancet. 2015; 385(9971):875–882

[34] Sundararaj GD, Babu N, Amritanand R, et al. Treatment of haematogenous pyogenic vertebral osteomyelitis by single-stage anterior debridement, grafting of the defect and posterior instrumentation. J Bone Joint Surg Br. 2007; 89(9):1201–1205

[35] Gorensek M, Kosak R, Travnik L, Vengust R. Posterior instrumentation, anterior column reconstruction with single posterior approach for treatment of pyogenic osteomyelitis of thoracic and lumbar spine. Eur Spine J. 2013; 22(3):633–641

[36] Mohamed AS, Yoo J, Hart R, et al. Posterior fixation without debridement for vertebral body osteomyelitis and discitis. Neurosurg Focus. 2014; 37(2):E6

[37] Mückley T, Schütz T, Schmidt MH, Potulski M, Bühren V, Beisse R. The role of thoracoscopic spinal surgery in the management of pyogenic vertebral osteomyelitis. Spine. 2004; 29(11):E227–E233

[38] Si M, Yang ZP, Li ZF, Yang Q, Li JM. Anterior versus posterior fixation for the treatment of lumbar pyogenic vertebral osteomyelitis. Orthopedics. 2013; 36(6):831–836

[39] Tannoury T, Haddadi K, Kempegowda H, Kadam A, Tannoury C. Role of minimally invasive spine surgery in adults with degenerative lumbar scoliosis: a narrative review. Iran J Neurosurg. 2017; 3(2):39–50

[40] An HS, Seldomridge JA. Spinal infections: diagnostic tests and imaging studies. Clin Orthop Relat Res. 2006; 444(444):27–33

[41] Lee KY. Comparison of pyogenic spondylitis and tuberculous spondylitis. Asian Spine J. 2014; 8(2):216–223

[42] Trecarichi EM, Di Meco E, Mazzotta V, Fantoni M. Tuberculous spondylodiscitis: epidemiology, clinical features, treatment, and outcome. Eur Rev Med Pharmacol Sci. 2012; 16 Suppl 2:58–72

[43] Jutte P, Wuite S, The B, van Altena R, Veldhuizen A. Prediction of deformity in spinal tuberculosis. Clin Orthop Relat Res. 2007; 455(455):196–201

[44] Kamara E, Mehta S, Brust JC, Jain AK. Effect of delayed diagnosis on severity of Pott's disease. Int Orthop. 2012; 36(2):245–254

[45] Thwaites G, Fisher M, Hemingway C, Scott G, Solomon T, Innes J, British Infection Society. British Infection Society guidelines for the diagnosis and treatment of tuberculosis of the central nervous system in adults and children. J Infect. 2009; 59(3):167–187

[46] Jain AK. Tuberculosis of spine: research evidence to treatment guidelines. Indian J Orthop. 2016; 50(1):3–9

[47] Chacko AG, Moorthy RK, Chandy MJ. The transpedicular approach in the management of thoracic spine tuberculosis: a short-term follow up study. Spine. 2004; 29(17):E363–E367

[48] Lee SH, Sung JK, Park YM. Single-stage transpedicular decompression and posterior instrumentation in treatment of thoracic and thoracolumbar spinal tuberculosis: a retrospective case series. J Spinal Disord Tech. 2006; 19(8):595–602

17 Inflammatory Spinal Disorders

Garrett K. Harada, Jannat M. Khan, and David F. Fardon

Abstract

Noninfectious inflammatory spinal diseases constitute a heterogeneous body of conditions that are frequently encountered by spine surgeons. While the need for surgical treatment of such diseases has diminished with the development of improved medical therapies, understanding the appropriate management of these conditions is important to prevent patients from having gross deformity and/or neurological deficits in terminal stages of their disease. Seronegative spondyloarthropathies, including ankylosing spondylitis (AS), have the potential to develop severe kyphotic deformities, requiring horizontal gaze assessments and, potentially, spinal osteotomy to restore sagittal balance. Enteropathic arthritides, reactive spondyloarthritis, psoriatic arthritis (PA), and other uncommon syndromes are recognized variations of spondyloarthritis. Rheumatoid arthritis (RA) is a common condition that has the potential to affect the spine, most often the upper and subaxial cervical spine, with uncommon involvement of the lumbar spine. Hypertrophic spine arthropathies include diffuse idiopathic skeletal hyperostosis (DISH) and Paget's disease. Arthropathic spine syndromes include those in which the predominant disease involves spinal ligament ossification, such as Ossification of the Posterior Longitudinal Ligament (OPLL) and Ossification of the Yellow Ligament (OYL). Though these conditions present with distinct pathophysiologies, many patients share similar signs and symptoms and pose challenges in making a timely diagnosis, pursuing appropriate surgical management, and coordinating care with other medical providers.

Keywords: spondyloarthritis, spondyloarthropathy, ankylosing spondylitis, rheumatoid arthritis, DISH, Paget's disease, OPLL, HLA-B27

17.1 Introduction

Inflammatory diseases include both infectious and noninfectious etiologies. These conditions can affect all levels of the spine. Recent improvements in medications and aggressive management by primary care providers have significantly changed the course of inflammatory arthropathies. Many patients with spondyloarthropathy, however, experience progression and chronicity of their symptoms.

Chapter 16 discusses spondylitis known to be due to infection. Degenerative and traumatic phenomena such as disc degeneration and stress-related hypertrophy of zygapophyseal and apophyseal bone, sometimes called "spondylosis," are not extensively covered in this discussion of primary inflammatory diseases, but should be included in the differential diagnosis of spinal pain. In this chapter, we discuss the presentation, evaluation, and management of inflammatory spondyloarthropathies that have not been shown to be directly caused by infection. Included are diseases such as ankylosing spondylitis (AS), psoriatic arthritis (PA), enteropathic arthritis (EA), and reactive arthritis (ReA). Diseases that resemble these conditions, such as diffuse idiopathic skeletal hyperostosis and rheumatoid arthritis (RA), and uncommon disorders, which are important to include in the differential diagnosis, will also be addressed.

17.2 Ankylosing Spondylitis

Also known as Marie-Strumpell or von Bechterew's disease, AS is a chronic autoimmune inflammatory spondyloarthropathy primarily affecting the entheses and discs of the spine. Among the inflammatory spondyloarthropathies, AS is the most common in the United States with an estimated prevalence of 5.2 per 1000 people.[1] While many patients have mild forms and respond to treatment, AS can cause joint ankylosis, with permanent deformity, disability, and fragility.

Focal inflammatory lesions at the entheses of the peripheral annulus and apophyseal bone cause erosion of the cortices and ossification of the marginal annular ligamentous tissue to form vertically oriented osteophytes, called syndesmophytes, and lead to replacement with brittle, lamellar bone. This predisposes the patient to microfractures and progressive kyphotic deformity of the spine, which can lead to loss of horizontal gaze, and difficulty in performing daily chores. These changes increase the risks of falling due to loss of agility and the risks of fractures and extension-type injuries, thereby resulting in higher morbidity and mortality late in the disease process.[2]

17.2.1 History and Examination

In young Caucasian males, AS presents in their third to fourth decades of life.[2] AS has a strong genetic predisposition and is associated with the allele HLA-B27. Sacroiliac (SI) joint involvement commonly causes buttock pain. Many patients have a relatively long history of low-grade back pain before becoming severe enough to seek medical care. The pain has an atypical character in contrast to common lumbar sprain/strain or discogenic pain. The SI areas are common foci, but, if inquiry is made, many patients confess to mid to upper thoracic pain. As with other types of inflammatory arthropathies, symptoms are worse in the morning and improve through activity or by the use of non-steroidal anti-inflammatory drugs (NSAIDs).

Pulmonary function might get compromised by impaired chest expansion due to arthritic involvement of costovertebral articulations. Shortness of breath may be an indicator of costovertebral joint involvement limiting chest wall expansion or leading to development of pulmonary fibrosis.[3]

Many associated conditions present in the AS patient such as: anterior uveitis, cardiac murmurs, and/or pulmonary crackles.[3] Some patients with severe AS suffer ankylosis of the hips, knees, and/or shoulders, so general orthopedic examination is indicated. Tape measure assessment of chest expansion is an important part of examination of patients with symptoms of spondyloarthropathy.

Importantly, acute onset of back or neck pain in a patient with AS should raise suspicion for vertebral fracture and warrant careful clinical and radiographic evaluation. An AS patient with acute pain, even after trivial or no injury, must be regarded as having a spinal fracture until proven otherwise by extensive advanced imaging and careful observation.

The examiner assesses range of motion of the cervical spine by measuring the "occiput-to-wall" distance, performed by instructing the patient to stand with heels against a wall and maximally extending the neck. The distance between the wall and the occiput quantifies cervical spine extension.

Schober test assesses the range of motion of the lumbar spine in AS patients. In the traditional Schober test, a horizontal line is drawn at the level of the lumbosacral junction (at the level of the "dimples of Venus"). A second horizontal line is then drawn 10 cm above this line. The patient is then instructed to bend forward, with knees in full extension. In a normal examination, the distance between both the horizontal lines should be greater than 15 cm. Some examiners use a modified Schober test, where the two horizontal lines are placed 10 cm above the lumbosacral junction, and 5 cm below. The amount of distraction between these two lines is recorded as a quantifiable measure of the patient's lumbar flexion.[4,5]

For lateral motion in the lumbar spine, the examiner instructs the patient to stand upright and bend laterally, sliding either hand down the leg without bending the knees. The distance from the third digit to the floor at the beginning and end positions should be greater than 10 cm in patients with normal mobility.

Assessing chest wall expansion is also indicated in examination of patients suspected of having AS. Measurements are performed at the level of the xiphisternum while the patient is instructed to inhale maximally. Less than 2.5 cm of chest expansion is considered abnormal and suggests restrictive lung disease and/or loss of costovertebral motion.[6]

Kyphotic deformity of the spine is often obvious in late stages of AS, as patients will have notable limitations in horizontal gaze and flexibility of the spine. In severe cases, patients may develop the "chin-on-chest" deformity. Such patients should also be evaluated for dysphagia. Care must be taken to rule out hip-flexion contractures as a possible cause for apparent sagittal imbalance. This is performed by observing the patient in supine and sitting positions to determine the relative contribution of spinal kyphosis and hip flexors on sagittal alignment.

Examples of provocative tests for SI joint pathology include elicitation of pain on flexion, abduction, and external rotation of the ipsilateral hip (FABER test) or the Gaenslen's test (one hip is maximally flexed while the opposite is maximally extended to elicit pain).[5]

17.2.2 Differential Diagnosis

Diagnosis of AS is based on the modified New York Classification Criteria, and requires radiographic evidence of sacroiliitis in combination with specific clinical examination findings (▶ Table 17.1).[7] Presence of HLA-B27 is highly sensitive in screening for AS and is positive in 90% of Caucasian AS

Table 17.1 Modified New York Classification Criteria for diagnosis of ankylosing spondylitis[7]

Diagnostic criterion
Radiographic
Grade ≥ II bilateral sacroiliitis
Grade III or IV unilateral sacroiliitis
Clinical
≥ 3 months of inflammatory back pain
Limited range of motion of lumbar spine in sagittal and coronal planes
Limited chest wall expansion relative to normal values for age and sex

Notes: Ankylosing spondylitis (AS) is definitively diagnosed if 1 of 2 radiographic and 1 of 3 clinical criteria are met. AS is probable if 1 of 2 radiographic or 3 of 3 clinical criteria are met.

patients in contrast to 10% of Caucasians without arthritis.[8] This prevalence is less pronounced in other ethnicities, although if positive, it raises suspicion for AS and warrants more aggressive investigation and management.

SI pathology is required to diagnose AS, although it is often not radiographically apparent at early stages of the disease. The alert interpreter of radiographs can occasionally recognize subtle changes such as "squaring off" of apophyseal beaks from bone resorption or vertical wisps of ligament calcification in early formation of syndesmophytes, as harbingers of more apparent disease to come, or as confirmation, when changes at the SI joints lead to concerns. Other early radiographic changes at the SI joints include juxtacortical rarefaction, superficial erosions (primarily on the iliac side of the joint), and progressive sclerosis of subchondral bone.[9]

17.2.3 Diagnostic Imaging

Basic imaging studies for AS (as with most other inflammatory spondyloarthropathies) include standing full-length anteroposterior (AP) and lateral views of the axial skeleton and Ferguson pelvic tilt views for the SI joints. These views provide clear evaluation of the intervertebral disc spaces, presence of syndesmophytes, SI inflammation, and sagittal balance.

Radiographic findings of AS, suggestive of spondylitis and SI joint inflammation, include marginal syndesmophyte formation (as inflammation occurs at the margin of the annulus fibrosus) and loss of disc height. In later stages of the disease,

continued inflammation can lead to complete ossification of the discs and scalloping of the vertebral bodies ("bamboo spine"). Sacroiliitis is often demonstrated by increased radiopacity bilaterally, at the level of the SI joints, and is graded (grades 0–4) based on the methods described by the New York Classification Criteria: (1) grade 0 = normal; (2) grade 1 = suspicious changes; (3) grade 2 = minimal abnormality (small localized areas with erosion or sclerosis, no joint space narrowing); (4) grade 3 = unequivocal abnormality (moderate to advanced sacroiliitis with erosions, sclerosis, and gross joint space abnormality); (5) grade 4 = severe abnormality (total ankylosis).[7]

Measurement of the chin-brow to vertical angle (CBVA) is performed on standing radiographs for assessment of the patient's "chin-on-chest" deformity. This is performed by measuring the angle between the vertical axis and a line drawn tangentially to the patient's chin and brow. This angle is an objective proxy for measuring loss of horizontal gaze and is crucial when planning operative correction of kyphosis.[10]

Computed tomography (CT) is particularly useful in detecting vertebral fractures. Magnetic resonance imaging (MRI) may often be combined with CT in instances where fractures are detected, so as to best rule out other injuries and to evaluate the spinal cord. In comparison with the general population, after a vertebral fracture, patients with AS have a 7.6-fold increase in risk of spinal epidural hematoma.[11] MRI also has additional utility in assisting in early diagnosis of AS, being the most sensitive modality for detecting early inflammation at the SI joints.

17.2.4 Treatment

AS patients have a tendency to develop severe osteopenia in later stages of the disease. As a result, many AS patients are at risk of significant vertebral fractures secondary to low-energy trauma. Most often, these injuries arise in mid-cervical and cervicothoracic segments, and if unstable, require surgery. Stable fractures can be treated by immobilization without surgery but only if carefully monitored in compliant patients.

Vertebral fractures in AS can be treated by multi-level posterior spinal fusion. Anterior, or anterior to posterior approaches carry increased risk of cardiopulmonary complications, longer hospital stays, and increased fusion failure rates.[12] For mid-cervical fractures, fusion involves the affected vertebra and levels above and below the injury. For increased stability, fusion may be extended from C2 to the thoracolumbar junction. This minimizes construct failure by allowing for multiple points of fixation to help combat the associated osteopenia and long lever arms of the ankylosed spine.

Often, surgical treatment of the deformity that arises in AS is performed by osteotomy at the apex of the kyphotic curve. Many types of osteotomies exist, including Smith-Petersen osteotomy (SPO), pedicle subtraction osteotomy (PSO), vertebral column resection (VCR), and cervical extension osteotomy (CEO) or cervical PSO. Selection of osteotomy largely depends on the following: (1) the amount of sagittal plane correction (in degrees) desired, (2) anatomy amenable to the procedure, (3) coincidence of coronal plane curvature, and (4) acceptable level of operative risk. The SPO, performed for treatment of kyphosis in AS, requires complete "cracking" of the bone at the intervertebral disc. Due to the inherent instability of the osteotomy site secondary to lack of bone in the anterior opening wedge space and the potential danger to vascular structures, it is rarely performed at present.

The PSO is a closing-wedge technique that involves the removal of the pedicles and associated posterior elements at the planned level of resection. This technique allows roughly 30 to 40 degrees of sagittal plane correction at each level it is performed, and is the preferred technique for management of kyphosis in AS. Frequently, due to the long lever arms of an ankylosed spine, these osteotomies are performed in the lower lumbar region to maximize correction. In addition, in cases where patients have concurrent coronal plane deformities, a PSO can be performed asymmetrically.

The VCR is performed by removing an entire vertebral body, posterior elements, and its superior and inferior facet joints and discs. Doing so allows for corrections of up to 50 degrees or more. Like the PSO, the VCR is technically demanding, and often requires longer operative times, incurs greater blood loss, and has higher risks of intra- and postoperative complications.[10,13]

CEOs directly treat cervical flexion abnormalities ("chin-on-chest" deformities) seen in AS. Indications for this surgery include loss of horizontal gaze and difficulty with activities of daily living (e.g., eating, personal hygiene). The CEO is an opening wedge osteotomy performed at the cervicothoracic junction by removing the lateral masses of C7 in addition to portions of the C7 and T1 pedicles to prevent spinal cord impingement.

Cervical PSO removes the C7 pedicle completely, followed by a closing wedge osteotomy. A study by Song et al revealed that patients are most satisfied with the results of their CEO when the CBVA is corrected to lie between 10 and 20 degrees.[14]

When addressing large spinal deformity, such as those that arise in AS, consideration should be given to concurrent hip joint pathology. Recent studies by Buckland et al have revealed that patients with previous lumbar spinal fusion have significantly higher rates of hip dislocation after undergoing a total hip arthroplasty.[15] They hypothesize that spinal fusions, especially those that involve the sacrum, limit pelvis mobility and prevent adequate retroversion of the pelvis to accommodate for the hip prosthesis. Implants with increased acetabular anteversion have helped address this issue, although patients with prosthetic hips *a priori* present challenges for future spinal deformity correction.

With AS and other multifocal diseases that result in deformity, loss of motion, and compromised ability to compensate, extra effort must be given to pre-operative planning. Normal horizontal gaze may be more important to some patients than others. Habits and requirements of daily living as well as personal tolerance for pain vis-à-vis stiffness must be carefully assessed to be sure the outcome of surgery will not just be one of technical success but also improvement in the life of the patient.

17.3 Enteropathic, Psoriatic, and Reactive Arthritis

Enteropathic, psoriatic, and reactive arthritis comprise the remainder of the seronegative spondyloarthropathies, and share many similar features regarding clinical presentation, diagnosis, and management. Though pathogenesis of these conditions largely remains unclear, genetics are thought to play a significant role, as HLA-B27 is found in 50–75% of cases.

EA is a chronic condition associated with inflammatory bowel disease (IBD) such as Crohn's disease and ulcerative colitis. Other gastrointestinal diseases such as Whipple's (gastrointestinal infection with *Tropheryma whipplei*) and celiac disease (gluten intolerance) also have a documented association with EA, although they are associated with spondyloarthritis much less frequently.[16] Conversely, PA is associated with active psoriatic lesions and typically causes asymmetric joint pathology. It is most frequently seen in patients with type I psoriasis and affects 0.3–1% of the world's population.[17] ReA, formerly known as Reiter's syndrome, is a rare condition that arises after a gastrointestinal or urogenital infection.

17.3.1 History and Examination

Patients with each of these diseases are most often young adults with complaints of specific oligoarticular pain, predominantly of the lower back, SI joints, and/or lower extremities. Men and women are equally affected by PA, although there is a slightly greater preponderance of EA and ReA in males. All patients will complain of inflammatory joint pain that worsens with long periods of immobility, although they improve with use of anti-inflammatory medications and/or control of the underlying disease. The clinician's careful inquiry of subtle nuances in the patient's history and examination allow distinction between these three conditions.

Patients with EA usually have a positive family history and/or previous diagnosis of IBD. Symptoms of EA may precede diagnosis of IBD; thus making important inquiry about recent gastrointestinal symptoms. Physical examination of the spine yields findings similar to those described for AS. Imaging changes depend upon the severity of the disease and can be negative in early stages. Laboratory observations of elevated inflammatory markers and presence of HLA-B27 are similar to AS—helpful but lacking specificity and sensitivity. Imaging, especially MRI, is sensitive to sacroiliitis, similar to AS though not likely to progress to "bamboo spine."

PA patients will often have first-degree relatives with psoriasis and will complain of inflammatory pain at joints of the appendicular skeleton, although many have complaints related to the spine and SI joints. PA has five major patterns based on the mode of joint involvement: (1) asymmetric oligo/monoarticular arthritis of the distal interphalangeal (DIP) proximal interphalangeal (PIP), and metacarpophalangeal (MCP) joints, (2) DIP-predominant arthritis, (3) symmetric rheumatoid factor (RF)-negative polyarthritis, (4) arthritis mutilans, and (5) psoriatic spondyloarthropathy. Inflammation at the entheses may also occur, which usually affects the plantar fascia, posterior tibialis, and Achilles tendons. Non-orthopedic symptoms such as nail-pitting, dactylitis, onycholysis, and uveitis also occur, and are classic findings in psoriatic patients.

Patients with ReA present with symptoms days to weeks after an antecedent infection of the gastrointestinal or urogenital tracts with typical causative microorganisms such as *Campylobacter*, *Shigella*, *Salmonella*, or *Chlamydia*. As such, patients may have symptoms associated with ongoing infection at the time of presentation such as fever, dysuria, and diarrhea. Given its systemic nature, ReA patients often have significant findings on examination of the eyes, skin or mucosa, cadiovascular, and genitourinary systems. Classic findings include conjunctivitis, uveitis, skin lesions on the palms or soles, and urethritis. Patients can also have other extra-articular manifestations, such as enthesitis, dactylitis, or nail changes such as onycholysis, nail-pitting, or subungual keratoses.

17.3.2 Differential Diagnosis

Distinction of spondyloarthropathy as enteropathic is usually driven by presence of Crohn's or ulcerative colitis. As many as 36% of IBD patients experience some form of spine involvement throughout their disease course, and may be exacerbated by concurrent treatment with corticosteroids.[18] Most misdiagnoses of EA occur when the patient has no formal diagnosis of IBD, and presents initially with non-specific back or SI pain.

In PA, the pattern of joint affliction, such as involvement of the hands, helps in the discernment. The location and morphology of syndesmophytes are predictable through understanding the pathophysiologies of the diseases. In AS, the bone along the margins of the vertebral bodies resorbs and ankylosis occurs from ossification of the ligamentous tissues—"marginal syndesmophytes." In contrast, the syndesmophytes of psoriatic spondyloarthritis usually extend 2–3 mm or more from the margins of the bone and may be oriented horizontally as well as vertically; hence, they are "non-marginal syndesmophytes."

For ReA, the diagnostician should consider febrile arthritides such as Still's disease, rheumatic fever, gonococcal arthritis, secondary syphilis, septic arthritis, and immunotherapy-related arthropathy. Additional considerations include asymmetrical oligoarticular conditions such as gout, PA, and RA. Though typically self-limited, up to 15–30% of patients with ReA can develop long-term joint abnormalities or complications related to sacroiliitis, cervical spine inflammation, or secondary AS.[19,20,21]

17.3.3 Diagnostic Imaging

Diagnostic imaging for each of these spondyloarthropathies is fairly similar. Standing AP and lateral views of the spine and imaging of the SI joints are most frequently indicated. MRI studies can be used to evaluate for early signs of inflammation. Additional flexion/extension and open-mouth views may be added for suspected cervical spine pathology.

17.3.4 Treatment

Treatment for these conditions is primarily medicinal in early stages of the disease. In the case of ReA, supportive therapy with NSAIDs or corticosteroids (in severe cases) is often sufficient. Antibiotics may also be considered if the source of infection is identified, although most cases of ReA are self-limited and will resolve without treatment. Treatment of EA and PA is primarily with the use of biologic agents and disease-modifying drugs to target the underlying disease.

EA presents a unique challenge in management for the spine surgeon given the morbidity of IBD. Patients will frequently be on high doses of corticosteroids during disease flares, and may have long-term consequences to the spine, in addition to pathology caused by EA. In cases where patients have a colostomy, spine surgery should be pursued cautiously, as recovery is often impeded by difficulties of postoperative therapy and bracing requirements. The treating physician should carefully review these complications with the patient when considering surgery.

For all of these conditions, indications for surgery arise late in the disease course, and include arthrodesis for refractory pain and correction and/or prevention of deformity. Procedures used in the treatment of these symptoms are as for other spondyloarthropathies and may include decompression, anterior or posterior instrumentation, osteotomy, and fusion.

17.4 Rheumatoid Arthritis

RA is an autoimmune inflammatory condition that causes polyarthritic erosive joint damage and impairment. RA can significantly damage the articulations of the cervical spine, and can lead to complications of instability, such as atlantoaxial subluxation, subaxial subluxation, and basilar invagination (cranial settling).

Atlantoaxial subluxation is caused by pannus formation between the odontoid and anterior arch of C1, causing instability through disruption of the transverse ligament. Similarly, subaxial subluxation is caused by pannus formation at the lower cervical vertebrae, disrupting uncovertebral and facet joints. Basilar invagination is defined as a cranial migration of the dens secondary to erosive bone loss at the occiput and C1 and/or C2. Together, these changes increase a patient's risk for myelopathy and associated disability, which, in turn, warrants urgent or emergent surgical intervention. Management of RA with drugs has improved since the introduction of methotrexate and biologic agents (e.g., TNF-a inhibitors, rituximab, and others) and has diminished the need for surgery.

17.4.1 History and Examination

RA presents in young adult to middle-aged women with fatigue, joint stiffness, swelling, and pain. Normally, joint complaints are symmetric and affect articulations of the upper and lower extremities, such as the MCP, PIP, and metatarsophalangeal (MTP) joints. Pain and stiffness are often worst in the morning, shortly after awakening, and improves with activity or with the use of NSAIDs. Distinguishing early stages of RA from other forms of inflammatory arthritis requires careful clinical observation and associated serologies (RF, anti-citrullinated peptide [anti-CCP]) and acute phase reactants (ESR, CRP). RA patients with cervical spine involvement, depending on the level of instability, complain of neck pain, loss of neck mobility, and other myelopathic symptoms, such as difficulty ambulating, weakness, incontinence, clumsiness, and spasticity. Up to 33–50% of RA patients with significant imaging findings in the cervical spine are asymptomatic.[22] As such, care must be taken to evaluate these latter symptoms, as an acute onset or rapid progression often warrants immediate surgical intervention.

Patients with RA exhibit tender and swollen joints with varying degrees of deformity and functional impairment. Classic findings of the hands include decreased grip strength, palmar erythema, ulnar deviation of the digits, and boutonniere and swan neck deformities. The knees, hips, elbows, wrists, and shoulders are all quite often victims of ravages of severe RA. Other findings include subcutaneous (rheumatoid) nodules, splenomegaly (Felty's syndrome), or an abnormal

Table 17.2 American College of Rheumatology Diagnostic Criteria for rheumatoid arthritis[23]

Diagnostic domain	Description	#	Points[a]
Joint involvement	Medium to large joints affected	1	0
		2–10	1
	Small joints affected	1–3	2
		4–10	3
		>10	5
Serologies	No positive RF or anti-CCP titer		0
	Low RF or anti-CCP titer[b]		2
	High RF or anti-CCP titer[c]		3
Duration of synovitis	>6 weeks duration		1
Acute phase reactants	Normal ESR and CRP		0
	Abnormal ESR or CRP		1

Notes: Patients receive the highest point total possible per diagnostic domain and require 6 out of 10 points for
[a] Diagnosis of rheumatoid arthritis (RA).
[b] Low titers are defined as being between 1 and 3 times the upper limit of normal.
[c] High titers are defined as being greater than 3 times the upper limit of normal.
Abbreviations: anti-CCP, anti-citrullinated peptide; RF, rheumatoid factor.

lung radiograph consistent with a pneumoconiosis (Caplan's syndrome).

Patients may present with tenderness at the craniocervical junction and may describe crepitation and/or the sensation of their head "falling forward" upon flexion. Palpation of the affected area may reveal a "clunking" when repeating movements.

17.4.2 Differential Diagnosis

Despite similarities in terms, the diseases AS, polymyalgia rheumatica, and RA are very different from one another. A peculiarity of RA is that, while the cervical spine is uniquely vulnerable, the lumbar spine is usually spared.

Diagnostic criteria for RA, revisited in 2010, include appropriate laboratory tests for the patient suspected of having RA (► Table 17.2). These include serologies such as RF and anti-citrullinated peptide (anti-CCP), as well as inflammatory markers such as ESR and CRP.[23]

17.4.3 Diagnostic Imaging

Imaging by conventional radiography is important to evaluate atlantoaxial instability, subaxial subluxation, or basilar invagination. AP, lateral, open-mouth, and flexion/extension views evaluate the atlantodental interval (ADI), spinal canal diameter, and indices for cranial settling.[14] CT or MRI may also be necessary as determined by clinical circumstances.

Atlantoaxial Instability

Measurement of the ADI has two components: the anterior atlantodental interval (AADI) and posterior atlantodental interval (PADI). The AADI is the distance from the posterior margin of the anterior arch of C1 to the anterior margin of the dens on a lateral view of the cervical spine. In normal healthy adults, the AADI is typically less than 3 mm and fixed with flexion-extension. Atlantoaxial instability is diagnosed with an AADI greater than 3 mm and increases with flexion and extension. The PADI is measured from the posterior border of the dens to the anterior margin of the posterior arch of C1. Normal values for the PADI are typically above 14 mm. Some studies report that the PADI is a more useful indicator of potential neurologic compromise, especially in the setting of concomitant cranial settling.[24]

Subaxial Subluxation

Subaxial subluxation is measured by evaluating for vertebral translation at affected cervical segments. A "shift" of 4 mm from the normal position indicates increased risks of cord compression. In smaller vertebral bodies (i.e., children), a shift of 20% of the total body width also indicates a similar increase in risk. The cervical height index can also be calculated to evaluate subaxial subluxation. This is performed by dividing the height of an affected vertebral body by its width. A cervical height index of less than 2 is highly sensitive and specific for neurologic compromise.

Basilar Invagination

Radiographic indices for basilar invagination include three scoring criteria: Clark station, Ranawat criterion, and Redlund-Johnell criterion, evaluated on lateral radiographs. Clark station divides the odontoid process into three equal stations (I, II, and III). This test is considered positive if the anterior arch of C1 lies in stations II or III. Ranawat criterion is met when a line drawn vertically through the pedicle of C2 intersects a horizontal line drawn through C1 at a length less than 15 mm in males or 13 mm in females. Redlund-Johnell criterion is evaluated by drawing a line from the midpoint of the caudal surface of the body of C2 to McGregor's line (a line drawn from posterior aspect of hard palate to caudal surface of occipital curve). Lengths less than 34 mm in males and 29 mm in females are considered positive. The combination of these three criteria is highly effective at screening for cranial settling (94% sensitivity) though they lack sufficient specificity.[25] CT or MRI should be considered to further evaluate these findings.

17.4.4 Treatment

Management of RA is primarily with medication to control progression of disease. Early detection and aggressive initiation of disease-modifying antirheumatic drugs (DMARDs) and biologic agents is both cost-effective and efficient at slowing the disease course.[26] Typical DMARDs used in the management of RA include methotrexate, leflunomide, sulfasalazine, and hydroxychloroquine. Biologic agents are often tumor necrosis factor inhibitors such as adalimumab and etanercept. Pharmacologic treatment has diminished the need for surgery, although many patients with refractory pain, neurologic deficits, and/or radiographic measures of instability still require operative intervention.

In cases where the radiographic measurements of the ADI are abnormal, various cutoffs have been reported as potential indications for surgery. For the AADI, cutoffs of 6 or 10 mm have been suggested, while for the PADI, values of 13 to 14 mm have been noted.[27,28,29,30] In either instance, the subluxation is considered unstable, and the risk of progression to spinal cord compression is increased, warranting arthrodesis of C1 and C2 (or occiput to C2 if basilar invagination is also present).[31]

Commonly employed techniques for fusion of C1–C2 include those of Magerl and of Goel-Harms. In Magerl's approach, C1 and C2 are approached posteriorly, with the use of transarticular screws to reduce instability. Invented in 1986, Magerl's technique quickly became the gold standard for C1–C2 arthrodesis given high fusion rates of 95–100% and elimination of post-operative immobilization with the halo vest.[32,33,34] In Goel-Harms technique, screws are placed into the lateral masses of C1 and the pars or pedicles of C2, followed by fixation with rods. A meta-analysis performed by Elliot et al in 2014 demonstrated no significant differences in fusion rates, 30-day post-operative mortality, or rates of neurologic injury between the two techniques.[35] Some studies report marginally increased rates of screw malalignment and vertebral artery injury in Magerl's technique.[35] Either approach is acceptable depending on the surgeon's experience and comfort. The peculiar anatomy and pathology of the patient must be considered to minimize risk of vertebral artery dissection. Pre-operative planning should include a pre-operative CT or CT angiogram to map out the path of the vertebral arteries, as a high-riding artery or narrow isthmus can prevent or preclude transarticular fixation.[31]

Often, posterior fusions are sufficient to reduce pannus formation and prevent further spinal cord compression. In rare instances, the pannus may not resolve following arthrodesis and may require odontoidectomy for residual ventral cord compression.

When basilar invagination is causing gross neurologic compromise, progressing with cranial settling > 5 mm, or if the cervicomedullary angle is < 135 degrees on MRI, occiput to C2 fusion is indicated, supplemented with resection of the odontoid in cases where there is significant brain stem compromise. Occipitocervical fixation is achieved by application of rigid plates from the occiput to at least C2, and may include resection of the C1 posterior arch. Resection of the posterior arch is performed in cases where atlantoaxial instability is also present.

Subaxial fusion is indicated for subluxation of 4 mm or > 20% of the width of the vertebral body in addition to intractable pain and/or neurologic compromise. The current technique of choice involves placement of lateral mass screws and rods. Three separate techniques, described by Magerl, Anderson, and An, differ with regards to screw entry point and orientation.[36] In one cadaveric study comparing these three approaches, the An technique was found to be the least likely to cause neurologic injury due to screw trajectory.[37] The An technique specifies screw direction should be ~30 degrees lateral and 15 degrees cephalad for C3 to C6, starting 1 mm medial to the center of the lateral mass.[37,38] At C7 to T2, the anterior-posterior diameter of the lateral mass is much smaller, and requires a more precise trajectory.[38]

17.5 Diffuse Idiopathic Skeletal Hyperostosis

Diffuse idiopathic skeletal hyperostosis (DISH) is a common systemic disease that preferentially affects the spine, and is often mistaken for AS due to its tendency to cause ossification of entheses and ligaments, leading to ankylosis. Some reports suggest that roughly 10% of people above the age of 50 are affected by DISH, pathogenesis remains unclear. Prevailing theories postulate that DISH may be caused by abnormal growth and function of osteoblasts in osteoligamentary binding.[39,40]

17.5.1 History and Examination

People diagnosed with DISH are frequently asymptomatic, the diagnosis having been made by distinctive incidental findings on imaging done for unrelated purposes. Symptoms may not appear until late middle or old age. In severe cases with large anterior osteophytes of the cervical spine, patients may also report dysphagia, hoarseness, sleep apnea, and/or stridor. As ossification progresses, the patient's spine stiffens, leading to increased risk of fractures from low-energy trauma. DISH is also associated with increased risk of spinal stenosis and neurogenic claudication.

DISH can also cause hyperostosis of peripheral articulations, including, but not limited to, the hands, knees, shoulders, and elbows. More distinctive entheses may be affected as well, including those of the Achilles or quadriceps tendons.

DISH is unique from other spondyloarthropathies in that it frequently occurs in patients with obesity, hypertension, diabetes mellitus, gout, and hyperlipidemia.[40] Accordingly, these patients will also have greater risk for stroke and coronary events.[41]

17.5.2 Differential Diagnosis

DISH most often occurs in the cervical and thoracolumbar segments and is diagnosed with the Resnick-Niwayama criteria: (1) ossification of the anterolateral aspects of four continuous vertebrae, (2) concurrent preservation of disc height, and (3) absence of features more characteristic of AS (facet joint ankylosis and SI joint degenerative changes) (▶ Fig. 17.1).[39]

Spondylosis and AS are perhaps the two most common conditions to be included in the differential diagnosis for DISH. Spondylosis is

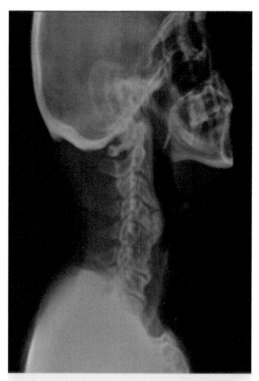

Fig. 17.1 Lateral extension-view conventional radiography (CR) of the cervical spine demonstrating significant anterior ossification of the anterior longitudinal ligament in diffuse idiopathic skeletal hyperostosis (DISH).

characterized by degenerative disc disease and stress-induced hypertrophy of vertebral column, although it differs from DISH due to lack of extensive ligamentous involvement. DISH classically causes ossification of the right side of the anterior longitudinal ligament on the thoracic spine. DISH rarely affects the SI joints and more frequently causes neurologic complications than AS.[42] Radiographic evaluation can also reveal differences between AS and DISH, including syndesmophyte appearance, preservation of disc height, and degree of ligamentous ossification.[43]

The clinician should also consider other ligamentous ossification diseases in the differential diagnosis of DISH: (1) ossification of the posterior longitudinal ligament (OPLL), (2) ossification of the ligamentum flavum (or ossification of the yellow ligament [OYL]), and (3) ossification of the nuchal ligament (ONL). While each condition is unique, each shares features of hypertrophic changes. Presence of one is an indication to assess the integrity of the entire spine, and a reason to consider full-length preoperative imaging.

OPLL is similar to DISH, although it has a predilection for the posterior longitudinal ligament in the cervical spine. OPLL is common among Asians, and has a high incidence of causing central stenosis and myelopathy. There are four subtypes of OPLL defined by their features on lateral radiographs: continuous, segmental, mixed-type, and localized. Continuous OPLL spans successive vertebral bodies and disc spaces while segmental is limited to ligamentous ossification posterior to the vertebral body alone. Mixed-type OPLL demonstrates features of both continuous and segmental phenotypes. Localized OPLL affects only the intervertebral disc spaces. Decompression is indicated for those that develop myelopathic symptoms and can be performed by laminectomy or laminoplasty and/or anteriorly by discectomy/corpectomy.

OYL occurs with ossification of the ligamentum flavum and can also cause myelopathy, although typically at the lower thoracic level.[44] OYL is sometimes not recognized in patients with concurrent lumbar spine pathology as symptoms between the two are clinically similar. This sometimes leads to disastrous consequences when undergoing decompression of the lumbar spine, as positioning may place significant pressure on the conus. Treatment of OYL is typically performed through posterior decompression and fusion at the affected level(s).

ONL, from its appearance and location, is not likely to be the source of symptoms, but, because it is frequently found in evaluations of patients with arthritic disease, its cause can be arguable. It has been noted to be present more frequently in patients who are diagnosed with DISH, OPLL, or OYL. It is sometimes misdiagnosed as an avulsion of the cervical spinous process(es) (clay-shoveler's fracture).

17.5.3 Diagnostic Imaging

AP and lateral radiographs of the affected region are helpful in evaluating for DISH. Characteristic findings include osteophyte formation primarily on the right side of the anterior longitudinal ligament along T7–T11 of the thoracic spine.[45] The reason for this asymmetry is unclear, although it is thought to be related to the position of the aorta in the thoracic cavity.[39]

The clinician can readily evaluate for enthesopathy or ossification with ultrasound or CT imaging, respectively. Furthermore, a history of neck pain or trauma should prompt the practitioner to order a CT and MRI to rule out fractures and/or epidural hematoma.

17.5.4 Treatment

Most cases of DISH can be managed conservatively with physical therapy, bracing, and activity modification. NSAIDs and bisphosphonate therapy may also be considered because they limit heterotopic ossification and osteophyte formation, respectively.[40] Stable fractures may be managed with cervical traction and bracing, although care must be taken to avoid over-distraction due to inherent ligamentous pathology. Unstable fractures, stenosis, deformity, and/or consequential myelopathy serve as indications for decompression and fusion.

17.6 Paget's Disease

Paget's disease (PD) is often considered a metabolic disease of the bone, and is characterized by increases in osteoblastic and osteoclastic activity. The vertebral column is the second most common site affected (pelvis is the first) by PD and can cause back pain, stenosis, and neural injury. Three phases describe the pathogenesis of PD: (1) an initial osteoclastic phase, (2) a last osteoblastic phase, and (3) a mixed osteoclastic/osteoblastic phase. Some report an additional fourth phase, where the bone is metabolically inactive and osteogenesis ceases temporarily.[46] Like DISH and other diseases of ligamentous ossification, PD can be considered a type of hypertrophic condition due to aberrancies in bone formation.

17.6.1 History and Examination

PD is a common disease that predominantly affects the bones of the skull, spine, pelvis, and appendicular skeleton. Patients will complain of symptoms based on the extent of their disease. Bone pain is due to osteolysis, and worsens at night or with weight-bearing. Bone enlargement may also be apparent, and gross deformity noticeable on examination. Due to the change in bone metabolic activity, the clinician may also feel increased warmth on palpation of affected area(s), often secondary to the increased vascularity of the region. After initial presentation, PD rarely spreads, as it is limited to the affected bones at the time of diagnosis.

PD also has a strong genetic component with high penetrance. First-degree relatives will often share the disease, although the pattern of involvement can differ. In addition, some studies report that PD may be a zoonosis, as antecedent paramyxoviral infection in dog, cat, bird, or cattle may trigger onset of PD in owners.[46]

Currently, there are four patterns of bone remodeling at the periosteal–endosteal interface that explain the anatomical changes seen on imaging: (1) periosteal apposition with normal endosteum, (2) periosteal apposition with endosteal resorption, (3) periosteal and endosteal apposition, and (4) focal periosteal apposition. In short, periosteal apposition is always present, although endosteal remodeling largely causes the anatomical heterogeneity seen in PD.

Skull involvement signals headaches and possible vision or hearing changes secondary to cranial nerve impingement. The patient may also have frontal bossing, causing complaints of an increasing hat size, or involvement of the facial bones, leading to lion-like facies. PD also affects the maxilla and mandible, and prompts the examiner to evaluate for changes in dentition. Excessive bone formation may cause symmetric enlargement of the alveolar ridge, spacing of teeth, ankylosis, and/or cementation and could warrant extraction.[47]

In limb involvement, progressive disease may lead to bowing of the femur or tibia, causing limb shortening and pain on ambulation or gait abnormalities. These findings are often only seen in late stages or poorly treated PD.

Hypertrophy of the vertebrae in PD can cause symptoms of back pain, spinal stenosis, radiculopathy, or myelopathy. When neurologic symptoms are present in PD, etiologies include: (1) compressive pagetic deformity secondary to remodeling, (2) vascular compromise, (3) trauma, or (4) compressive malignant transformation.[46] Neurologic symptoms are more common in the cervical and/or thoracic spine, and will present clinically distinct from lumbar spinal stenosis.

17.6.2 Differential Diagnosis

Due to diffuse deformity and sclerosis on imaging, the clinician should consider other metabolic diseases of bone and/or malignancies. Isolated sclerotic lesions may include enchondromas, bone infarcts, and enostoses. More diffuse involvement may signal hyperparathyroidism or malignancy (metastatic disease, leukemia, lymphoma). Appropriate laboratory studies and imaging assist in early detection of PD. Abnormalities detected on labs include elevated hemoglobin and high urine hydroxyproline, ALP, and/or calcium.

17.6.3 Diagnostic Imaging

The examiner should consider most imaging modalities in the evaluation of PD. Bone scans may detect unsuspected active PD, calling for further assessment. Characteristic findings are often present on plain radiographs, although CT and MRI can further evaluate the extent of disease and its sequelae.

Radiographs should include multiple views of symptomatic areas. Depending upon the phase of disease, bone density will often fluctuate and appear differently on plain films. During the lytic phase, diffuse focal lucencies and thinned cortices are often present. Conversely, blastic phases will demonstrate enlarged cortices. Mixed phases are a combination of the blastic phase with the lytic, accompanied by sclerotic lesions. The combination of lysis and thickening of trabeculae in PD results in a "honeycomb" appearance on conventional radiographs, and is easily confused with the more common vertebral hemangioma. PD can be distinguished by looking for evidence of thickened cortices and overall bone enlargement not seen in hemangiomas.

Regarding the spine, vertebral body changes are detectable on radiographs, and demonstrate increase in circumferential width. There are rarely increases in height as vertebral endplates do not truly form periosteal–endosteal junctions.[48] The earliest evidence of PD is seen during the mixed phase—trabecular bone hypertrophies in parallel to the endplates with concurrent periosteal–endosteal changes at the anterior and posterior borders. This collectively gives the vertebra a "picture frame" appearance.

CT allows for more sensitive evaluation of vertebral body and posterior element changes. Narrowing of the cortices and decreases in marrow content can easily be detected on axial cuts of affected vertebrae, allowing for characterization of the appositional changes that occur in remodeling of the spine. Reconstructions have utility in better depicting hypertrophic changes, especially in the early phase of the disease.

MRI has particular utility in studying the trabecular changes in the vertebral bodies. Frequently, signal intensities are heterogeneous on both T1- and T2-weighted images secondary to marrow changes. Less frequently, in severe sclerosis, the vertebral body may have significant signal dropout (corresponding with an "ivory vertebra" appearance on conventional radiographs). MRI also allows for sensitive evaluation of the soft tissues, and may be able to detect ossification of the epidural fat. Neuropathic symptoms also warrant the use of MRI as axial imaging can identify pagetic changes leading to compression of the spinal cord.

17.6.4 Treatment

PD is primarily treated conservatively (with NSAIDs) or with bisphosphonate therapy to inhibit osteoclastic activity. Calcitonin can be used as a second-line agent in refractory cases. Most patients experience relatively good control of PD with these medications. Parathyroid agents, such as teriperatide, are contraindicated in PD due to increased risk of osteosarcoma formation.

Surgical indications for PD are secondary to consequences of remodeling and hypertrophy in the spine. Stenosis and myelopathy are addressed with posterior decompression and fusion. In rare instances, Paget's lesions may also undergo malignant transformation to sarcoma, warranting excision. Due to the increased metabolic activity of bone in PD, pre-operative treatment with calcitonin or bisphosphonates is recommended to decrease vascularity, and limit intraoperative bleeding.[46]

17.7 Other Inflammatory Spine Disorders

17.7.1 Oligoarthritis

Oligoarthritis is a name applied to a specific syndrome of Juvenile Idiopathic Arthritis (JIA) that includes ocular, flu-like, and occasionally spinal pain manifestations. The syndrome should not be confused with the more familiar use of the term "oligoarthritis" meaning involving two to four joints.

17.7.2 Gout and Pseudogout

Gout rarely involves the spine, but when it does, it may cause inflammatory and mass-effect radiculopathy. The diagnosis should be suspected in the patient with acute spinal or radicular pain, an established diagnosis of gout, and an elevated uric acid. Gout tophi in the spinal canal may be observed as hypointense on T1 lesions. The diagnosis is confirmed if surgical specimen or aspirate from the site of pain generation reveals negatively birefringent needle-shaped monosodium urate crystals.

Pseudogout, another form of crystal inflammatory joint disease, can cause arthritic pain from facet joints and cord or root symptoms from mass effect of the inflamed periarticular tissues. Calcium pyrophosphate crystals are present in the inflamed tissues and appear as positively birefringent rhomboids under microscopy.

17.7.3 Synovitis, Acne, Pustulosis, Hyperostosis, and Osteitis Syndrome

Synovitis, Acne, Pustulosis, Hyperostosis, and Osteitis (SAPHO) syndrome is a rare inflammatory disease that shares many features with the spondyloarthropathies. The pathogenesis of SAPHO syndrome is believed to be a combination of genetic and environmental factors, as it also has a high prevalence of HLA-B27 and has been associated with low-grade infections with *Cutibacterium acnes, Staphylococcus aureus, Actinomyces, Treponema pallidum, Veillonella,* and *Eikenella*.[49,50] SAPHO syndrome primarily affects young adults, and as its name suggests, "synovitis, acne, pustulosis, hyperostosis and osteitis syndrome" presents with hyperostosis, osteitis, and synovitis, in addition to a number of dermatologic changes. It may also present with enthesitis and arthropathy, and primarily affects the sternocostal and sternoclavicular joints of the chest wall. SAPHO syndrome also affects the spine and may cause thoracic and lumbar pain correlated with unique patterns of signal changes on MRI.[51] Chronic Refractory Multifocal Osteomyelitis (CRMO) is a syndrome of recurrent osteomyelitis that presents patterns similar to SAPHO but is less likely to involve the spine.

17.7.4 Ochronosis (Alkaptonuria)

Ochronosis is a rare autosomal recessive metabolic disorder characterized by the inability to metabolize homogentisic acid. This leads to accumulation and damage of the body's connective tissues, and can cause quite striking imaging effects, especially of the intervertebral discs. Ochronotic spondyloarthropathy can also cause osteoporosis of the vertebral bodies and ossification of spinal ligaments. Surgical intervention may be required in cases of severe disc degeneration leading to herniation or spondylosis.

17.7.5 Additional Inflammatory Disorders

Many disorders not addressed in this chapter because they are not inflammatory diseases of the spine, must be included in the differential diagnosis of patients with inflammatory disorders of the spine because of shared features. Polymyalgia rheumatica (PMR), which is primarily a muscular disease, presents with back and shoulder pain, is accompanied by elevated inflammatory lab markers, and often responds dramatically to systemic corticosteroids. About 10% of people with PMR also have temporal arteritis and risk of cerebrovascular events. "Baastrup's Disease" refers to focal inflammatory reaction of soft tissue around contact areas of enlarged spinous processes. Radiation osteitis is most often due to bone damage and/or reaction to radiation therapy. Scheuermann's disease is a developmental disorder of unknown etiology, resulting in kyphosis. Infectious and noninfectious diseases of the meninges and spinal cord, such as multiple sclerosis, Guillain-Barre, and various forms of meningitis, all may have spinal pain and neurologic dysfunctions that cross over with symptoms of the musculo-skeletal spine. It is important that they be included in the differential diagnosis.

Though mentioned in the introduction to this chapter, it is worth repeating that considerations of infection of the spine are covered in Chapter 17 and to note that osteomyelitis and discitis are often not diagnosed early because of absence of fever and other classic signs of infectious disease.

17.8 Conclusion

Noninfectious inflammatory diseases of the spine are relatively common conditions that differentially affect components of the axial and peripheral skeleton. They affect the young, and many have a strong genetic association with the allele HLA-B27. Introduction of biologics and DMARDs has drastically improved the prognosis of these conditions, and has reduced the need for surgical intervention. However, in some circumstances, some patients may respond poorly to conservative therapy, and require surgery for refractory symptoms of pain, deformity, trauma, and/or to prevent disability. Such techniques include osteotomies (SPO, PSO, VCR, CEO) and single- or multi-level decompressions and fusions. Taken together, the spine surgeon requires a deep understanding of the inflammatory spondyloarthropathies to best diagnose and manage patients with spinal disorders.

Pearls

- The 20 to 30 something years old Caucasian males with non-mechanical low back pain should be specifically questioned regarding thoracic pain, morning stiffness, and family history. Their examination should include assessment of provocation of pain by sacroiliac (SI) stress and measurement of chest expansion. HLA-B27 antigen testing and response to anti-inflammatories, while not specific, may help with odds on correct identification of the pain generator.
- AS is a common disease. It may cause buttock and post-axial pain and cause straight leg raising intolerance. It may coexist with disc herniation, spondylolisthesis, and other conditions that may be treated surgically. BEWARE: operating for disc pathology when the source of pain was occult AS makes for a bad result—and it won't go away.
- The thoracic spine contains 12 intervertebral disc articulations, 24 facet joints, and 48 costovertebral articulations. That makes 84 joints. Have you ever wondered why patients with polyarticular joint disease have thoracic pain?
- When the complaint is pain in movement of the neck and examination shows that rotation hurts more than flexion and extension, be sure conventional radiographic assessment includes a good open mouth (OM) view. In an office setting, the OM is often OMitted, which can result in unforced error in the diagnosis of atlantoaxial pathology. The clue is pain worse with rotation.
- The surgeon's array of possible ways to decompress and/or correct deformity is as mind-boggling as the complexities of the patient's suffering and functional incapacities. With the exception of emergency, there should not be a rush to the operating room.
- The anatomy and pathology of the patient are considered to minimize risk of vertebral artery dissection in posterior fusions of C1 and C2.
- As medical therapies continue to improve, the number of surgeries has decreased in spondyloarthropathies. While it is generally good to be able to avoid surgery, the goal is to make and/or keep the patient better. Sometimes, surgery is conservative care.
- Just because it is an orthopedic spine clinic does not mean the patient's symptoms aren't from multiple sclerosis, polymyalgia rheumatica, or Parkinson's disease.
- Cervical spine imaging dimensions and effects of motion should accompany a pertinent history and physical examination to assess risks for patients with RA who are anticipating general anesthesia.

17.9 Case Examples

17.9.1 Case 1

A previously healthy 37-year-old male presents with 3 months of persistent, moderate, mildly progressive midthoracic back pain, worsened with exercise. The patient denied any other symptoms, although he notes a distant history of two episodes of skin sloughing from his hands in his early 20 s. On examination, the patient appears healthy, with findings notable for thoracic tenderness to palpation, as well as pain on forward flexion and extension of the thoracolumbar spine. Neurologic examination and laboratory studies were normal. CT and MRI are shown (▶ Fig. 17.2).[51] Two biopsies and positron emission tomography (PET) scans were subsequently unremarkable, leading ultimately to suspicion for spondyloarthritic findings of SAPHO syndrome.

17.9.2 Case 2

A 36-year-old male comes in for evaluation after a motor vehicle accident. The patient notes a distant history of bilateral uveitis and periodic swelling and pain in his knees and shoulders. On examination, the patient shows significant limitations in flexion, extension, and rotation of his neck, and can only bring his gaze parallel to the floor. Movement of his shoulders and hips results in moderate pain, although the range of motion appears within normal limits. He has no range of motion of the lumbar spine, although he can bring his fingertips down to his shins when bending laterally. Imaging of the lumbar spine is shown (▶ Fig. 17.3). CT and MRI were negative for occult fracture. The patient was diagnosed with AS, given celecoxib for pain, and referred to rheumatology.

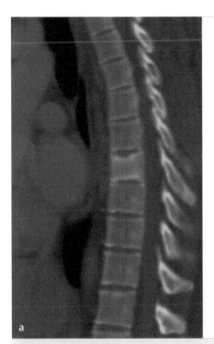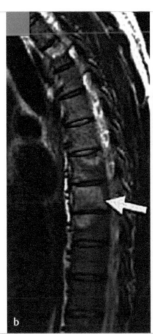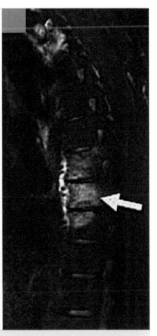

Fig. 17.2 (a, b) Computed tomography (CT) and magnetic resonance imaging (MRI) of the thoracic spine showing mild sclerosis and endplate irregularities at the T8 vertebral body. T2-weighted and short-T1 inversion recovery (STIR) images showing hyperintense bone marrow edema. Note the reverse C-pattern of signal changes in contiguous vertebrae (*arrows*) typical of synovitis, acne, pustulosis, hyperostosis, and osteitis (SAPHO).

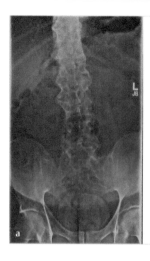
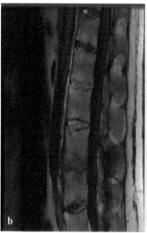

Fig. 17.3 Anteroposterior (AP) CR of the lumbar spine showing advanced arthropathic changes with loss of definition of the intervertebral disc, facet, and sacroiliac (SI) joints **(a)**. Lateral magnetic resonance imaging (MRI) of the lumbar spine demonstrating prominent squaring off of the vertebral bodies with marginal syndesmophyte formation spanning disc spaces **(b)**. Replacement of disc soft tissues and joint lining creates symmetrically spaced nodularity of a rigid spine, the pattern of bamboo, hence occasionally called "bamboo spine", typical of advanced ankylosing spondylitis (AS).

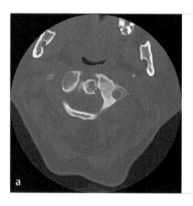
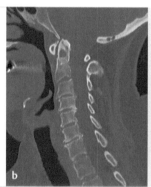

Fig. 17.4 (a, b) Axial and sagittal computed tomography (CT) views of C1–C2 showing a large lytic lesion of the dens. The eccentric positioning of the dens on axial CT is indicative of instability. No specific diagnosis was reached in the evaluation of this patient.

17.9.3 Case 3

A 78-year-old female presents with complaints of a left-sided posterior headache for over a year. The pain radiates up into her scalp on the left side of her head and is associated with stiffness and pain with neck movement. She denies radiation of pain into her arms, clumsiness, loss of sensation, or weakness. She was treated with anti-inflammatories, physical therapy, and numerous steroid injections without any relief. On examination, her neck motion was found to be grossly limited secondary to pain. Her temporal arteries are palpable and non-tender, and neurologic examination was unremarkable. Plain radiographs revealed loss of C1–C2 joint space with sclerotic endplates. CT of the cervical spine was ordered and revealed significant left-sided C1–C2 arthritis, evidence of rotational instability (dens sitting eccentrically toward the right), and erosive lesion of the dens (▶ Fig. 17.4). Treatment-resistant pain led to a C1–C4 posterior fusion, which gave her very satisfying relief.

17.9.4 Case 4

A 48-year-old obese male presents with 4 months of right chest wall and right lower back pain after a ground level fall. At the time of injury, he was found to have a fracture of the right tenth rib, although he notes his pain has never improved. On examination, the patient was non-tender to palpation and percussion around the ribs, and demonstrated no difficulty with breathing or reaching overhead. Radiographs of the chest revealed large osteophytes along the right side of his thoracic spine suggestive of DISH (▶ Fig. 17.5). CT imaging of the thoracic spine showed ossification of the ligamentum flavum (yellow ligament) extending beneath the T5 and T6 laminae on both sides (▶ Fig. 17.6). MRI showed effacement of the thecal sac. There were no signal changes within the cord.

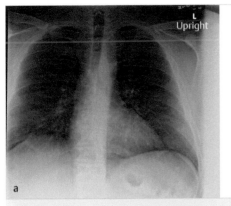
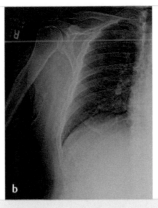
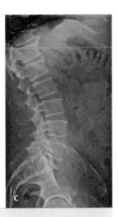

Fig. 17.5 (a–c) Anteroposterior (AP) radiographs of the chest and lumbar spine showing diffuse osteophyte formation along the right side of the thoracic spine and non-marginal syndesmophyte formation at the thoracolumbar junction, suggestive of diffuse idiopathic skeletal hyperostosis (DISH).

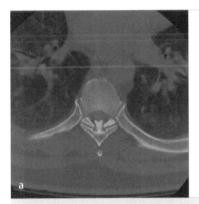
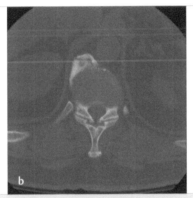
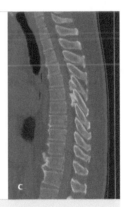

Fig. 17.6 (a–c) Axial and sagittal cuts showing the thoracic spine, revealing ossification of the ligamentum flavum at T5–T6 and right-sided anterior osteophyte formation at T12–L1.

He is being evaluated every 6 months and urgently if symptoms of myelopathy arise. He understands his situation, is compliant with restrictions, and wishes to avoid surgery. His findings demonstrate that the permutations of spinal and paraspinal heterotopic ossification are in some, as yet, undefined way related.

17.9.5 Case 5

A 30-year-old man presents with a chief complaint of 10 years of episodic, severe back pain that acutely worsened 2 weeks ago. The pain has improved, although he now notes radiation of symptoms down the left buttock and lower extremity. His pain is bilateral in the lumbar spine, crossing midline, although without symptoms of radiation

down the right lower extremity. On examination, the patient was reluctant to sit down due to pain, although he had no localizing signs of motor or sensory dysfunction. Paraspinal muscles were tense and range of motion in the lumbar spine was significantly decreased. Chest expansion measured between 1 and 1½ inches. Radiographs of the lumbar spine and pelvis revealed questionable sclerotic changes at the SI joints and absorption of the apophyseal beaks. MRI revealed subtle evidence of inflammation at the SI joints (▶ Fig. 17.7). The patient was subsequently found to have elevated inflammatory markers (ESR, CRP), and positive HLA-B27. The patient was diagnosed with an undifferentiated spondyloarthropathy, with greatest concern for AS, and referred to rheumatology for medical management.

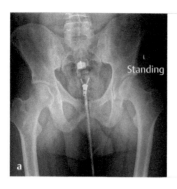
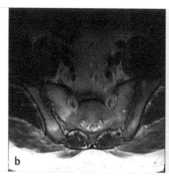

Fig. 17.7 (a, b) CR and T2-weighted magnetic resonance imaging (MRI) demonstrating questionable sclerotic changes and increased signal intensity of the sacroiliac (SI) joints.

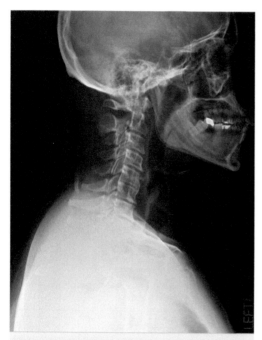

Fig. 17.8 Lateral CR of the cervical spine showing spondylosis primarily at C5–C6 and ossification of the nuchal ligament, *not* an avulsion fracture of a cervical spinous process ("clay-shoveler's" fracture).

17.9.6 Case 6

A 51-year-old man was referred to the orthopedic clinic. He came wearing a soft cervical collar. He said he had slipped and fallen and had some neck pain but did not think he was badly injured. He had no symptoms of neurological dysfunction and no past history of significant neck injury. Imaging at the walk-in clinic on the day of injury caused the examining doctor to be concerned for fracture (▶ Fig. 17.8). The patient wanted to stop using the collar. He was permitted normal functions without the collar and was asymptomatic in a few days.

17.9.7 Case 7

A 37-year-old male presents after a work-related injury 5 months ago when hauling heavy machinery. At that time, he heard a crack in his back, followed by intense pain. The patient has since been unable to return to work despite anti-inflammatory medications and physical therapy. His pain is constant, sharp, worsens with activity, and is primarily mid-thoracic with radiation to the anterior chest wall. Examination was notable for decreased spinal range of motion secondary to pain primarily centered at the thoracolumbar junction. Radiographs at the time of injury were notable for mild anterior disc protrusion at T10–T11. HLA-B27 was found to be negative, and the patient was initially advised to follow-up as needed. His symptoms persisted in the following year, warranting reevaluation. CT revealed advanced left T8 costovertebral joint arthritis, probably due to injury (▶ Fig. 17.9). Surgical treatment, such as by costo-transversectomy, was obviated by injections of corticosteroids into the area. He gradually improved.

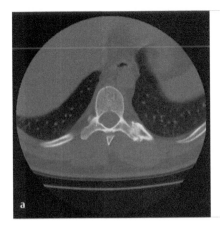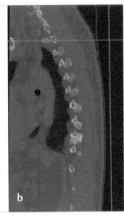

Fig. 17.9 (a, b) Axial and sagittal computed tomography (CT) images of T8 demonstrating left-sided costovertebral posttraumatic arthropathy.

17.10 Board-style Questions

1. A 65-year-old woman with AS presents with acute onset of neck pain after being involved in a low-speed motor vehicle accident. The patient denies any other injuries and has a grossly normal motor and neurologic examination. A CT scan of the cervical spine shows a stable extension-type fracture of the C6 vertebral body with diffuse formation of bridging syndesmophytes across adjacent segments. The patient is placed in a cervical orthosis and admitted for monitoring. What is the most appropriate next step in management?
   a) Discharge if asymptomatic for 6 hours with plans for follow-up
   b) Place patient in Gardner-Wells traction
   c) Schedule for anterior cervical discectomy and fusion of C6–C7
   d) Schedule for posterolateral decompression and fusion of C6–C7
   e) Obtain additional MRI studies

2. A 55-year-old woman with RA presents to clinic for follow-up. At her last visit, the patient was found to have an anterior atlantodens interval (AADI) of 4.4 mm (7 and 3.6 mm on flexion-extension, respectively). Today the patient is asymptomatic, and clinical examination is normal. Repeat radiographs of the cervical spine reveal an AADI of 11 (13 and 8 mm on flexion-extension, respectively). Clark station was III. The patient is scheduled for surgery and preoperative imaging is obtained. On CT, the patient is found to have narrow cervical isthmuses bilaterally and a high-riding vertebral artery. Which of the following is the most appropriate surgical technique for this patient?

   a) Magerl's technique for C1–C2 fusion
   b) Goel-Harms technique for C1–C2 fusion
   c) An technique for C1–C2 fusion
   d) Occiput to C2 fusion
   e) Occiput to C3 fusion

3. A 53-year-old man, with a medical history of heart failure, diabetes, and obesity, comes in with complaints of 6 months of low back pain and stiffness that is at its worst in the early morning. Radiographs of the lumbar spine reveal non-marginal formation of syndesmophytes from L1 to L5 vertebrae. What is the next most appropriate step in management?
   a) Conservative management
   b) Referral to rheumatology for evaluation of possible AS
   c) Conduct advanced imaging to inspect for occult fracture
   d) Schedule for lumbar decompression and fusion
   e) Test for HLA-B27

4. A 44-year-old male with history AS comes in to the emergency department with acute onset of neck pain after experiencing a fall down a flight of stairs. On examination, the patient is found to have weakness of the upper extremities bilaterally. Advanced imaging of the cervical spine reveals an unstable extension-type fracture of C4 and evidence of a compressive anterior epidural hematoma. What is the next most appropriate step in management?
   a) Posterior fusion of C3–C5
   b) Posterior fusion of C3–C7
   c) Occipitocervical fusion to C5
   d) Anterior cervical discectomy/corpectomy and fusion of C3–C5
   e) Conservative management

Answers

1. e
2. e
3. a
4. d

References

[1] Reveille JD. Epidemiology of spondyloarthritis in North America. Am J Med Sci. 2011; 341(4):284–286

[2] El Maghraoui A. Osteoporosis and ankylosing spondylitis. Joint Bone Spine. 2004; 71(4):291–295

[3] Momeni M, Taylor N, Tehrani M. Cardiopulmonary manifestations of ankylosing spondylitis. Int J Rheumatol. 2011; 2011:728471

[4] Rezvani A, Ergin O, Karacan I, Oncu M. Validity and reliability of the metric measurements in the assessment of lumbar spine motion in patients with ankylosing spondylitis. Spine. 2012; 37(19):E1189–E1196

[5] Raychaudhuri SP, Deodhar A. The classification and diagnostic criteria of ankylosing spondylitis. J Autoimmun. 2014; 48–49:128–133

[6] Fisher LR, Cawley MI, Holgate ST. Relation between chest expansion, pulmonary function, and exercise tolerance in patients with ankylosing spondylitis. Ann Rheum Dis. 1990; 49(11):921–925

[7] van der Linden S, Valkenburg HA, Cats A. Evaluation of diagnostic criteria for ankylosing spondylitis: a proposal for modification of the New York criteria. Arthritis Rheum. 1984; 27(4):361–368

[8] Kubiak EN, Moskovich R, Errico TJ, Di Cesare PE. Orthopaedic management of ankylosing spondylitis. J Am Acad Orthop Surg. 2005; 13(4):267–278

[9] Grigoryan M, Roemer FW, Mohr A, Genant HK. Imaging in spondyloarthropathies. Curr Rheumatol Rep. 2004; 6(2):102–109

[10] Suk K-S, Kim K-T, Lee S-H, Kim JM. Significance of chin-brow vertical angle in correction of kyphotic deformity of ankylosing spondylitis patients. Spine. 2003; 28(17):2001–2005

[11] Thumbikat P, Hariharan RP, Ravichandran G, McClelland MR, Mathew KM. Spinal cord injury in patients with ankylosing spondylitis: a 10-year review. Spine. 2007; 32(26):2989–2995

[12] Kurucan E, Bernstein DN, Mesfin A. Surgical management of spinal fractures in ankylosing spondylitis. J Spine Surg. 2018; 4(3):501–508

[13] Gill JB, Levin A, Burd T, Longley M. Corrective osteotomies in spine surgery. J Bone Joint Surg Am. 2008; 90(11):2509–2520

[14] Song K, Su X, Zhang Y, et al. Optimal chin-brow vertical angle for sagittal visual fields in ankylosing spondylitis kyphosis. Eur Spine J. 2016; 25(8):2596–2604

[15] Buckland AJ, Puvanesarajah V, Vigdorchik J, et al. Dislocation of a primary total hip arthroplasty is more common in patients with a lumbar spinal fusion. Bone Joint J. 2017; 99-B(5):585–591

[16] Holden W, Orchard T, Wordsworth P. Enteropathic arthritis. Rheum Dis Clin North Am. 2003; 29(3):513–530, viii

[17] Sankowski AJ, Lebkowska UM, Cwikla J, Walecka I, Walecki J. Psoriatic arthritis. Pol J Radiol. 2013; 78(1):7–17

[18] Peluso R, Di Minno MND, Iervolino S, et al. Enteropathic spondyloarthritis: from diagnosis to treatment. Clin Dev Immunol. 2013; 2013:631408

[19] Cheeti A, Ramphul K. Arthritis, Reactive (Reiter Syndrome). In: StatPearls. Treasure Island, FL: StatPearls Publishing; 2018

[20] Resnick D. Inflammatory disorders of the vertebral column: seronegative spondyloarthropathies, adult-onset rheumatoid arthritis, and juvenile chronic arthritis. Clin Imaging. 1989; 13(4):253–268

[21] Reiter MF, Boden SD. Inflammatory disorders of the cervical spine. Spine. 1998; 23(24):2755–2766

[22] Gillick JL, Wainwright J, Das K. Rheumatoid arthritis and the cervical spine: a review on the role of surgery. Int J Rheumatol. 2015; 2015:252456

[23] Aletaha D, Neogi T, Silman AJ, et al. Rheumatoid arthritis classification criteria: an American College of Rheumatology/European League Against Rheumatism collaborative initiative. Arthritis Rheum. 2010; 62(9):2569–2581

[24] Heidari B. Rheumatoid arthritis: early diagnosis and treatment outcomes. Caspian J Intern Med. 2011; 2(1):161–170

[25] Riew KD, Hilibrand AS, Palumbo MA, Sethi N, Bohlman HH. Diagnosing basilar invagination in the rheumatoid patient: the reliability of radiographic criteria. J Bone Joint Surg Am. 2001; 83(2):194–200

[26] Sizova L. Approaches to the treatment of early rheumatoid arthritis with disease-modifying antirheumatic drugs. Br J Clin Pharmacol. 2008; 66(2):173–178

[27] Papadopoulos SM, Dickman CA, Sonntag VK. Atlantoaxial stabilization in rheumatoid arthritis. J Neurosurg. 1991; 74(1):1–7

[28] Boden SD, Dodge LD, Bohlman HH, Rechtine GR. Rheumatoid arthritis of the cervical spine: a long-term analysis with predictors of paralysis and recovery. J Bone Joint Surg Am. 1993; 75(9):1282–1297

[29] Oda T, Yonenobu K, Fujimura Y, et al. Diagnostic validity of space available for the spinal cord at C1 level for cervical myelopathy in patients with rheumatoid arthritis. Spine. 2009; 34(13):1395–1398

[30] Kawaida H, Sakou T, Morizono Y, Yoshikuni N. Magnetic resonance imaging of upper cervical disorders in rheumatoid arthritis. Spine. 1989; 14(11):1144–1148

[31] Mallory GW, Halasz SR, Clarke MJ. Advances in the treatment of cervical rheumatoid: less surgery and less morbidity. World J Orthop. 2014; 5(3):292–303

[32] Magerl F, Seemann P-S. Stable Posterior Fusion of the Atlas and Axis by Transarticular Screw Fixation. In: Kehr P, Weidner A, eds. Cervical Spine I: Strasbourg 1985. Vienna: Springer Vienna; 1987:322–327

[33] Fielding JW, Hawkins RJ, Ratzan SA. Spine fusion for atlanto-axial instability. J Bone Joint Surg Am. 1976; 58(3):400–407

[34] Sen MK, Steffen T, Beckman L, Tsantrizos A, Reindl R, Aebi M. Atlantoaxial fusion using anterior transarticular screw fixation of C1-C2: technical innovation and biomechanical study. Eur Spine J. 2005; 14(5):512–518

[35] Elliott RE, Tanweer O, Boah A, et al. Outcome comparison of atlantoaxial fusion with transarticular screws and screw-rod constructs: meta-analysis and review of literature. J Spinal Disord Tech. 2014; 27(1):11–28

[36] Mohamed E, Ihab Z, Moaz A, Ayman N, Haitham AE. Lateral mass fixation in subaxial cervical spine: anatomic review. Global Spine J. 2012; 2(1):39–46

[37] Xu R, Haman SP, Ebraheim NA, Yeasting RA. The anatomic relation of lateral mass screws to the spinal nerves: a comparison of the Magerl, Anderson, and An techniques. Spine. 1999; 24(19):2057–2061

[38] An HS, Gordin R, Renner K. Anatomic considerations for plate-screw fixation of the cervical spine. Spine. 1991; 16 (10) Suppl:S548–S551

[39] Nascimento FA, Gatto LAM, Lages RO, Neto HM, Demartini Z, Koppe GL. Diffuse idiopathic skeletal hyperostosis: a review. Surg Neurol Int. 2014; 5 Suppl 3:S122–S125

[40] Mader R, Verlaan J-J, Eshed I, et al. Diffuse idiopathic skeletal hyperostosis (DISH): where we are now and where to go next. RMD Open. 2017; 3(1):e000472

[41] Kiss C, Szilágyi M, Paksy A, Poór G. Risk factors for diffuse idiopathic skeletal hyperostosis: a case-control study. Rheumatology (Oxford). 2002; 41(1):27–30

[42] Vaishya R, Vijay V, Nwagbara IC, Agarwal AK. Diffuse idiopathic skeletal hyperostosis (DISH)—a common but less known cause of back pain. J Clin Orthop Trauma. 2017; 8(2):191–196

[43] Tsukamoto Y, Onitsuka H, Lee K. Radiologic aspects of diffuse idiopathic skeletal hyperostosis in the spine. AJR Am J Roentgenol. 1977; 129(5):913–918

[44] Park DA, Kim SW, Lee SM, Kim CG, Jang SJ, Ju CI. Symptomatic myelopathy caused by ossification of the yellow ligament. Korean J Spine. 2012; 9(4):348–351

[45] Toyoda H, Terai H, Yamada K, et al. Prevalence of diffuse idiopathic skeletal hyperostosis in patients with spinal disorders. Asian Spine J. 2017; 11(1):63–70

[46] Hadjipavlou AG, Gaitanis LN, Katonis PG, Lander P. Paget's disease of the spine and its management. Eur Spine J. 2001; 10(5):370–384

[47] Sabharwal R, Gupta S, Sepolia S, et al. An insight in to Paget's disease of bone. Niger J Surg. 2014; 20(1):9–15

[48] Dell'Atti C, Cassar-Pullicino VN, Lalam RK, Tins BJ, Tyrrell PN. The spine in Paget's disease. Skeletal Radiol. 2007; 36(7): 609–626

[49] Rozin AP, Nahir AM. Is SAPHO syndrome a target for antibiotic therapy? Clin Rheumatol. 2007; 26(5):817–820

[50] Arnson Y, Rubinow A, Amital H. Secondary syphilis presenting as SAPHO syndrome features. Clin Exp Rheumatol. 2008; 26(6):1119–1121

[51] Basques BA, Kontzialis M, Fardon DF. Vertebral osteitis as the manifestation of SAPHO syndrome: a case report and review of the literature. Rush Orthop J. 2018:26–9

18 Management of Early Onset Scoliosis

Daniel J. Miller and Patrick J. Cahill

Abstract

Early onset scoliosis (EOS) describes a structural lateral curvature of the spine in a young child. Although defined based on coronal plane parameters, EOS represents a complex three-dimensional deformity with sagittal and/or axial plane abnormalities as well. By definition, EOS occurs during critical periods of thoracic maturation. As such, progressive EOS has the potential for deleterious effects on cardiopulmonary development and function if left untreated. EOS has numerous etiologies with idiopathic, neuromuscular, syndromic, and congenital forms being the most prevalent. Children with EOS represent a heterogeneous population with significant variability in severity of spinal deformity, age, function, cognition, and medical comorbidities. Because of this variability, a patient-centered approach to care is critical. Treatment options for EOS include observation, serial casting, bracing, and surgery. Observation is indicated in mild and/or nonprogressive deformities. Serial casting has demonstrated success in curing cases of infantile idiopathic scoliosis (IIS), particularly if initiated early. Bracing may prevent curve progression in patients with EOS, although the literature regarding outcomes of bracing in EOS is sparse. Surgery is indicated for severe and/or progressive deformities that are not amenable to nonoperative modalities. Surgical options for EOS include distraction-based constructs, guided growth systems, and compression-based techniques. Although these techniques vary in their approach, all share a common goal of controlling spinal deformity while maximizing growth and development of the spine and thorax. Spinal fusion is avoided in patients with significant growth remaining because of the potential for iatrogenic thoracic insufficiency syndrome. Despite recent advances in the care of EOS, complications are frequent and long-term outcomes reveal numerous areas for process improvement.

Keywords: scoliosis, kyphosis, Mehta casting, magnetically controlled growing rods (MCGR)

18.1 Introduction

Early onset scoliosis (EOS) is defined as a structural lateral curvature of the spine measuring greater than 10 degrees on a posteroanterior (PA) radiograph diagnosed in a patient less than 10 years old. Although the exact incidence of EOS is not known, it represents approximately 4–10% of patients with idiopathic scoliosis.[1]

EOS is a heterogeneous condition associated with multiple etiologies including neuromuscular, idiopathic, structural, syndromic, and congenital forms. Treatment of congenital scoliosis is specifically tied to the underlying defects in vertebral formation and/or segmentation and is outside the scope of this chapter.[2,3]

Because EOS occurs during critical periods of cardiopulmonary maturation, untreated progressive spinal and thoracic deformity has potential for substantial morbidity and an increased rate of mortality in the long term.[4,5]

18.2 History and Examination

Evaluation of the child with EOS consists of a complete history, physical examination, and multisystem review of systems. Typically, patients have a known underlying medical diagnosis by the time of referral. Careful scrutiny is required to evaluate for any occult neuromuscular, syndromic, and/or congenital condition in a patient with presumed idiopathic scoliosis. Review of the patient's birth and developmental history is for events and/or items that may suggest perinatal brain injury. Caregivers should be queried regarding the patient's qualitative pulmonary function. The assisted ventilation rating (AVR) may be used to quantify the degree of external respiratory support patients require on a regular basis. The Early Onset Scoliosis Questionnaires (EOSQ-24) is a validated disease-specific instrument that evaluates health-related quality of life for patients with EOS and the burden of the disease on their caregivers.[6]

Physical examination should include assessment of the child's spinal balance, seating posture, and standing posture (when able). The Adam's forward bend test is used to evaluate the degree of axial spinal deformity. Dermatological examination should be attentive to hairy patches, sacral dimples, and/or café au lait spots that may be suggestive of spinal dysraphism. A complete neurologic examination, including assessing for ankle clonus and abdominal reflex asymmetry, is essential.

Prior to surgery, multidisciplinary medical optimization with careful attention to the patient's nutrition status is critical toward minimizing the risk of perioperative complications such as surgical site infection.

18.3 Diagnostic Imaging

Plain radiographs (AP and lateral views) of the entire spine are the first line modality for evaluating deformity in EOS. Upright standing or sitting films should be utilized when able as these images incorporate the influence of gravity on the spine. The degree of spinal deformity is quantified using the Cobb technique. Measures of spinal balance include pelvic obliquity, coronal balance, and sagittal balance. Numerous measures have been described to quantify the thoracic volume including the space available for lung (SAL)[7] and the thoracic height.[8] In patients with IIS, the Rib Vertebra Angle Difference (RVAD), originally described by Mehta, has been demonstrated to predict curve progression and resolution.[9] In her series of 138 patients with IIS, ~80% of the cases of progressive case were associated with an RVAD of> 20 degrees, whereas ~80% of spontaneously resolving cases were associated with an RVAD of< 20 degrees.[9] Overlap of the rib head on the vertebral body due to rotation at the apex of a curve (e.g., a phase 2 rib) is associated with an increased rate of progression in IIS when compared patients with no such overlap (e.g., phase 1 rib).[9]

Stress radiograph films in the form of supine, side bending, fulcrum bending, and/or traction may be used to help determine curve flexibility, level selection, and correction maneuvers. Preoperative magnetic resonance imaging (MRI) is recommended prior to surgical intervention to evaluate for neuraxial abnormality, which has an increased incidence in several forms of EOS. A computed tomography (CT) scan with three-dimensional reconstruction and/or modeling may be obtained to better understand the osseous anatomy and to assist with instrumentation in patients with EOS. All radiographs and advanced imaging should be evaluated closely for evidence of congenital vertebral abnormalities, such as occult spina bifida, that may complicate surgical treatment.

18.4 Treatments

Given the heterogeneous nature of EOS, no simple recipe exists for management of spinal deformity in this unique and diverse patient population. Recent research has demonstrated significant variability in management of EOS among experienced surgeons.[10,11] Despite this, universal treatment principles are well agreed upon. Management of EOS should aim to control spinal deformity and maximize spinal, thoracic, and cardiopulmonary growth while minimizing complications and negative effects of treatment on the patient's quality of life.[12]

Treatment options for EOS include observation, bracing, casting, and surgery. Observation is indicated in cases of mild deformity. Bracing may be utilized in patients with moderate deformity (e.g., 20–45 degrees); however, bracing is typically unable to correct existing spinal deformity and it is unclear whether bracing can positively influence the natural history of curve progression in EOS. Furthermore, some patients are unable to tolerate bracing secondary to pulmonary and/or skin related issues.

Serial casting has demonstrated success in curing several cases of IIS, particularly if initiated early.[9] Although serial casting is not associated with complete resolution of spinal deformity in patients with neuromuscular, syndromic, and/or congenital scoliosis, it may have a beneficial role in delaying the need for surgical intervention in children with EOS.[13,14]

Indications for surgical treatment of EOS include severe (e.g., > 50 degrees) and/or progressive spinal deformity in patients on whom nonoperative management has either failed or is likely to fail. Contraindications to surgical intervention include patients with active infection, soft tissue compromise, insufficient bone stock, and those who are medically unfit for surgery and/or anesthesia secondary to comorbid medical conditions.

Surgical options for EOS include distraction-based constructs, guided growth systems, and compression-based techniques.[15] Spinal fusion, the typical surgical treatment for severe spinal deformity in patients at or near skeletal maturity, is avoided in patients with EOS because of the association with iatrogenic thoracic insufficiency syndrome.[4,8,16] We typically avoid definitive spinal fusion in patients less than 10 years old or in those with a thoracic height of less than 22 cm, although these cutoffs vary based on the metabolic and functional demands of the patient.

Compression-based techniques (e.g., vertebral body stapling) rely on gradual deformity correction by growth inhibition on curve convexity via compressive forces and are typically reserved for patients with juvenile idiopathic scoliosis.[15] Guided growth systems (e.g., Shilla) involve limited apical fusion and segmental spinal instrumentation that is fixed posteriorly to stainless steel rods, allowing for continued spinal growth and deformity correction without the need for surgical lengthening.[17] Unfortunately, this technique is associated with a high rate of complications and has not been widely accepted nationally or internationally.[18,19] Furthermore, compression-based techniques such as vertebral body stapling or tethering are only indicated in idiopathic deformities and have limited utility in patients less than 9 years of age given the possibility of overcorrection.

Distraction-based systems apply tensile forces posteriorly to correct and control spinal deformity. These forces are applied directly or indirectly to the spine via anchors that are connected with intervening telescoping and/or linked rods. The intervening rod(s) segments are periodically lengthened over time, allowing for growth of the spine and thorax while controlling spinal deformity.[20]

Traditional growing distraction-based systems required lengthening every 4–12 months via an open surgical procedure. Newly developed magnetically controlled growing rods (MCGR) allow for transcutaneous lengthening via a handheld magnetic external remote controller. Because of the decreased need for lengthening procedures (and the associated risks with each of those procedures), we typically prefer MCGR for surgical treatment of EOS, unless contraindicated by patient size, sagittal alignment, curve rigidity, underlying condition that may require MRI of the spine, chest, or abdomen (such as neurofibromatosis), or co-existing implanted magnetic devices (including magnetically gated ventriculoperitoneal shunts).

Dual rod constructs are associated with fewer complications and improved deformity correction when compared to single rod constructs and should be utilized when possible.[21] Proximal anchors, either spine based or rib based, are placed at the proximal portion of the spinal deformity, typically in the proximal thoracic spine. Our current practice is to use multiple proximal anchors (e.g., ≥ 4) in order to distribute load, thereby decreasing the risk of proximal anchor failure. Distal anchors are placed at the distal aspect of the spinal deformity. In ambulatory patients, this is typically in the mid-lumbar spine. Pelvic instrumentation (in the form of hooks or screws) is typically utilized in non-ambulatory patients with significant pelvic obliquity. Postoperatively, a cast or brace is generally not necessary. Transcutaneous lengthening of MCGR is performed in the outpatient setting after wound healing. Surgeon preference regarding the amount and frequency of lengthening varies. We typically aim to lengthen each rod 5 mm every 3 months for patients 5–10 years of age. Lengthening every 3–6 months is associated with a decreased rate of reoperation compared to more frequent lengthening.[22] At or near skeletal maturity, MCGR are removed and patients are treated with spinal fusion.

18.5 Outcomes

The heterogeneous nature of EOS presents a dilemma when evaluating the efficacy of MCGR or other treatment modalities. Multiple studies have demonstrated that MCGR are effective at maintaining or improving deformity correction in patients with EOS.[23,24,25,26,27,28] Compared to traditional growing rods, MCGR are associated with a higher overall caregiver satisfaction and avoid the need for repeated lengthening surgeries.[29] Despite this, complications in patients managed with MCGR are common, and nearly half of all patients will require at least one unplanned operation for a variety of reasons including failure of rod distractions, proximal anchor failure, rod breakage, and/or infection.[22,23,26] Additionally, actual increases in MCGR length frequently appear to be less than programmed distraction (particularly in children with larger soft tissue envelopes), and are susceptible to a decreased lengthening, and/or failure to lengthen over time.[30,31,32] Furthermore, there are numerous reports of significant metallosis surrounding the implants at mid- to long-term follow-up; however, the long-term ramifications of this metallosis is unknown.[33,34]

- Obtain a screening spine MRI in all patients with idiopathic EOS to evaluate for neuraxial abnormality.
- Scrutinize preoperative imaging for anatomic variants.
- Multidisciplinary preoperative medical optimization is essential to decrease the risk of perioperative complications.
- Counsel families on the high rate of complications with long-term growth-sparing constructs.
- Avoid performing long spinal fusions in skeletally immature patients with EOS to prevent iatrogenic thoracic insufficiency syndrome.
- Use fluoroscopy to localize incisions for proximal and distal anchors to minimize exposure and soft tissue dissection.
- Use multiple proximal anchors (e.g., ≥ 4) in distraction-based construct to decrease the risk of proximal anchor failure.
- Use pelvis anchors in non-ambulatory patients with significant pelvic obliquity.
- A temporary rod can provisionally achieve deformity correction and allow for precise measurement of MCGR.
- Contour implants to maintain a low-profile position, particularly in patients with limited soft tissue coverage.

18.6 Case Example

A 7-year-old male presented with a long-standing history of idiopathic spinal deformity. He denied any pain or neurologic symptoms. A screening MRI of the spine and neural axis demonstrated no significant neuraxial abnormality. He trialed bracing with a thoracic lumbar sacral orthosis (TLSO) but was noted to have continued deformity progression.

Plain radiographs of the entire spine show a right main thoracic curvature measuring 51 degrees without any associated congenital abnormalities (▶ Fig. 18.1, ▶ Fig. 18.2, and ▶ Fig. 18.3).

He subsequently underwent insertion of bilateral MCGR from T3 to L1 with bilateral rib anchors between T3 and T5 and bilateral pedicle screw fixation distally at T12 and L1.

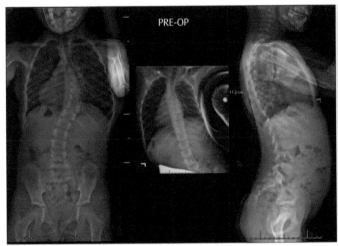

Fig. 18.1 Preoperative posteroanterior (PA), fulcrum bending, and lateral radiographs show significant thoracic spinal deformity in without evidence of congenital anomalies.

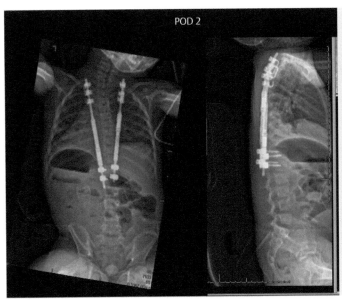

POD 2

Fig. 18.2 Initial postoperative PA and lateral images show the dual magnetically controlled growing rod construct with improved alignment.

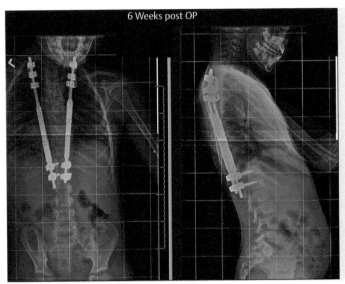

6 Weeks post OP

Fig. 18.3 PA and lateral images 6 weeks following surgery show maintained alignment without evidence of implant complication.

18.7 Board-style Questions

1. A 5-year-old male presents for follow-up evaluation of IIS. The deformity was first noticed at age 2. He has been managed with a TLSO brace which he wears only part time. A previous screening spine MRI demonstrated no neuraxial abnormalities. New X-rays demonstrate a double major curve that has progressed to over 60 degrees. Physical examination is normal save for coronal decompensation and a positive Adam's forward bend test. Which of the following treatment modalities is contraindicated?
a) MCGR in a rib to spine construct
b) MCGR in a spine to spine construct
c) Traditional growing rods in a rib to spine construct
d) Traditional growing rods in a rib to spine construct
e) Posterior spinal fusion T2–L3

2. A 6-year-old female is referred to you for evaluation of juvenile idiopathic scoliosis. The deformity was first noticed at age 4 and has progressed to 55 degrees over the course of 2 years despite physical therapy and bracing. The patient denies any back pain or neurologic symptoms. There is no family history of spinal deformity. On physical examination, she is well appearing and breathing comfortably on room air. Spine examination reveals a large thoracic prominence. Skin examination is unremarkable. Neurologic examination demonstrates asymmetric abdominal reflexes but is otherwise normal. X-rays demonstrate a 55-degree right thoracic scoliosis without congenital vertebral abnormalities. Which of the following additional tests is required prior to considering surgical intervention?
   a) Renal ultrasound
   b) MRI of spine and neural axis
   c) Bone scan
   d) Echocardiography
   e) C-reactive protein

3. A 15-month-old male presents for evaluation after his pediatrician noted a prominence in his back on a well child examination. He is the product of a full-term normal spontaneous vaginal delivery and has been growing and developing normally as per his pediatrician. There is no family history of spinal deformity. On physical examination, he is well appearing and breathing comfortably on room air. Spine examination reveals a left thoracic prominence which is accentuated with Adam's forward bend test. Skin and neurologic examination are within normal limits. X-rays reveal a thoracic scoliosis without congenital vertebral or chest wall abnormalities. Which of the following findings would be most suggestive of future curve progression?
   a) Left thoracic curve
   b) Curve magnitude of 17 degrees
   c) RVAD of 26 degrees
   d) Age 15 months
   e) Phase 1 rib-vertebral relationship

Answers ✔

1. e
2. b
3. c

References

[1] Riseborough EJ, Wynne-Davies R. A genetic survey of idiopathic scoliosis in Boston, Massachusetts. J Bone Joint Surg Am. 1973; 55(5):974–982

[2] Hedequist D, Emans J. Congenital scoliosis. J Am Acad Orthop Surg. 2004; 12(4):266–275

[3] Hedequist DJ. Surgical treatment of congenital scoliosis. Orthop Clin North Am. 2007; 38(4):497–509, vi

[4] Vitale MG, Matsumoto H, Roye DP, Jr, et al. Health-related quality of life in children with thoracic insufficiency syndrome. J Pediatr Orthop. 2008; 28(2):239–243

[5] Pehrsson K, Larsson S, Oden A, Nachemson A. Long-term follow-up of patients with untreated scoliosis: a study of mortality, causes of death, and symptoms. Spine. 1992; 17 (9):1091–1096

[6] Matsumoto H, Williams B, Park HY, et al. The Final 24-Item Early Onset Scoliosis Questionnaires (EOSQ-24): validity, reliability and responsiveness. J Pediatr Orthop. 2018; 38(3): 144–151

[7] Campbell RM, Jr, Smith MD, Mayes TC, et al. The characteristics of thoracic insufficiency syndrome associated with fused ribs and congenital scoliosis. J Bone Joint Surg Am. 2003; 85(3):399–408

[8] Karol LA, Johnston C, Mladenov K, Schochet P, Walters P, Browne RH. Pulmonary function following early thoracic fusion in non-neuromuscular scoliosis. J Bone Joint Surg Am. 2008; 90(6):1272–1281

[9] Mehta MH. The rib-vertebra angle in the early diagnosis between resolving and progressive infantile scoliosis. J Bone Joint Surg Br. 1972; 54(2):230–243

[10] Williams BA, Asghar J, Matsumoto H, Flynn JM, Roye DP, Jr, Vitale MG. More experienced surgeons less likely to fuse: a focus group review of 315 hypothetical EOS cases. J Pediatr Orthop. 2013; 33(1):68–74

[11] Corona J, Miller DJ, Downs J, et al. Evaluating the extent of clinical uncertainty among treatment options for patients with early-onset scoliosis. J Bone Joint Surg Am. 2013; 95(10):e67

[12] Gomez JA, Lee JK, Kim PD, Roye DP, Vitale MG. "Growth friendly" spine surgery: management options for the young child with scoliosis. J Am Acad Orthop Surg. 2011; 19(12): 722–727

[13] Baulesh DM, Huh J, Judkins T, Garg S, Miller NH, Erickson MA. The role of serial casting in early-onset scoliosis (EOS). J Pediatr Orthop. 2012; 32(7):658–663

[14] Fletcher ND, McClung A, Rathjen KE, Denning JR, Browne R, Johnston CE, III. Serial casting as a delay tactic in the treatment of moderate-to-severe early-onset scoliosis. J Pediatr Orthop. 2012; 32(7):664–671

[15] Skaggs DL, Akbarnia BA, Flynn JM, Myung KS, Sponseller PD, Vitale MG, Chest Wall and Spine Deformity Study Group, Growing Spine Study Group, Pediatric Orthopaedic Society of North America, Scoliosis Research Society Growing Spine Study Committee. A classification of growth friendly spine implants. J Pediatr Orthop. 2014; 34(3):260–274

[16] Karol LA. Early definitive spinal fusion in young children: what we have learned. Clin Orthop Relat Res. 2011; 469(5): 1323–1329

[17] McCarthy RE, Luhmann S, Lenke L, McCullough FL. The Shilla growth guidance technique for early-onset spinal deformities at 2-year follow-up: a preliminary report. J Pediatr Orthop. 2014; 34(1):1–7

[18] McCarthy RE, McCullough FL. Shilla growth guidance for early-onset scoliosis: results after a minimum of five years of follow-up. J Bone Joint Surg Am. 2015; 97(19):1578–1584

[19] Sucato DJ. Guiding growth is promising but can it compare with growth promotion? Commentary on an article by Richard E. McCarthy, MD, and Frances L. McCullough, MNSc: "Shilla Growth Guidance for Early-Onset Scoliosis. Results After a Minimum of Five Years of Follow-up". J Bone Joint Surg Am. 2015; 97(19):e66

[20] Akbarnia BA, Marks DS, Boachie-Adjei O, Thompson AG, Asher MA. Dual growing rod technique for the treatment of progressive early-onset scoliosis: a multicenter study. Spine. 2005; 30(17) Suppl:S46–S57

[21] Thompson GH, Akbarnia BA, Kostial P, et al. Comparison of single and dual growing rod techniques followed through definitive surgery: a preliminary study. Spine. 2005; 30(18): 2039–2044

[22] Kwan KYH, Alanay A, Yazici M, et al. Unplanned reoperations in magnetically controlled growing rod surgery for early onset scoliosis with a minimum of two-year follow-up. Spine. 2017; 42(24):E1410–E1414

[23] Lebon J, Batailler C, Wargny M, et al. Magnetically controlled growing rod in early onset scoliosis: a 30-case multicenter study. Eur Spine J. 2017; 26(6):1567–1576

[24] Thompson W, Thakar C, Rolton DJ, Wilson-MacDonald J, Nnadi C. The use of magnetically-controlled growing rods to treat children with early-onset scoliosis: early radiological results in 19 children. Bone Joint J. 2016; 98-B(9):1240–1247

[25] Yılmaz B, Ekşi MS, Işık S, Özcan-Ekşi EE, Toktaş ZO, Konya D. Magnetically controlled growing rod in early-onset scoliosis: a minimum of 2-year follow-up. Pediatr Neurosurg. 2016; 51(6):292–296

[26] Choi E, Yaszay B, Mundis G, et al. Implant complications after magnetically controlled growing rods for early onset scoliosis: a multicenter retrospective review. J Pediatr Orthop. 2017; 37(8):e588–e592

[27] Hosseini P, Pawelek J, Mundis GM, et al. Magnetically controlled growing rods for early-onset scoliosis: a multicenter study of 23 cases with minimum 2 years follow-up. Spine. 2016; 41(18):1456–1462

[28] Cheung KM, Cheung JP, Samartzis D, et al. Magnetically controlled growing rods for severe spinal curvature in young children: a prospective case series. Lancet. 2012; 379(9830): 1967–1974

[29] Doany ME, Olgun ZD, Kinikli GI, et al. Health-related quality of life in early-onset scoliosis patients treated surgically: EOSQ scores in traditional growing rod versus magnetically controlled growing rods. Spine. 2018; 43(2):148–153

[30] Ahmad A, Subramanian T, Panteliadis P, Wilson-Macdonald J, Rothenfluh DA, Nnadi C. Quantifying the "law of diminishing returns" in magnetically controlled growing rods. Bone Joint J. 2017; 99-B(12):1658–1664

[31] Gilday SE, Schwartz MS, Bylski-Austrow DI, et al. Observed length increases of magnetically controlled growing rods are lower than programmed. J Pediatr Orthop. 2018; 38(3): e133–e137

[32] Cheung JPY, Yiu KKL, Samartzis D, Kwan K, Tan BB, Cheung KMC. Rod lengthening with the magnetically controlled growing rod: factors influencing rod slippage and reduced gains during distractions. Spine. 2017

[33] Rushton PRP, Siddique I, Crawford R, Birch N, Gibson MJ, Hutton MJ. Magnetically controlled growing rods in the treatment of early-onset scoliosis: a note of caution. Bone Joint J. 2017; 99-B(6):708–713

[34] Teoh KH, von Ruhland C, Evans SL, et al. Metallosis following implantation of magnetically controlled growing rods in the treatment of scoliosis: a case series. Bone Joint J. 2016; 98-B (12):1662–1667

19 Thoracic Disc Disorders

Colin B. Harris and Jacob R. Ball

Abstract

Thoracic disc disorders are an uncommon and often overlooked condition that may have a varied clinical presentation including axial back pain, radicular symptoms, or myelopathy with spinal cord involvement. Given wide variations in clinical presentation, a high index of suspicion must be present when evaluating patients with potential thoracic disc pathology. A detailed history and physical examination including neurologic examination and evaluation for myelopathic signs is mandatory for all such patients. Although most patients can be treated successfully with nonoperative treatment measures including physical therapy, anti-inflammatory pain medication, and less commonly, interventional pain management, a small subset of patients will benefit from surgery. Surgical intervention is generally reserved for patients with myelopathy or spinal cord compression given the significant morbidity associated with surgery. Commonly used approaches include anterior thoracotomy or minimally invasive transthoracic decompression using tubular retractors, as well as posterior approaches, including transpedicular decompression, costotransversectomy, and lateral extracavitary, in order of increasing midline exposure. Fusion may be necessary when spinal stability is compromised or in the presence of spinal deformity. Patients with ossification of the posterior longitudinal ligament and higher degrees of thoracic kyphosis are challenging to treat and historically have experienced poorer outcomes with surgical intervention. As newer and less invasive treatment methods continue to evolve, patient outcomes should continue to improve and become more reliable with surgical intervention.

Keywords: thoracic spine, thoracic disc herniation, myelopathy, transthoracic, discectomy, transpedicular, costotransversectomy

19.1 Introduction

Thoracic disc disorders are a rare clinical entity, comprising less than 5% of all symptomatic disc herniations and accounting for less than 2% of all surgical procedures performed for herniated discs.[1] The vast majority of patients can be treated nonoperatively, with surgical intervention limited to those rare patients with myelopathic symptoms, neurological deficits or intractable radicular pain despite appropriate conservative treatment. Diagnosis can be difficult, as classic dermatomal radicular patterns seen in cervical and lumbar disc herniations are often absent, and a high index of suspicion is necessary. Although surgery has been classically associated with poor outcomes and potential for neurologic decline in the past, modern surgical techniques have greatly improved the ability to treat thoracic disc herniations successfully and with much lower complication rates.

19.2 Pathogenesis

The vast majority of thoracic disc herniations are thought to be degenerative in nature, although a minority of patients report a history of trauma antecedent to the onset of symptoms. Links to adolescent Scheuermann's disease have been suggested but definitive evidence is lacking. In addition to disc pathology, thoracic spinal stenosis and its associated symptoms can also be caused by thoracic ossification of the ligamentum flavum, ossification of the posterior longitudinal ligament (OPLL), and spondylosis secondary to hypertrophic facet changes. These pathologic conditions can be challenging to treat and may require surgical strategies different from thoracic disc herniation, to be discussed later in this chapter. The thoracic spinal cord has a limited ability to tolerate compression given the narrow thoracic canal and tenuous blood supply in this region, and patients may develop neurological deficit secondary to both direct mechanical compression and vascular insult. In contrast to lumbar disc herniations, thoracic disc herniations have a tendency to be located centrally in the canal and have calcified components, further complicating management.

19.3 Clinical Presentation

Patients with thoracic disc disorders may present with a variety of symptoms, often without an easily identifiable clinical syndrome. In addition to back pain which may be midline or paraspinal in cases of more lateral disc herniations, patients may present with sensory disturbances below the level of pathology, motor weakness, or bowel and bladder dysfunction, which is generally a late finding. Radiation of pain to the anterior chest wall at the level of pathology can be present, as well as abdominal pain, chest pain, and periscapular pain. Primary complaints of chest pain should be expeditiously evaluated by an internist or cardiologist, and if a cardiac workup is negative then thoracic disc pathology may be included in the differential diagnosis. Patients may present with more classic symptoms of myelopathy, including gait disturbance and balance problems, which can be distinguished from cervical myelopathy by the absence of upper extremity long tract signs and normal hand function.

Thoracic ossification of the ligamentum flavum can also be easily misidentified due to its slow progression and frequent presence of additional lumbar pathology. Patients typically present with gait disturbance, but there is also an association with progressive loss of vibratory sensation and proprioception (posterior cord syndrome) followed by upper motor neuron signs in the lower extremities as the cord compression worsens.[2] OPLL conversely presents with upper motor neuron signs earlier in the course of disease than it typically occurs in ossification of the ligamentum flavum.[3]

In physical examination, in addition to evaluation of the patient's gait and global alignment in the coronal and sagittal planes, a thorough neurologic examination should be performed. This should include motor and sensory testing including the chest and abdomen to evaluate for a thoracic sensory level, in addition to reflex testing and noting the presence of any pathologic reflexes, including brisk or absent deep tendon reflexes, upgoing Babinski sign, and sustained clonus. The presence of Hoffman's sign or hyper-reflexia in the upper extremities should alert the clinician to a cervical, rather than thoracic, etiology; although in rare instances, spinal cord compression in both regions can be present, a variation of cervical and lumbar tandem stenosis is more common. The abdomen should be examined for any masses, guarding, and abnormal bowel sounds, and a thorough vascular examination including peripheral pulses should be performed.

19.4 Imaging Findings

Although rarely diagnostic for this condition, standing orthogonal radiographs of the thoracic spine are the most appropriate initial imaging modality (▶ Fig. 19.1a, b). The presence of degenerative disc

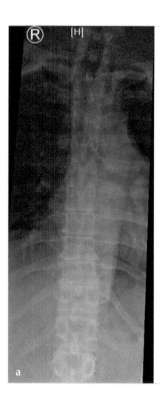
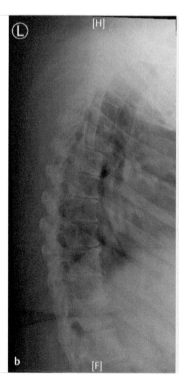

Fig. 19.1 Anteroposterior (AP) **(a)** and lateral **(b)** standing radiographs of the thoracic spine for patient with T11–T12 thoracic disc herniation. Note nonspecific findings of spinal asymmetry and multilevel degenerative findings.

changes, disc space calcifications, scoliosis or kyphosis, and an ossification pattern consistent with either Diffuse Idiopathic Skeletal Hyperostosis (DISH) or Ankylosing Spondylitis (AS) can have treatment implications and also help establish a differential diagnosis for thoracic pain syndromes. The suggestion of a calcified disc in the spinal canal on a lateral plain radiograph can be helpful in establishing the diagnosis of a disc herniation but should be followed by advanced imaging. Magnetic resonance imaging (MRI) is the gold standard test for diagnosis of thoracic disc disease and thoracic disc herniation. No radiation is involved, and both the disc pathology and neural elements including the spinal cord, thecal sac and exiting nerve roots can be clearly identified (▸ Fig. 19.2a–c). Multilevel disc herniations are noted on MRI in approximately 25–40% of cases, and determining which level is causing a specific symptom pattern can be challenging.[4] In cases of a suspected calcified disc herniation or in patients with stainless steel implants, pacemakers, or other contraindications to MRI, a computed tomography (CT) myelogram can be helpful. Despite the more invasive nature of the CT myelogram, better delineation of disc calcification is possible which can be helpful for surgical planning in patients with spinal cord compression. Provocative discography has been reported in the thoracic spine but is not commonplace and its role is limited in the evaluation of these disorders.

19.5 Classification Systems

Thoracic disc herniations have been classified as central, centrolateral (paracentral), or lateral (foraminal), with the majority being central or centrolateral.[5] Although several original studies were done using CT myelography, the findings are consistent with MRI findings, and no reliable imaging characteristics have been found to correlate with symptoms; therefore, imaging findings alone should not guide treatment. Lateral herniations are more likely to cause root compression and thoracic radicular symptoms, while disc herniations at T11–T12 and T12–L1 can cause conus medullaris compression with resultant bowel and bladder disturbances or pain referred to the lower extremities.[6] The presence of calcification within a thoracic disc herniation is not uncommon and should be noted, as calcified discs may require wider exposure to remove and have specific surgical implications. Likewise, OPLL has been associated with poorer outcomes following surgical intervention, although it can be easily identified preoperatively by CT reconstructions.[7] The severity of OPLL can be estimated by the occupancy ratio measured on CT imaging. Occupancy ratios greater than 30% and lateral OPLL are the most common signs present in patients with myelopathy.[3] Thoracic ossification of the ligamentum flavum can be graded by the Sato classification system (A–E) and

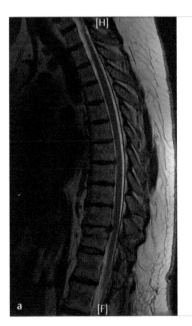
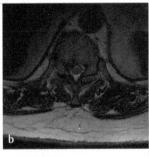
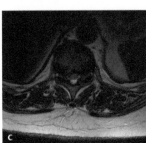

Fig. 19.2 Mid-sagittal (a) and axial (b, c) T2-weighted magnetic resonance imaging (MRI) images of the same patient depicted in ▸ Fig. 19.1, showing right T11–T12 disc herniation and facet hypertrophy causing right-sided thoracic radicular pain without myelopathy.

worsening of ossification can lead to increased stenosis and, ultimately, cord infarction.[2] Intradural disc herniations are rare and can be difficult to identify on MRI preoperatively due to cerebrospinal fluid (CSF) flow void sign, a phenomenon related to the pulsatile flow of CSF during MRI examination. They are more often associated with neurologic deficits and if suspicion is high, a preoperative CT myelogram is recommended to better delineate the pathoanatomy.

19.6 Treatment

19.6.1 Conservative Treatment

The majority of thoracic disc herniations are asymptomatic and may be found incidentally or associated with acute or subacute axial back pain syndromes. While no treatment may be necessary for the majority of patients, anti-inflammatory pain medication, muscle relaxants, and a directed exercise program to improve posture and spinal extensor strength are appropriate for them. Bracing plays little role in the treatment of thoracic disc disorders but can be helpful for patients with concomitant scoliosis or Scheuermann's disease. For patients with persistent and disabling pain, despite a reasonable conservative treatment course, referral to interventional pain management for diagnostic or therapeutic intercostal or trigger point injections can be helpful. Thoracic interlaminar epidural injections can be performed safely but are not utilized as commonly as lumbar injections due to the increased risk of injections at cord level and lack of clear-cut radicular patterns present in the lumbar spine that often guide treatment. It should be noted that neither thoracic OPLL nor thoracic ossification of the ligamentum flavum typically respond well to conservative management due to the late stage of presentation in many patients, as well as association with neurologic symptoms.

19.6.2 Indications for Surgery

Broadly speaking, indications for surgery include thoracic disc herniation confirmed with MRI or CT myelogram and presence of myelopathy of moderate to severe degree, progressive lower extremity neurologic deficit, bowel or bladder involvement, or disabling thoracic radicular pain that persists despite extensive conservative treatment. Surgical

indications are similar for thoracic stenosis secondary to OPLL, ligamentum flavum ossification, or spondylosis. There is reasonable consensus that axial thoracic back pain in the absence of any of the above criteria should be treated conservatively except in rare circumstances. Concomitant disorders such as thoracic scoliosis, Scheuermann's disease, or prior lumbar fusion with flat-back syndrome may necessitate surgical treatment which would otherwise not be recommended for an isolated thoracic disc problem; however, a thoracic discectomy may need to be incorporated as part of the surgical plan. The size of the thoracic disc herniation is not a reliable predictor of the need for surgery, as a subset of small herniations have been associated with neurologic deficits and should not be ignored, and some large herniations can be asymptomatic.[8]

19.6.3 Surgical Considerations

Intraoperative localization is the first challenge to be considered in all surgical cases addressing thoracic disc pathology. The reasons for this include lack of easily identifiable pathology on fluoroscopy, difficulty counting from the first or twelfth rib especially in the mid-thoracic spine, and kyphosis or large body habitus leading to difficulty interpreting imaging. Strategies to minimize the risk of wrong-level surgery include use of intraoperative CT navigation, placement of a metallic fiducial marker preoperatively under CT guidance, and full-length preoperative spine x-rays and MRI of the entire neural axis, so that true disc spaces can be counted from the sacrum to the level of disc pathology and matched to a plain radiograph.[9,10]

Laminectomy via midline approach and disc excision were commonly performed in the past for thoracic disc disorders; however, this is of historical value only due to the high rate of postoperative neurologic decline most likely caused by the manipulation of the thoracic cord (▶ Fig. 19.3). With a greater understanding of thoracic disc disorders and surgical anatomy, both anterior and posterior approaches are now widely accepted and can result in excellent outcomes when applied appropriately. It is best to tailor the treatment approach to each individual patient as no one approach can be considered a panacea to all clinical situations; for example, posterior approaches may be favored in older patients or those with restrictive lung

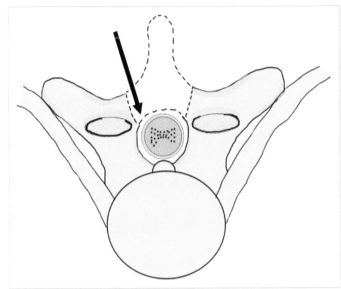

Fig. 19.3 Image showing bone resection and relationship to spinal cord and facets with a thoracic laminectomy via midline approach. *Arrow* indicates path of instruments necessary to perform disc resection. (Reproduced with permission, from Currier BL, Eck JC, Eismont FJ, Green BA. Thoracic Disc Disease. In: Garfin SR, Eismont FJ, Bell GR, Fischgrund JS, Bono CM, eds. Rothman-Simeone and Herkowitz's The Spine. New York, NY: Elsevier; 2018:787–805.)

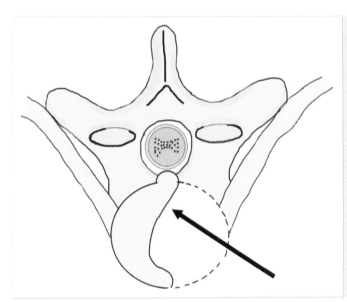

Fig. 19.4 Image showing partial disc resection accomplished through transthoracic (left-sided) approach to thoracic disc herniation, with *arrow* indicating access to central and centrolateral portions of disc. (Reproduced with permission, from Currier BL, Eck JC, Eismont FJ, Green BA. Thoracic Disc Disease. In: Garfin SR, Eismont FJ, Bell GR, Fischgrund JS, Bono CM, eds. Rothman-Simeone and Herkowitz's The Spine. New York, NY: Elsevier; 2018:787–805.)

disease that are unlikely to tolerate a thoracotomy. Open transthoracic approaches have the advantage of direct access to the central portions of the disc and do not require fusion if the disc can be resected unilaterally and no postoperative instability is anticipated; however, they require rib resection, lung retraction, and postoperative chest tube placement, and carry significant risk of approach-related morbidity (▶ Fig. 19.4). Minimally invasive

lateral approaches using tubular retractors offer a similar midline exposure and with less soft tissue trauma and morbidity; however, the learning curve can be steep, similar to other minimally invasive techniques including endoscopic and thoracoscopic discectomies.[11] Video-assisted thoracoscopic surgery (VATS) has the advantage of avoiding rib resection with less postoperative pain and respiratory issues. However, it is technically

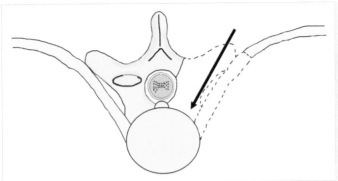

Fig. 19.5 Image showing pedicle, facet, and rib resection secondary to left-sided costotransversectomy, with *arrow* indicating access to lateral and paracentral portions of disc. (Reproduced with permission, from Currier BL, Eck JC, Eismont FJ, Green BA. Thoracic Disc Disease. In: Garfin SR, Eismont FJ, Bell GR, Fischgrund JS, Bono CM, eds. Rothman-Simeone and Herkowitz's The Spine. New York, NY: Elsevier; 2018:787–805.)

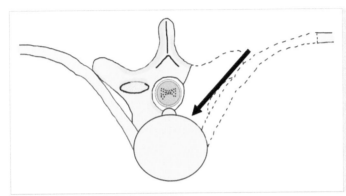

Fig. 19.6 Image showing pedicle, facet, and rib resection secondary to left-sided lateral extracavitary approach, with *arrow* indicating wider access to central portions of disc compared to costotransversectomy. (Reproduced with permission, from Currier BL, Eck JC, Eismont FJ, Green BA. Thoracic Disc Disease. In: Garfin SR, Eismont FJ, Bell GR, Fischgrund JS, Bono CM, eds. Rothman-Simeone and Herkowitz's The Spine. New York, NY: Elsevier; 2018:787–805.)

challenging and is associated with many of the same risks as open transthoracic approaches. Posterior approaches have gained wide favor in recent years and can be thought of as a continuum with transpedicular, costotransversectomy (▶ Fig. 19.5), and lateral extracavitary (▶ Fig. 19.6) approaches, offering progressively greater midline exposure but at the expense of greater soft tissue dissection and rib resection. Transpedicular approaches are the least invasive and can offer exposure of foraminal and some paracentral disc herniations but would require cord manipulation for central or calcified discs, which are best approached through a more lateral extracavitary or transthoracic approach (▶ Table 19.1). As minimally invasive techniques continue to be refined, they will likely play a greater role in optimizing patient outcomes with less approach-related morbidity. Other considerations for the addition of fusion with instrumentation to decompression include patients with large calcified transdural discs, herniation at the thoracolumbar junction, spinal deformities, multiple contiguous herniations, and significant bone resection leading to instability.[12]

19.6.4 Surgical Techniques and Postoperative Care

When undertaking an anterior (transthoracic) approach, the patient is placed in the lateral decubitus position to expose the side of pathology in more lateral disc herniations, while central disc herniations can generally be approached from either side. Upper thoracic discs are often best approached from the right to avoid the heart and great vessels, while lower thoracic discs are often approached from the left to avoid the more friable vena cava and liver.[13] Single lung ventilation is generally performed and communication with the anesthesiologist prior to intubation is necessary. Rib resection is performed based on radiographic marking of the pathologic disc, usually 1–2 ribs above the level of interest. The pleura can be bluntly dissected

Table 19.1 Summary of various surgical approaches to thoracic disc herniations

Approach	Indications	Advantages	Disadvantages
Transthoracic (Thoracotomy)	Central or calcified disc herniations	Wide access to disc can address calcified discs and OPLL	Rib resection and lung retraction required Postoperative pain, respiratory issues
Minimally invasive lateral transthoracic	Same as transthoracic, lateral discs	Retropleural Less trauma to lung Central and lateral access	Steep learning curve Postoperative pneumothorax
Transpedicular	Lateral and some paracentral disc herniations	Limited morbidity Not destabilizing if performed unilaterally	Limited access to central disc without cord manipulation
Costotransversectomy	Lateral and paracentral disc herniations	Greater midline exposure than transpedicular	Generally requires fusion, central disc difficult to access
Lateral extracavitary	Central, paracentral, and lateral disc herniations	Greater midline exposure than costotransversectomy	Requires fusion Larger bone and soft tissue dissection

Abbreviation: OPLL, ossification of the posterior longitudinal ligament.

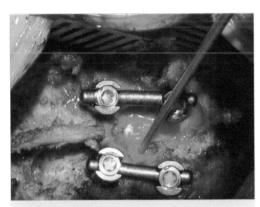

Fig. 19.7 Image demonstrating left transpedicular approach to the T9–T10 disc space, with left T9–T10 complete facetectomy, resection of superior pedicle and bilateral T9–T10 pedicle screw instrumentation. Surgical instrument is pointing to the disc space. Cephalad is to the left of the image and caudal to the right. (Image courtesy of Ira Goldstein, MD, with permission.)

along the chest wall until the spine is visible, and the lung is retracted while the disc space is accessed. Limited or complete discectomy as well as partial corpectomies can be performed to visualize across midline and decompress the thoracic cord, followed by fusion with rib graft or structural cages, if necessary. Closure is performed after placing a chest tube, although extrapleural and minimally invasive tubular approaches may not require chest tube placement.

Transpedicular approaches involve unilateral or bilateral facetectomy and the resection is then based on the pedicle of the caudal level (T10 for a T9–T10 discectomy), which is resected with a high-speed burr, allowing access to the lateral third of the disc space (▶ Fig. 19.7). Costotransversectomy is often performed through a paramedian incision on the side of the pathology, followed by excision of the transverse process, facet, and pedicle in addition to the head and neck of the rib. The pleura is then bluntly retracted to expose the disc space, making visualization of the lateral and paracentral regions of the disc possible. Lateral extracavitary approaches involve greater rib resection and a more lateral to medial trajectory, with increased soft tissue dissection and bone removal, but greater access to the central portion of the disc. Subtotal and total discectomies generally require fusion, and laminectomy as well as pedicle screw instrumentation can be performed concomitantly (▶ Fig. 19.8a, b). Reverse-angled curettes and a high-speed burr are helpful in managing central or calcified disc herniations. Intradural disc herniations present unique challenges, and they may be missed on preoperative imaging unless a high index of suspicion is present. Dural repair is routinely necessary in these cases prior to closure, and they often require grafting as primary repair which is generally not feasible. Surgical drains are placed, and a meticulous closure is necessary to avoid wound compromise and late pseudomeningocele formation, with patients mobilized postoperatively without the need for a brace in most cases.

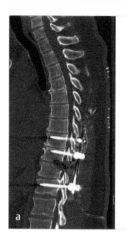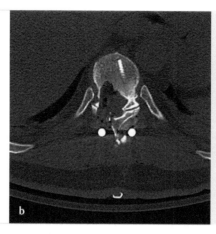

Fig. 19.8 Postoperative sagittal (**a**) and axial (**b**) computed tomography (CT) images of a patient who underwent right transpedicular decompression at T8–T9 and T7–T10 posterior instrumented fusion using image navigation for right T8–T9 disc herniation, causing spinal cord compression and myelopathy. (Images courtesy of Simon Hanft, MD, and M. Omar Iqbal, MD, with permission.)

19.7 Outcomes

Given the often-vague presenting symptoms and lack of a clear dermatomal pain distribution in many cases as well as expectation of limited improvement of myelopathic symptoms following surgical decompression, symptom relief following surgery for thoracic disc disorders can be less predictable than that for cervical and lumbar pathologies. In general, early decompression is recommended in patients with myelopathy or progressive neurologic deficit and has been associated with superior outcomes in comparison to a delayed approach.[14] In addition, patients with soft disc herniations and more lateral pathology have been found to have better results, presumably due to less dural retraction or manipulation. Conversely, the presence of disc calcification and OPLL have been associated with suboptimal outcomes following surgical decompression, with higher rates of intraoperative CSF leaks and postoperative neurologic decline. These operations are technically difficult and should always be performed without manipulation of the thoracic cord, with anterior approaches preferred in cases of central disc pathology. Minimally invasive and transpedicular approaches have been compared and found to have similar rates of postoperative neurologic improvement, with 50% of patients in each group improving at least one American Spinal Injury Association (ASIA) grade postoperatively.[15] Hyper-reflexia, spasticity, sensory changes, and pain have been found to improve in over 80% of patients undergoing surgery for thoracic disc herniations, while motor dysfunction and bowel and bladder dysfunction are associated with less predictable recovery following surgery.[1] In summary, despite outcomes that are generally considered less predictable than similar operations for cervical and lumbar pathology, significant symptom improvement is possible as long as good indications and sound surgical principles are adhered to in the treatment of these patients.

- Thoracic disc herniations are largely asymptomatic, which masks their true prevalence. Studies using MRI have shown that up to 50% of subjects have thoracic disc herniations, but the vast majority extended less than 2 mm past the vertebral bodies.
- Proper diagnosis requires a high degree of clinical suspicion due to atypical presentations that may mimic visceral organ pathology. Failure to find evidence of thoracic or abdominal organ pathology may warrant a workup for thoracic disc disorders.
- The most common presenting symptom for patients with thoracic disc disorders is sensory disturbance below the level of the pathology followed by motor weakness, with bowel and bladder dysfunction often found only as a late finding.
- Neurologic deficits in thoracic spine disorders are thought to be the result of a combined insult of mechanical cord compression and vascular compromise.
- The majority of thoracic disc herniations are central or centrolateral, but the location and size are generally not helpful for categorizing symptomatic and asymptomatic patients.
- MRI is considered the gold standard for the identification of thoracic disc herniations but it has limited ability to correctly identify intradural disc herniation. If suspicion for intradural pathology is sufficiently high, CT myelogram may be indicated.
- In both asymptomatic patients and those with radicular pain, conservative treatment with non-steroidal anti-inflammatory drugs (NSAIDs), muscle relaxants, and physical therapy are first line treatment options which are generally successful.
- Patients with moderate to severe myelopathy, worsening lower extremity motor or sensory dysfunction, or bowel and bladder involvement should be considered for surgery.
- Localization can be difficult, especially in patients with mid-thoracic pathology and absence of anatomic cues such as osteophytes or compression fractures. Helpful strategies include placement of a radiopaque fiducial marker in an adjacent pedicle under CT guidance in interventional radiology preoperatively, as well as intraoperative CT navigation where this is available.
- Midline laminectomy with discectomy is contraindicated in patients with thoracic disc disorders due to the high rate of postoperative decline. Costotransversectomy and lateral extracavitary approaches can provide better outcomes by avoiding cord manipulation.
- VATS and minimally invasive lateral retropleural techniques are associated with less postoperative pain and pulmonary compromise when compared to traditional open trans-thoracic approaches; however, their role continues to evolve and a steep learning curve is present.
- Lateral extracavitary approaches involve greater rib resection, increased soft tissue dissection, and more bone removal, but offer greater access to the central portion of the disc. True central disc herniations may be better accessed through anterior approaches.
- Dural repair commonly requires grafting as primary suture repair is difficult, especially in cases of OPLL or ligamentum flavum ossification. Postoperative subarachnoid drain and flat bedrest can be considered if watertight repair is not feasible.
- In cases of thoracic ossification of the ligamentum flavum, the decompression is challenging as it is not safe to place Kerrison rongeurs or curettes directly ventral to the ossified mass to remove it due to high risk of neurologic injury. Instead, the authors recommend using a high-speed burr to detach the periphery of the mass after facetectomies are complete, followed by leaving a thin rim of bone dorsally, if necessary, to avoid dural injury and CSF leak, similar to the approach used ventrally for OPLL in the cervical spine.
- Rather than performing an inadequate decompression of ventral or central pathology, it is generally best to apply a higher grade of resection and instrumented fusion, if necessary, to avoid any manipulation of the thoracic cord.

19.8 Case Example

A 50-year-old male presented with a 6-week history of progressive difficulty ambulating, subjective leg weakness, and gait imbalance. He had tried anti-inflammatory pain medication and physical therapy without benefit and presented to the emergency department with worsening leg weakness. On physical examination, the patient was noted to have hyper-reflexia in both lower extremities, sustained clonus, and 4/5 motor function. MR imaging, sagittal and axial T2-weighted images, showed a large left T9–T10 disc herniation with cord compression and associated cord signal change (see top row three images). The patient underwent a T9–T10 left facetectomy and transpedicular decompression with discectomy as well as posterior pedicle screw instrumentation in T9–T10. Images show intraoperative photograph of discectomy and instrumentation (see bottom left image) and anteroposterior (AP) and lateral fluoroscopic images of final construct (see bottom right two images). (Images courtesy of Ira Goldstein, MD, with permission)

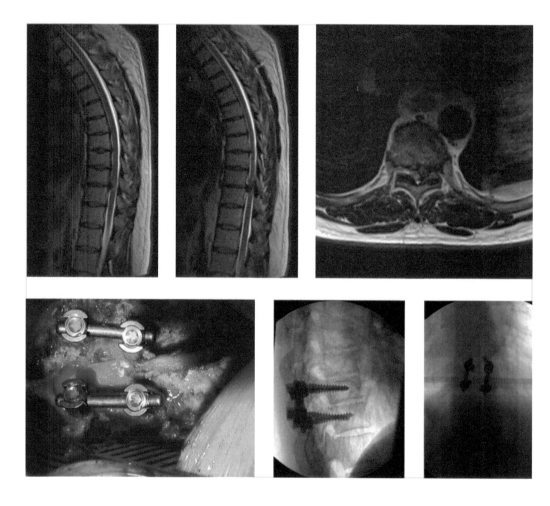

19.9 Board-style Questions

1. A 54-year-old male presents with a 3-month history of worsening bandlike chest pain, followed by lower extremity weakness, and ultimately bladder incontinence. What is the most sensitive imagining modality for detection of potential intradural thoracic disc herniation?
   a) Contrast enhanced MRI
   b) Plain radiograph
   c) CT myelogram
   d) Contrast enhanced CT

2. During lung cancer evaluation of a 73-year-old female, MRI revealed a large T4–T5 centrolateral disc herniation. She has no neurologic deficits on examination and gait is normal. What initial treatment is most appropriate?
   a) NSAIDs, physical therapy, and observation
   b) Laminectomy with disc removal due to high probability of disease progression
   c) Transthoracic cord decompression due to high risk of vascular compromise
   d) VATS with decompression due to 5 mm size of disc herniation

3. During an uncomplicated surgical repair of a T8–T9 disc herniation, several vessels were ligated within the neural foramina. Upon completion of the surgery, the patient developed paraplegia. What precautions could have been taken to avoid this adverse event?
   a) Opt for transthoracic decompression to minimize cord manipulation.
   b) Perform angiography or transient occlusion intraoperatively to identify the artery of Adamkiewicz prior to ligation.
   c) Assess patient for risk of global ischemic injury prior to surgical intervention.
   d) No precautions could have prevented this adverse event.

4. A 46-year-old male with a suspected disc herniation has a upgoing Babinski sign, Hoffman's sign, and bladder incontinence along with motor and sensory abnormalities. What part of the spine is most likely to have the herniated disc?
   a) Cervical
   b) Thoracic
   c) Lumbar
   d) Sacral

5. A 63-year-old female presents with recent onset of urinary and fecal incontinence in addition to progressive lower back pain radiating to the groin, pain radiating to the lower extremities, and lower extremity hyper-reflexia. What is the most likely location of disc herniation that could cause these symptoms?
   a) C2–C3
   b) T4–T6
   c) T11–T12
   d) S4–S5

6. Which of the following patients is the best candidate for surgical repair of a herniated thoracic disc?
   a) Incidental finding of a T1–T2 central herniation
   b) T3–T4 lateral herniation improving with physical therapy
   c) T11–T12 central herniation with gait instability
   d) T19–T10 lateral herniation with unilateral radiating pain

7. A 58-year-old male with a month-long history of periscapular pain radiating to the right arm presents to the emergency room with new onset right-sided ptosis, miosis, and anhidrosis. Which of the following best explains this condition?
   a) Right internal carotid artery dissection that compresses sympathetic plexus
   b) T1–T2 disc herniation that impinges the right oculosympathetic pathway and spinal nerve root
   c) Right-sided Pancoast tumor that compresses the sympathetic ganglion but spares the brachial plexus
   d) Intracranial mass that compresses the sympathetic fibers within the cavernous sinus

8. Which of the following patients deserves a higher level of suspicion for thoracic disc herniation?
   a) 65-year-old female with osteoporosis and vertebral compression fractures
   b) 18-year-old male who was recently in a motor vehicle accident
   c) 72-year-old female with long-standing spinal stenosis
   d) 40-year-old man with wedge-shaped vertebrae and kyphosis

9. In a patient with suspected thoracic disc herniation with calcification, which of the following imaging modalities is most appropriate to assess the degree of pathology and guide treatment?
   a) MRI
   b) Plain orthogonal radiographs
   c) Whole body bone scan with single-photon emission computed tomography (SPECT)
   d) CT imaging

10. A 67-year-old woman with a T3–T4 thoracic disc herniation requires surgery for symptom relief. Which of the following conditions is an absolute contraindication for performance of VATS?

a) Extensive calcification of the herniated disc
b) Previous lung cancer and pneumectomy
c) Minimal collateral circulation in the location of herniation
d) History of chronic obstructive pulmonary disease

Answers ✓

1. c
2. a
3. b
4. a
5. c
6. c
7. b
8. d
9. c
10. b

References

[1] Stillerman CB, Chen TC, Couldwell WT, Zhang W, Weiss MH. Experience in the surgical management of 82 symptomatic herniated thoracic discs and review of the literature. J Neurosurg. 1998; 88(4):623–633

[2] Ahn DK, Lee S, Moon SH, Boo KH, Chang BK, Lee JI. Ossification of the ligamentum flavum. Asian Spine J. 2014; 8(1): 89–96

[3] Abiola R, Rubery P, Mesfin A. Ossification of the posterior longitudinal ligament: etiology, diagnosis and outcomes of nonoperative and operative management. Global Spine J. 2016; 6(2):195–204

[4] Wood KB, Garvey TA, Gundry C, Heithoff KB. Magnetic resonance imaging of the thoracic spine: evaluation of asymptomatic individuals. J Bone Joint Surg Am. 1995; 77 (11):1631–1638

[5] Awwad EE, Martin DS, Smith KR, Jr, Baker BK. Asymptomatic versus symptomatic herniated thoracic discs: their frequency and characteristics as detected by computed tomography after myelography. Neurosurgery. 1991; 28 (2):180–186

[6] Currier BL, Eck JC, Eismont FJ, Green BA. Thoracic Disc Disease. In: Herkowitz H, Garfin S, Eismont FJ, Balderston R, eds. Rothman-Simeone: The Spine. 6th ed. Philadelphia, PA: Elsevier; 2011

[7] Aizawa T, Sato T, Sasaki H, et al. Results of surgical treatment for thoracic myelopathy: minimum 2-year follow-up study in 132 patients. J Neurosurg Spine. 2007; 7(1): 13–20

[8] Lesoin F, Rousseaux M, Autricque A, et al. Thoracic disc herniations: evolution in the approach and indications. Acta Neurochir (Wien). 1986; 80(1–2):30–34

[9] Madaelil TP, Long JR, Wallace AN, et al. Preoperative fiducial marker placement in the thoracic spine: a technical report. Spine. 2017; 42(10):E624–E628

[10] Holly LT, Foley KT. Intraoperative spinal navigation. Spine. 2003; 28(15) Suppl:S54–S61

[11] Snyder LA, Smith ZA, Dahdaleh NS, Fessler RG. Minimally invasive treatment of thoracic disc herniations. Neurosurg Clin N Am. 2014; 25(2):271–277

[12] Oppenlander ME, Clark JC, Kalyvas J, Dickman CA. Indications and techniques for spinal instrumentation in thoracic disc surgery. Clin Spine Surg. 2016; 29(2): E99–E106

[13] Currier BL, Eck JC, Eismont FJ, Green BA. Thoracic Disc Disease. In: Garfin SR, Eismont FJ, Bell GR, Fischgrund JS, Bono CM, eds. Rothman-Simeone and Herkowitz's The Spine. New York, NY: Elsevier; 2018:787–805

[14] Cornips EM, Janssen ML, Beuls EA. Thoracic disc herniation and acute myelopathy: clinical presentation, neuroimaging findings, surgical considerations, and outcome. J Neurosurg Spine. 2011; 14(4):520–528

[15] Arts MP, Bartels RH. Anterior or posterior approach of thoracic disc herniation? A comparative cohort of mini-transthoracic versus transpedicular discectomies. Spine J. 2014; 14(8):1654–1662

Index

Note: Page numbers set in bold indicate headings.